PROMOTING HEALTH AND ACADEMIC SUCCESS

The Whole School, Whole Community, Whole Child Approach

David A. Birch, PhD, MCHES
The University of Alabama

Donna M. Videto, PhD, MCHES
SUNY College at Cortland

EDITORS

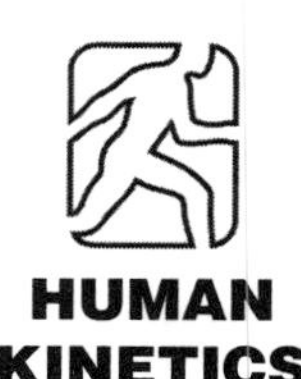

HUMAN
KINETICS

Library of Congress Cataloging-in-Publication Data

Birch, David A.
Promoting health and academic success : the whole school, whole community, whole child approach / [David A. Birch and Donna M. Videto]
pages cm
Includes bibliographical references and index.
1. School health services--United States. 2. Health education--United States. 3. Health promotion--United States. I. Videto, Donna M. II. Title.
LB3409.U5B57 2015
371.7'1--dc23

2014032303

ISBN: 978-1-4504-7765-9 (print)

The web addresses cited in this text were current as of October 2014, unless otherwise noted.

Acquisitions Editor: Ray Vallese; **Developmental Editor:** Jacqueline Eaton Blakley; **Managing Editor:** Elizabeth Evans; **Copyeditor:** Bob Replinger; **Indexer:** Nan N. Badgett; **Permissions Manager:** Dalene Reeder; **Graphic Designer:** Fred Starbird; **Cover Designer:** Keith Blomberg; **Photograph (cover):** Reprinted from ASCD, 2014, *Whole school, whole community, whole child: A collaborative approach to learning and health.*; **Photographs (interior):** Chapter 1: © Jim West/imageBROKER/age fotostock; chapter 2: AP Photo/Ernest K. Bennett; chapter 3: © Savannah1969 / Dreamstime.com; chapter 4: © Shannon Fagan / Dreamstime.com; chapter 5: Laurence Gough; chapter 6: © Monkey Business Images / Dreamstime.com; chapter 7: Monkey Business; chapter 8: © Human Kinetics; chapter 9: © Norma Jean Gargasz/age fotostock; chapter 10: Comstock; chapter 11: © Corbis. All Rights Reserved.; chapter 12: © Jim West/age fotostock; chapter 13: Edie Layland; **Photo Asset Manager:** Laura Fitch; **Visual Production Assistant:** Joyce Brumfield; **Photo Production Manager:** Jason Allen; **Art Manager:** Kelly Hendren; **Associate Art Manager:** Alan L. Wilborn; **Illustrations:** © Human Kinetics, unless otherwise noted; **Printer:** Sheridan Books

Printed in the United States of America 10 9 8 7 6 5 4 3 2 1

The paper in this book is certified under a sustainable forestry program.

Human Kinetics
Website: www.HumanKinetics.com

United States: Human Kinetics
P.O. Box 5076
Champaign, IL 61825-5076
800-747-4457
e-mail: humank@hkusa.com

Canada: Human Kinetics
475 Devonshire Road Unit 100
Windsor, ON N8Y 2L5
800-465-7301 (in Canada only)
e-mail: info@hkcanada.com

Europe: Human Kinetics
107 Bradford Road
Stanningley
Leeds LS28 6AT, United Kingdom
+44 (0) 113 255 5665
e-mail: hk@hkeurope.com

Australia: Human Kinetics
57A Price Avenue
Lower Mitcham, South Australia 5062
08 8372 0999
e-mail: info@hkaustralia.com

New Zealand: Human Kinetics
P.O. Box 80
Torrens Park, South Australia 5062
0800 222 062
e-mail: info@hknewzealand.com

E6224

This book is dedicated to Diane Demuth Allensworth and Lloyd J. Kolbe for their vision, commitment, and leadership related to the well-being of children and youth.

Contents

Foreword

I grew up in a family that was rich in spirit although somewhat poor in possessions. We were helped in everlasting ways by the schools we attended. I remember an evening in first grade when I regained consciousness in a hospital room to learn that, earlier in the day, I had fallen from the top of a sliding board onto the school playground. I was told that our school nurse and several teachers had picked me up and helped transport me to the emergency room. In second grade, I waited with my classmates to get the newly developed polio vaccination that our school provided, which saved us from ever suffering the effects of the disease. In third grade, I ambled through the school cafeteria line to be greeted and served lunch by the cafeteria ladies and men, as we called them. The daily welcome and food they provided sustained me and my classmates throughout our school years. All these events helped shape my life.

In the United States, 130,000 public and private schools employ more than 5 million teachers and other school staff to nurture and educate more than 55 million students, usually for the 13 most formative years of their lives. All of our schools help shape the short- and long-term health and well-being of students at least as much as they help shape their education. In turn, the health of students determines their ability to regularly attend school, to be engaged with others in the tasks at hand, to think, to learn, and to become successful. And all schools influence the well-being and productivity of teachers and other school staff.

You might be interested in learning about what you could do to improve both the education and health of young people in your school and in your community. In the United States there is more racial, cultural, and economic diversity now than there was in the past. One in five lives in poverty. Many live with only one or neither parent. Many are immigrants, many are transient, and many have special education and health needs. They have a range of health threats: hunger and neglect; asthma; obesity and consequent diabetes, heart disease, and cancer; toxic stress, anxiety, and depression; attention-deficit/hyperactivity disorder and autism spectrum disorders; and potential threats in the school environment such as noroviruses, pesticides, and violence. Still, most children today enter kindergarten healthy and resilient. Our schools and communities could do much to ensure students remain that way throughout their school years—healthy, safe, supported, engaged, and challenged to do their very best.

Early in the 20th century, educators and health professionals began to develop means that schools could employ to improve both education and health concomitantly. During the latter part of the 20th century these means began to be aggregated into what some have called coordinated school health programs and others have called healthy schools. This book presents a compendium of those means. *Promoting Health and Academic Success: The Whole School, Whole Community, Whole Child Approach* explains a collaborative approach for implementing these various means of improving both education and health outcomes. Implementing this approach requires a joint effort of those responsible for the well-being of students: administrators and teachers; parents and students; education, health, and social service organizations and their respective boards; nurses and physicians; counselors, psychologists, and social workers; food service staff; health educators; physical educators and coaches; custodians and safety personnel; community workers and legislators; and health coordinators charged with orchestrating the critical but otherwise scattered interdependent efforts of these professionals and community members. Each has a decisive and integrated role to play.

If you are a professional or a concerned community member—or aspire to be—this book will be instrumental in developing your ability to improve both the education and health of young people in your community. This is a textbook to be used in colleges and universities that provide preservice and in-service training for school and community professionals in order to improve education and health. It's also a resource for schools and communities interested in improving the education and health of their students with or without the assistance of a college or university. Accordingly, the book also might serve as a means of bringing together faculty from various departments to work more collaboratively to improve both education and health. In doing so, the otherwise disconnected colleges of education, health, nursing, medicine, social work, and others might learn from and with one another, support one another, more effectively train their own students, move forward with a more unified voice and agenda, and thus model more collaborative means to improve both the education and health of young people.

The editors and authors are recognized as some of the foremost leaders in concomitantly improving both education and health in the United States. They have woven together theory with practice, policy with program, planning with implementation across the spectrum of professional disciplines. In effect, this book does much to explain and advance an evolving national strategy to improve both education and health during the early decades of the 21st century. Whether we label this strategy as coordinated school health programs, healthy schools, or a Whole School, Whole Community, Whole Child Approach matters less. What matters more is increasing our capacity to make this evolving approach available to a rapidly growing number of schools and communities that have expressed interest in using it. Although the book is based largely on U.S. experiences in implementing this approach, the approach might be applicable to other nations as well.

We now have the means for schools and communities to collaboratively improve both education and health. Regardless of your profession or role in your school or community, you have an integral part to play. I hope you choose to become a part of this evolving approach to improving both education and health. And if you do, I hope you pass along to the editors of this book the methods you found to make this approach progressively better. Surely the editors and authors will update this next edition as we learn more.

Lloyd J. Kolbe, PhD
Professor Emeritus of Applied Health Science
Indiana University School of Public Health
Bloomington, Indiana
Founding director (1988-2003)
Division of Adolescent and School Health
U.S. Centers for Disease Control and Prevention
Atlanta, Georgia

Preface

Parents, educators, and community members want children to experience optimal health and academic success. The relationship between the health of students and their academic achievement is becoming increasingly evident. Students who engage in healthy behaviors at school, at home, and in the community are more likely to come to school focused on learning and less likely to miss school or not complete their education.

Healthy kids and ultimately healthy adults are the product of their school, family, and community influences. Schools have the potential to serve as centers for health promotion not only for students but also for families and communities. In the mid-1980s a model eventually known as Coordinated School Health (CSH) was introduced by two leaders in school health, Diane Allensworth and Lloyd Kolbe (both contributors to this book). This model was designed to coordinate various school programs to maximize health promotion for students. The basic idea behind the model is that schools should address the health of students through coordinated activities, policies, and programs that involve the following components:

- Health education
- Health services
- Physical education
- Nutrition services
- Counseling and psychological and social services
- Healthy school environment
- Parent, family, and community involvement
- Health promotion for faculty and staff

The release of this book comes at an opportune time. In 2014 a new version for coordinated school health, the Whole School, Whole Community, Whole Child (WSCC) approach was developed by the Centers for Disease Control and Prevention and ASCD. The development process for the new model involved both a consultation and a review team consisting of leaders in education and health. Several of our chapter authors, including Diane Allensworth, David Birch, and Robert Valois, served as members of these teams. Leadership for the overall process was provided by Sean Slade, an author of two chapters in this book.

The new WSCC model places a high level of emphasis on the potential of promoting both health and learning. The WSCC approach highlights the idea that healthy kids are more likely to be academically successful students. From a structural standpoint, WSCC increased the number of components from 8 to 10 and highlighted the importance of five whole child tenets: healthy, safe, engaged, supported, and challenged. In addition, the concept of community is presented as an overarching feature of the new approach (see figure 1.3, p. 9). The 10 components of WSCC are the following:

- Health education
- Physical education and physical activity
- Nutrition environment and services
- Health services
- Counseling and psychological and social services
- Social and emotional climate
- Physical environment
- Employee wellness
- Family engagement
- Community involvement

This book, *Promoting Health and Academic Success: The Whole School, Whole Community, Whole Child Approach*, has two specific purposes: (1) to serve as a textbook for college and university undergraduate and graduate courses that emphasize topics such as CSH or WSCC, health promotion for youth, and school health programs, and (2) to serve as a resource for school districts involved in initiating, maintaining, and improving efforts in health promotion for students. The authors of each chapter, many of whom are recognized as leaders in school health, all have experience working with school districts in coordinated school health.

The experiences and many resources that are described in the book are related to CSH, but because of the similarities between CSH and WSCC, these experiences and resources are relevant to WSCC. You will also find examples of guidelines and approaches that relate directly to WSCC. We believe that the book will provide the direction necessary to help readers transition from CSH to WSCC.

The book is organized into five parts. The chapters in the first part (chapters 1–3), "Moving From Coordinated School Health to the Whole School, Whole Community, Whole Child Approach," provide readers with a description of the WSCC approach, the rationale and history of CSH, the evolution to WSCC, and the best practices within each content area. The second part (chapters 4–5), "Putting the Focus on the Child," focuses on the ASCD Whole Child Initiative and the link between health and academic success and the importance of cultural competence in addressing health disparities and meeting the needs of our diverse student population. Part III (chapters 6–8), "Building Partnerships and Support," present strategies for securing the support and engagement of school administrators, parents, and family members along with strategies for addressing the diverse assets and needs of our diverse student, family, and community population. In part IV (chapters 9–11), "Planning, Implementation, and Evaluation," detailed content is presented related to specific considerations, strategies, and tools for the planning, implementation, and evaluation of the WSCC approach. Part V (chapters 12–13), "The Path Forward," presents an examination of the future of education and school health promotion. Chapter 13 includes the perspectives regarding the future of school health from leaders in both education and school health. The book also includes an appendix that presents useful tools that have been developed by U.S. governmental agencies and nongovernmental organizations. While developed for use with the CSH approach, they can be useful resources for the WSCC model.

Beyond the content, at the end of each chapter application activities are included that provide students and other readers with the opportunity to apply information to simulations based on WSCC scenarios. Each chapter also contains a list of important resources including relevant articles, books, websites, and blogs.

We believe that *Promoting Health and Academic Success: The Whole School, Whole Community, Whole Child Approach* will be an invaluable resource for college and university faculty members, students, and professionals in education and health who are working with schools and school districts to improve academic achievement and student health. Ultimately, we believe that this resource can play an important role in planning, implementing, and evaluating initiatives designed to promote education and health for students through meaningful engagement of their parents and other family members, community members, and school faculty and staff members. We believe that these coordinated initiatives will not only improve health but also increase the likelihood of academic success.

David A. Birch
Donna M. Videto

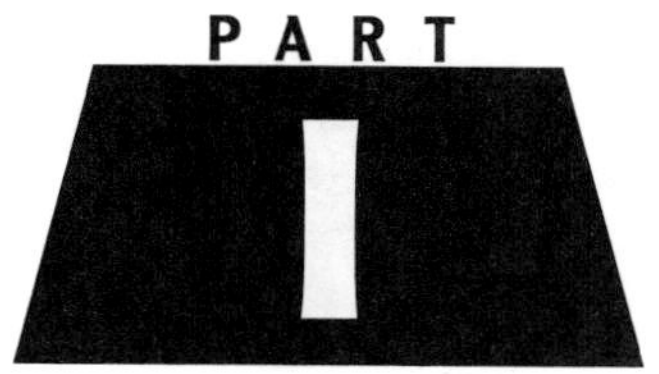

PART I

Moving From Coordinated School Health to the Whole School, Whole Community, Whole Child Approach

1

Whole School, Whole Community, Whole Child: A New Model for Health and Academic Success

DAVID A. BIRCH • DONNA M. VIDETO

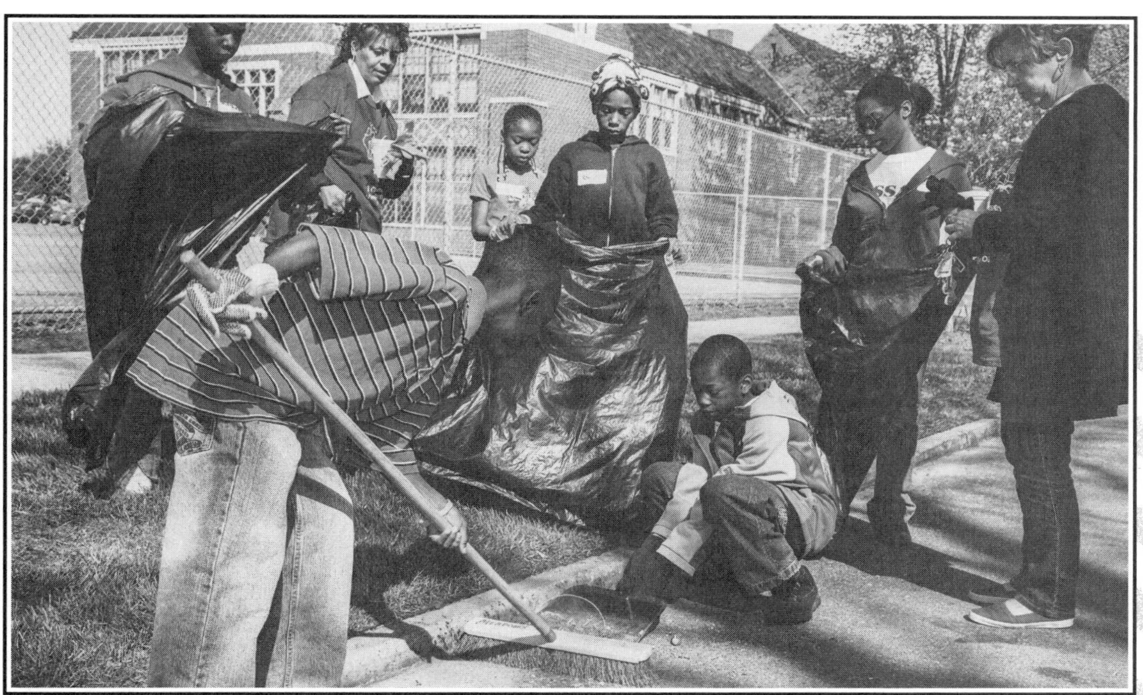

Since the early part of the 20th century, promoting the health of students has been recognized as a responsibility of schools. The model for school health that was used for most of the 20th century was a three-component model that included health education, the school environment, and health services. In the 1980s Diane Allensworth and Lloyd Kolbe developed an expanded approach, Coordinated School Health (CSH), that included eight components. The intent of CSH was that it would serve not only as a vehicle for promoting the health of students but also as a strategy for promoting academic success (Allensworth & Kolbe, 1987). Implementation of CSH in schools, however, was limited (Basch, 2010). In 2014 ASCD (formerly known as the Association for Supervision and Curriculum Development) and the Centers for Disease Control and Prevention (CDC) collaborated on the development of a new, 10-component model titled Whole School, Whole Community, Whole Child (WSCC) (ASCD, 2014). This chapter presents a brief historical overview of school health before the introduction of WSCC. A more detailed history is presented in chapter 2. The primary focus of this chapter is the presentation of WSCC, including a description of the of the new model, the ten components, the tenets of the whole child approach, and important considerations related to advocacy and implementation.

EVOLUTION OF SCHOOL HEALTH MODELS

The role of schools in promoting the health of students has been recognized since the early 1900s. In the early part of the 20th century, a primary focus of school health was the prevention of communicable diseases. At that time, a school health program was expected to include three components: school health education, the school health environment, and school health services. Although the prevention of communicable diseases is still a responsibility of schools, in the last 30 years greater emphasis has been placed on the prevention of risk behaviors that can increase the likelihood of present and future morbidity and mortality (Allensworth & Kolbe, 1987). Examples of these behaviors include not using tobacco products, maintaining a healthy diet, being physically active, and avoiding the use of alcohol and other drugs.

Coordinated School Health

In the late 1980s, to provide direction for better addressing the health priorities of school-age children, Diane Allensworth and Lloyd Kolbe, prominent leaders in school health, proposed a new eight-component model for health promotion, the **Comprehensive School Health program** (CSH). The term *comprehensive* was later replaced by *coordinated* when referring to CSH. The eight CSH components included

- school health services,
- school health education,
- school health environment,
- integrated school and community health promotion efforts,
- school physical education,
- school food service,
- school counseling, and
- school site health promotion programs for faculty and staff.

The importance of CSH was emphasized through the publication of a special issue of the *Journal of School Health* in December 1987. This special publication was funded by the Metropolitan Life Foundation. Allensworth and Kolbe coauthored the introductory article in the issue, which presented an overview of the new approach to school health. Invited national leaders in the relevant areas wrote articles related to each of the eight components. Two important principles were presented in the overview article: the importance of collaboration by professionals involved in the various components of CSH in the planning and implementation of health programs for students, and the linkage of positive health behaviors to students' cognitive performance and educational achievement (Allensworth & Kolbe, 1987).

Although CSH received increased national recognition in the late 1980s and funding was provided by the Centers for Disease Control and Prevention (CDC), Division of Adolescent and School Health (DASH) to selected state departments of education and departments of health, implementation in local school districts was less than optimal. McKenzie and Richmond in 1998 stated, "The promise of Coordinated School Health program thus far outshines its practice" (p. 10). Findings from the 2006 CDC **School Health Policies and Program Studies** (**SHPPS**) indicated that most schools in the United States did not spend sufficient time on health education (Kann et al., 2007) and physical education (Lee et al., 2007), provided less than recommended levels of nursing (Brener et al, 2006) and mental health services (Brener et al., 2007), and provided access to high-calorie, low-nutrient foods and beverages (O'Toole et al., 2007). Basch (2010) described the situation by stating, "Though rhetorical support is increasing, school health is currently not a central part of the fundamental mission of schools in America, nor has it been well integrated into the broader national strategy to reduce the gaps in educational opportunity and outcomes." One possible contributing reason for this lack of acceptance is that educators have viewed CSH as a health program focused only on health outcomes rather than an initiative that would also contribute to improved academic outcomes (ASCD, 2014).

ASCD Whole Child Initiative

ASCD, a global community dedicated to excellence in learning, teaching, and leading, has been a leader in the 21st century in illuminating the connection between health and education. In 2007 ASCD implemented its **Whole Child Initiative**. The initiative focuses on the long-term development and success of children rather than only on a narrowly defined version of academic achievement (ASCD, 2014). One goal of the initiative is to help educators, families, community members, and policy makers engage in sustainable, collaborative action related to educating the whole child. Numerous partner organizations from education, arts, health, and the policy and community sectors have joined ASCD in the Whole Child effort.

CREATION OF WSCC

ASCD, in collaboration with CDC, moved forward in 2013 to develop a new model that builds on both the Whole Child Initiative and the original eight-component CSH approach. The development of the new model, titled **Whole School, Whole Community, Whole Child (WSCC)**, involved a consultation group that developed the documents and frameworks related to the new model and a review group that periodically reviewed and provided feedback to the work of the consultation group. Members of both groups were selected because of their role as leaders in both education and health. The new WSCC model was introduced at two national conferences, the ASCD conference in Los Angeles in March 2014 and the **Society for Public Health Education (SOPHE)** conference in Baltimore, also in March 2014. WSCC incorporates and builds on CSH and the ASCD Whole Child Initiative (ASCD, 2014).

WSCC is designed to promote alignment, integration, and collaboration between education and health and is intended to enhance health outcomes and academic success. Support and engagement of the whole community should be an important aspect of the implementation of WSCC (ASCD, 2014).

An important aspect of the new model is the expansion from 8 to 10 components. One original component, healthy and safe school environment, has been expanded to two separate components, physical environment and social and emotional climate. Another original component, family and community involvement, has been expanded to two components, community involvement and family engagement (see figure 1.1) (ASCD, 2014). The evolution of the school health models is presented in figure 1.2.

Following are brief descriptions of all 10 WSCC components:

- **Health education**: Health education provides students with opportunities to acquire the knowledge, attitudes, and skills necessary for making health-promoting decisions, achieving health literacy, adopting health-enhancing behaviors, and promoting the health of others. Health education should be provided sequentially from pre-K through grade 12. Health education curricula should address important health topic areas through instruction based on the National Health Education Standards (NHES) (CDC, 2013).
- **Physical education and physical activity**: Physical education is a school-based instructional opportunity for students to gain the necessary skills and knowledge for lifelong participation in physical activity. Physical education is characterized by a planned, sequential K through 12 curriculum that assists students in achieving the national standards for K through 12 physical education. The outcome of a quality physical education program is a physically educated person who has the knowledge, skills, and confidence to enjoy a lifetime of healthful physical activity (CDC, 2013).
- **Health services**: These services are designed to ensure access or referral to primary health care services; foster appropriate use of primary health care services; prevent and control communicable disease and other health problems; provide emergency care for illness or injury; promote and provide optimum sanitary conditions for a safe school facility and school environment; and provide educational and counseling opportunities for promoting and maintaining individual, family, and community health (CDC, 2013).
- **Nutrition environment and services**: Schools should provide access to a variety of nutritious and appealing meals that accommodate the health and nutrition needs of all students. School nutrition programs should reflect *U.S. Dietary Guidelines for Americans* and other criteria to achieve nutrition integrity. The school nutrition services should offer students a learning laboratory for classroom nutrition and health education and serve as a resource for linkages with nutrition-related community services (CDC, 2013).
- **Counseling, psychological, and social services**: These services are provided to improve students' mental, emotional, and social health and include individual and group assessments, interventions,

CSH
WSCC
Healthy and safe school environment
Social and emotional climate
Physical environment
Family/Community involvement
Community involvement
Family engagement

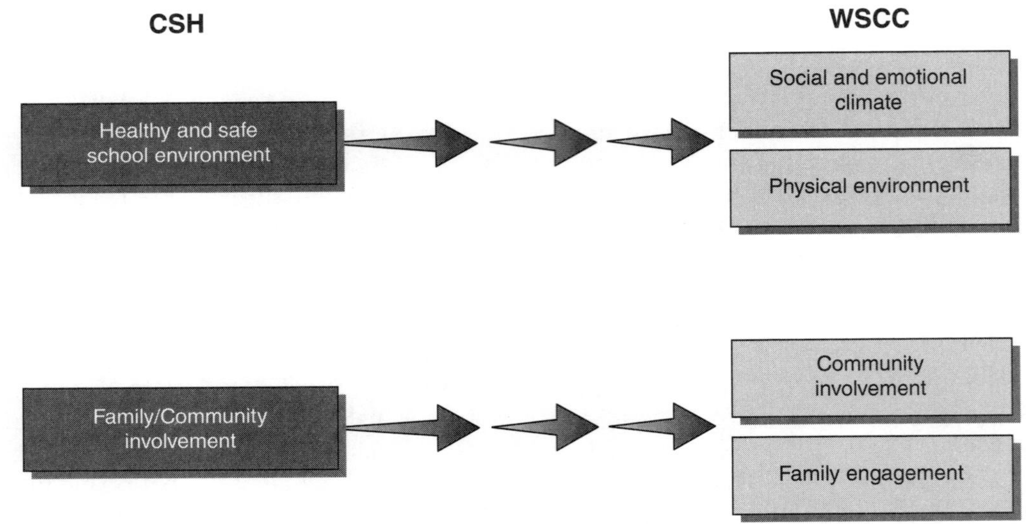

Figure 1.1 Two components of the CSH model have been translated into four components in the WSCC model.
Reprinted from CDC, *Expanding the coordinated school health approach*, 2014. Available: http://www.cdc.gov/healthyyouth/wscc/approach.htm.

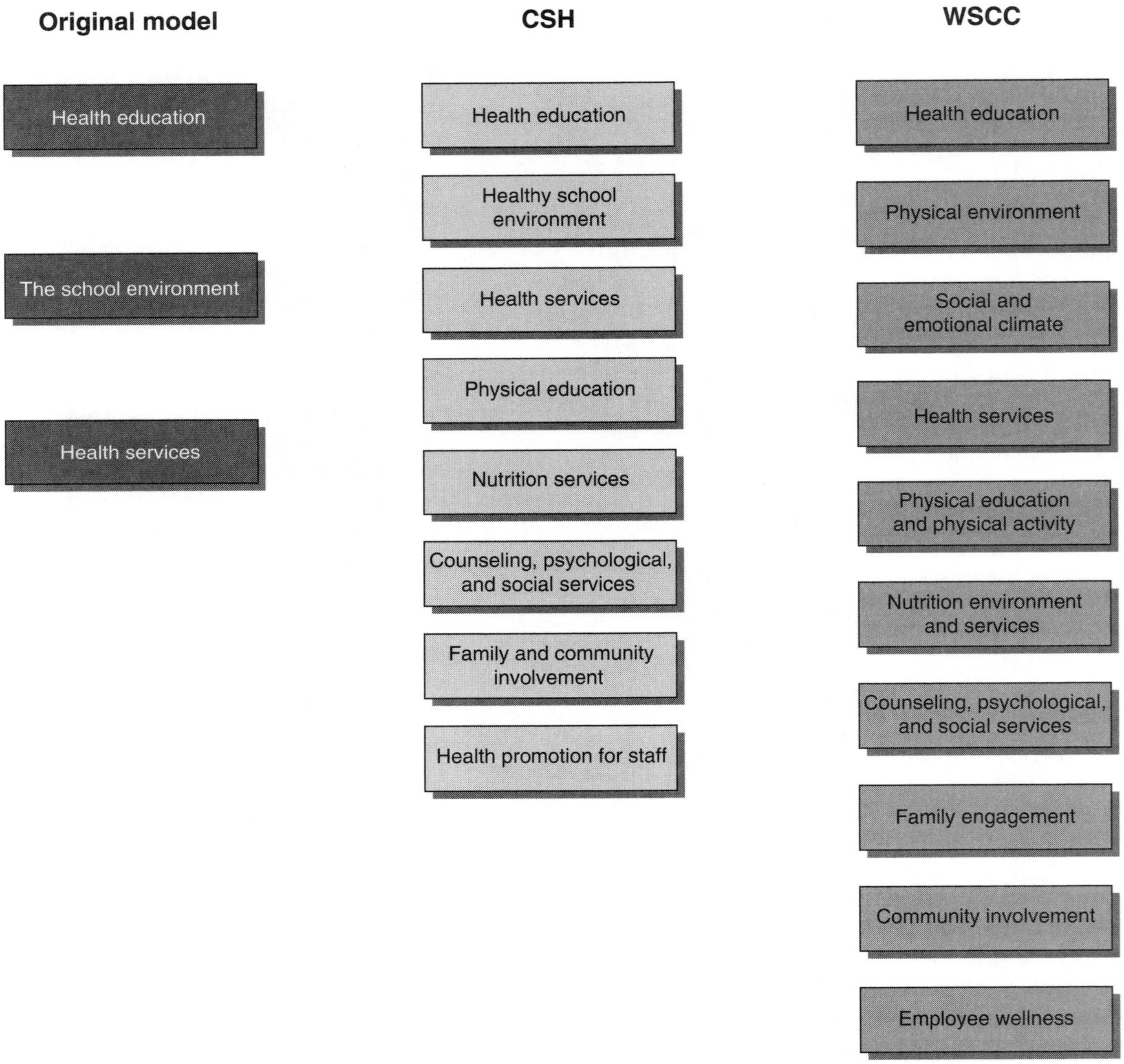

Original model
CSH
WSCC
Health education
The school environment
Health services
Health education
Healthy school environment
Health services
Physical education
Nutrition services
Counseling, psychological, and social services
Family and community involvement
Health promotion for staff
Health education
Physical environment
Social and emotional climate
Health services
Physical education and physical activity
Nutrition environment and services
Counseling, psychological, and social services
Family engagement
Community involvement
Employee wellness

Figure 1.2 Evolution of components in school health models.

School Health *in Action*

An Early Step Forward in Promoting WSCC at the Local Level

Upon the March 2014 unveiling of the Whole School, Whole Community, Whole Child model, a local school district in upstate New York introduced WSCC to the district's faculty and administration across their rural school district. A faculty member from a local college was asked to introduce the new WSCC model and then work with the district health and wellness coordinator to oversee 25 breakout sessions focused on the theme of incorporating wellness into learning. One goal for the day was to provide participants with knowledge and skills to adjust the physical, social, and emotional climate in their classrooms to improve the learning environment for each student. In an attempt to achieve the workshop goal, the WSCC model was introduced and compared with the CSH model. The ASCD video that provides an overview of the WSCC model was shown to the audience. Following the video a discussion was held on how a collaborative approach can have a positive effect on health and learning in the school district.

At the conclusion of the opening session, breakout sessions with small groups were held. An example of a breakout session was one titled "Healthy and Wise: Preparing Students for the World Beyond Formal Schooling." In this session, the facilitator went into detail about the collaborative WSCC approach while putting a strong focus on the ASCD Whole Child concept. The goal of this breakout session was to challenge the participants to produce a comprehensive health and academic plan in which the faculty and staff become leaders in the quest to reinvent, refocus, and recharge the health and academic status of the school district.

At the conclusion of the workshop it was decided to begin an initiative to implement the WSCC approach in the school district. The name of the first effort is "Optimize the Year with Healthy Habits: Incredible You, Incredible Year." In this effort the wellness committee will begin by addressing the wellness of the faculty and staff for the upcoming school year as a way to develop health and wellness leaders for the work to follow.

and referrals. Organizational assessment and consultation skills of counselors and psychologists should contribute not only to the health of students but also to the health of the school environment (CDC, 2013).

- **Physical environment**: The physical environment of the school includes buildings, school grounds, playground equipment, and athletic fields. The physical environment within the school includes building design, adequate space, cleanliness, noise level, heating and cooling, ventilation, and restrooms. These interior and exterior areas should be clean; safe; free from environmental hazards, tobacco, drugs, weapons, and violence; and appropriately secure from unauthorized access (Allensworth, Lawson, Nicholson, & Wyche, 1997; ASCD, 2014).
- **Social and emotional climate**: The social and emotional climate should provide a supportive culture conducive to enabling students, families, and staff members to feel safe, secure, accepted, and valued. Important factors in the social and emotional climate of a school include an attractive, comfortable physical environment; appreciation and respect for individual differences and cultural diversity; value placed on equity and social justice; high expectations and supportive actions for learning; size and structure of classes and organizations; and a general sense of comfort and safety (Allensworth, Lawson, Nicholson, & Wyche, 1997).
- **Health promotion for staff**: Schools can provide opportunities for school staff members to improve their health status through activities such as health assessments, health education, and health-related fitness activities. These opportunities should encourage staff members to pursue a healthy lifestyle that contributes to their improved health status, improved morale, and a greater personal commitment to the school's overall coordinated health approach (CDC, 2013).

- **Family engagement**: Epstein et al. (2009) identified six types of involvement necessary for successful school and family partnerships: (1) providing parenting support, (2) communicating with parents, (3) providing diverse volunteer opportunities, (4) supporting at-home learning, (5) encouraging parents to engage in decision-making opportunities in schools, and (6) collaborating with the community. Engaging family members often involves overcoming challenges such as family time conflicts, lack of transportation to school, and lack of comfort among family members in engaging in school activities. In addition, teachers and school staff may lack adequate time and resources to work with families.
- **Community involvement**: Meaningful community involvement in the WSCC approach is characterized by systematic collaboration among individuals and organizations within the school community. This systematic collaboration involves the engagement of individuals and organizations representing various segments of the community in the planning, implementation, and evaluation of programs, structures, and systems designed to create and sustain WSCC. The collaboration also involves the sharing of both community and school resources.

The following considerations are important to the new WSCC model (ASCD, 2014).

- Regular practices within each component should be examined for possible collaboration opportunities with other components.
- All stakeholders should have an understanding of the interconnectedness between health and learning.
- The focus of the new model is on the child rather than on a subject or other sector.
- Learning, health, and schools are a part of and reflection of the local community.
- Every adult and every child has a role in the growth and development of self, peers, and the school.
- The school is not only a hub but also a reflection of the local community; it requires community input, resources, and collaboration to support students.
- Although community strengths can support schools, community needs are often reflected in schools and thus must be addressed to promote health and academic success.
- The connection between learning and health is essential.
- All children in all communities deserve to be healthy, safe, engaged, supported, and challenged.

The new model is presented in figure 1.3. The child is in the center—at the focal point and surrounded by the Whole Child tenets: healthy, safe, engaged, supported, and challenged. The school surrounds the child, acting as the hub that provides the full range of learning and health support systems to each child, in each school, in each community. The community is on the periphery, demonstrating that although the school may be a hub, it remains a reflection of its community and requires community input, resources, and collaboration to support its students.

Many leaders in both education and health believe that the new model presents great promise for helping decision makers understand the connection between the health of students and their ability to learn. This increased understanding will enable schools to emphasize WSCC as part of their overall plan for promoting students' health and academic achievement.

Dr. Gene R. Carter, recently retired ASCD chief executive officer, stated,

> The WSCC model developed by ASCD and the CDC takes the call for greater collaboration over the years and puts it firmly in place. For too long, entities have talked about collaboration without taking the necessary steps. This model puts the process into action. (ASCD, 2014, p. 8)

Wayne H. Giles, MD, director of the CDC Division of Population Health, added to Dr. Carter's observations by stating,

> Schools, health agencies, parents, and communities share a common goal of supporting the health and academic achievement of children and adolescents. Research shows that the health of students is linked to their academic achievement,

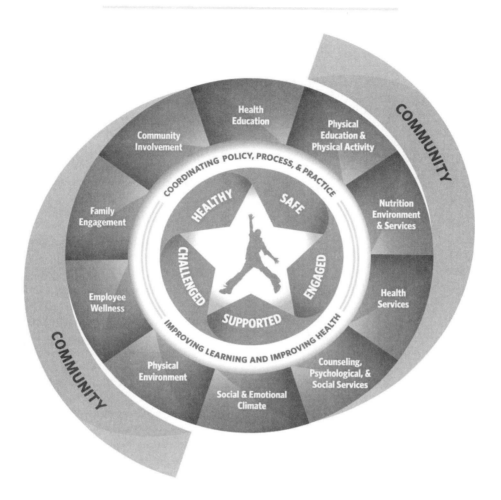

Figure 1.3 Whole School, Whole Community, Whole Child model.
Reprinted from ASCD, 2014, *Whole school, whole community, whole child: A collaborative approach to learning and health.*

> so by working together, we can ensure that young people are healthier and ready to learn. (ASCD, 2014)

CDC will be integrating this new model into its school health initiatives, placing ASCD's Whole Child framework at the center of health and education alignment in school settings. For more information about CDC's school health initiatives, visit www.cdc.gov/healthyyouth.

For more information about ASCD's Whole Child Initiative, visit www.ascd.org/wholechild. To find out about ASCD's focus on integrating learning and health, visit www.ascd.org/learningandhealth.

SUMMARY

School health has evolved from focusing on health education, the school environment, and health services to the current 10-component WSCC model. The WSCC model was developed collaboratively by an education organization, ASCD, and the federal Centers for Disease Control and Prevention (CDC). This collaboration symbolizes the potential of WSCC as an education and health model designed to promote better health and academic success. For WSCC to reach its full potential, stakeholders in local school will need to understand the connection between health and learning; the importance of focusing on the needs of the child in addressing this connection; and the necessity of collaboration among schools, families, and communities.

Glossary

ASCD—Founded in 1943, ASCD (formerly the Association for Supervision and Curriculum Development) is the global leader in developing and delivering innovative programs, products, and services that empower educators to support the success of each learner.

Comprehensive School Health Education—Defined by CDC as a course of study, or curriculum, for students in pre-K through grade 12 that addresses a variety of topics such as alcohol and other drug use and abuse, healthy eating and nutrition, mental and emotional health, personal health and wellness, physical activity, safety and injury prevention, sexual health, tobacco use, and violence prevention.

Coordinated School Health program—An eight-component model designed to promote health and learning in schools. The eight components include health education, physical education, health services, nutrition services, counseling and psychological services, healthy and safe school environment, health promotion for staff, and family and community involvement. This approach is being phased out in favor of the new Whole School, Whole Community, Whole Child (WSCC) approach.

Division of Adolescent and School Health (DASH)—Unit in the Centers for Disease Control and Prevention that focuses its activities on improving the health and quality of life of all children and adolescents.

School Health Policies and Programs Study—A national survey periodically conducted to assess school health policies and practices at the state, district, school, and classroom levels.

Society for Public Health Education—A professional organization for health educators working in all health education sections and health education students enrolled in professional preparation programs at the undergraduate and graduate levels.

Whole Child Initiative—The initiative started in 2007 by ASCD that aims to focus greater attention on a holistic, well-rounded education that caters to each child's social, emotional, mental, physical, and cognitive development.

Whole School, Whole Community, Whole Child (WSCC)—A collaborative approach to promoting health and academic success. It is an expanded 10-component model of the coordinated school health approach. It integrates the components of the model with the tenets of the whole child approach developed by ASCD.

Application Activities

1. The WSCC model is going to be presented at a school health conference in your region of the state. The rationale, components, and important considerations related to the model will be included in the presentation. You have been asked to be part of a respondents' panel to provide your thoughts on the WSCC model. The panel members will provide their response after the WSCC presentation. You will have 10 minutes to provide your response. It should include your thoughts on the model and your perception of its applicability for students, schools, and the community. Perhaps you might have other ideas for the model; if so, identify anything that you think should be added to the WSCC model or something that might be eliminated from the model. Develop a detailed outline for your 10-minute response.
2. Conduct a literature search of newspapers, magazines, or electronic media for a story (or several stories) of a student whose academic progress was affected by a health or safety issue. Identify any positive actions that were taken in this situation or make recommendations on how this situation could have been addressed in a more productive way.

Resources

ASCD and CDC Announce Whole School, Whole Community, Whole Child Model. www.ascd.org/news-media/Press-Room/News-Releases/ASCD-and-CDC-announce-whole-child-model.aspx

Expanding the Coordinated School Health Approach. www.cdc.gov/healthyyouth/wscc/approach.htm

Health and Academics. www.cdc.gov/healthyyouth/health_and_academics/index.htm

Learning and Health. www.ascd.org/programs/learning-and-health.aspx

Whole Child Initiative. www.ascd.org/whole-child.aspx

Whole School, Whole Community, Whole Child. www.cdc.gov/healthyyouth/wscc/index.htm

References

Allensworth, Diane D., & Kolbe, Lloyd. 1987. The Comprehensive School Health Program: Exploring and Expanded Concept. *Journal of School Health*, *57*, 409–412.

ASCD. 2014. *Whole School, Whole Community Whole Child: A Collaborative Approach to Learning and Health.* Alexandria, VA: ASCD.

Basch, Charles E. 2010. Healthier Students Are Better Learners: A Missing Link in School Reforms to Close the Achievement Gap. *Equity Matters: Research Reviews*, No. 6.

Brener, Nancy D., Wheeler, Lani, Wolfe, Linda C., Vernon-Smiley, Mzry, & Caldert Olsen, Linda. 2007. Health Services: Results From the School Health Policies and Programs Study 2006. *Journal of School Health*, *77*, 464–485.

Centers for Disease Control and Prevention (CDC). 2013. *Components of Coordinated School Health.* www.cdc.gov/healthyyouth/cshp/components.htm

Epstein, Joyce L., Sanders, Mavis G., Sheldon, Steven B., Simon, Beth S., Salinas, Karen C., Jansorn, Natalie R., Van Vooris, Frances L., Martin, Cecelia S., Thomas, Brenda G., Greenfield, Marsha D., Hutchins, Darcy J., & Williams, Kenyatta J. 2009. *School, Family, and Community Partnerships: Your Handbook for Action* (3rd ed.). Thousand Oaks, CA: Corwin Press.

Institute of Medicine. 1997. *Schools and Health: Our Nation's Investment.* Diane Allensworth, Elaine Lawson, Lois Nicholson, & James Wyche (Eds.). Washington, DC: National Academy Press.

Kann, Laura, Telljohann, Susan, & Wooley, Susan, F. 2007. Health Education: Results from the School Health Policies and Programs Study 2006. *Journal of School Health*, *77*, 408–434.

Lee, Sarah M., Burgeson, Charlene R., Fulton, Janet E., & Spain, Christine G. 2007. Physical Education and Physical Activity: Results from the School Health Policies and Programs Study 2006. *Journal of School Health*, *77*, 435–463.

O'Toole, Terry P., Anderson, Susan, Miller, Claire, & Guthrie, Joanne. 2007 Nutrition Services and Foods and Beverages Available at School: Results From the School Health Policies and Programs Study 2006. *Journal of School Health*, *77*, 500–521.

2

Historical Overview of Coordinated School Health

DIANE DEMUTH ALLENSWORTH

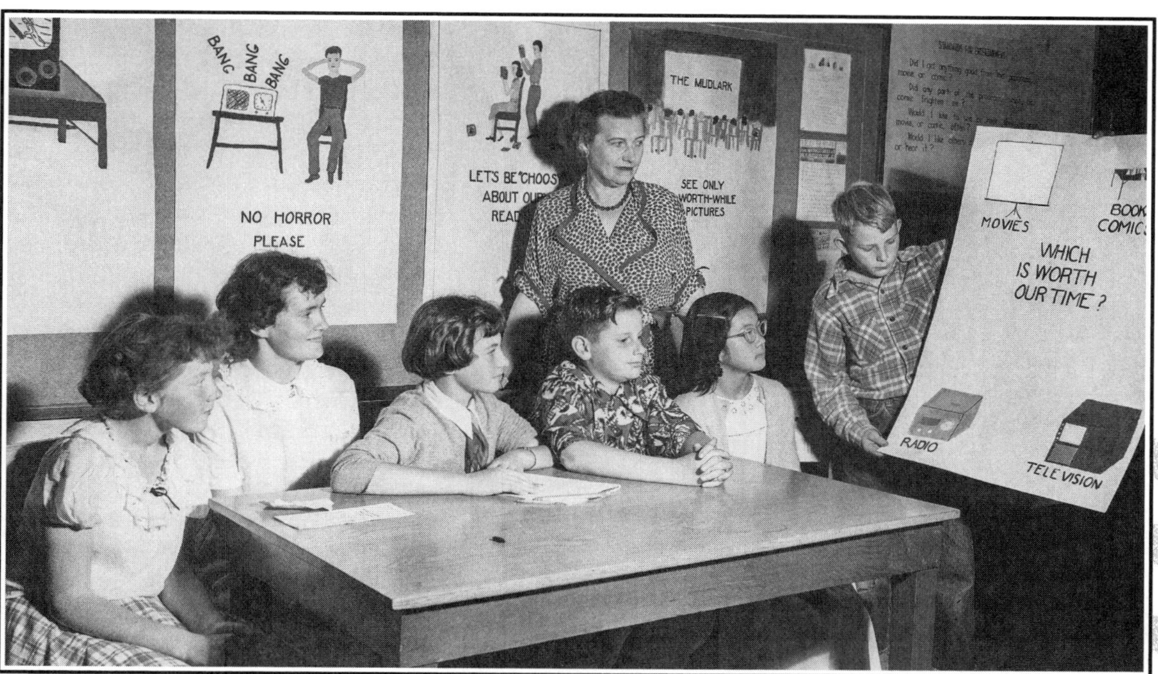
BANG
BANG
BANG
NO HORROR
PLEASE
THE MUDLARK
SEE ONLY
WORTH-WHILE
PICTURES
MOVIES
BOOK
WHICH
IS WORTH
OUR TIME?
RADIO
TELEVISION

Education and health are inextricably intertwined. Ensuring the maturation of children and youth into productive and contributing members of society is a complex endeavor requiring the collaborative efforts of families, schools, and community agencies as well as the youth themselves. In the United States, approximately 49 million young people attend 99,000 elementary and secondary schools for about 6 hours of classroom time each day for 13 of the most formative years of their lives. Although the major focus for the education sector is learning and achievement, recent research has documented the value of addressing the health of students as a means to improve achievement (Bryk et al., 2010; ICF International, 2010; Blank et al., 2004; Walsh, 2013). In turn, students who complete high school live 6 to 9 years longer than those who drop out of school (Wong, et al., 2002). Better educated people are generally healthier and will have healthier children (Murray et al., 2006).

In this chapter we explore the evolution of the school health program from its early beginning to its current practices. We describe how the eight Coordinated School Health (CSH) components replaced the original three-component model and how that model is now being replaced by the Whole School, Whole Community, Whole Child (WSCC) 10-component model. The context for how the school health program has evolved will be placed within the context for health promotion and public health. Finally, we make the case that school health programming is needed today as much as at any time in the past even though the health problems facing students have changed dramatically.

The history of school health programming closely follows the historical context for **health promotion**. We may think of this history as having three evolutionary stages in the quest to promote healthy people living in healthy communities (Kickbush & Payne, 2003). The first stage, which focused on addressing sanitary conditions and infectious diseases, occurred from the mid-19th century to the mid-20th century. The initiating event occurred in 1854 when a physician in London traced the source of cholera in a community to its water source. By removing the pump handle on the community's water supply, he prevented the cholera bacteria from infecting other community members. This discovery not only led to the development of the modern science of epidemiology but also helped governments around the world recognize the need to address infectious diseases. The second stage began approximately one hundred years later with the Lalonde report in 1974 when health promotion began to address the behavioral or root causes of diseases and injury. The third and final stage occurred around the beginning of the 21st century as the focus shifted from premature illness and death to the **social determinants of health**.

FIRST STAGE OF HEALTH PROMOTION: ADDRESSING INFECTIOUS DISEASES

> Every child should be taught early in life, that, to preserve his own life and his own health and the lives and health of others, is one of the most important and constantly abiding duties . . .
>
> *—Lemuel Shattuck, Sanitary Commission of Massachusetts, 1850*

School health programming in the United States often is traced to the 1850 report by the Sanitary Commission of Massachusetts (the Shattuck report, cited in the quotation above) that has become a classic in the field of public health and has had a significant influence on school health. Soon after the release of the Shattuck report, the medical and public health sectors recognized that schools could play a major role in controlling communicable disease with their "captive audience" of children and youth. Medical inspections of children for specific infectious diseases became the forerunner of the current health services component provided by school nurses. Although medical inspections by school physicians continued into the 1930s, the 1930 White House Conference on Child Health and Protection, which called for the elimination of medical treatments in schools, had the effect of ultimately ensuring that the primary provider of health services in the school would become the school nurse. The school's role was to refer students in need of medical care to their private physicians. It was not until the Robert Wood Johnson Foundation began its work in 1986 to support school-based health clinics that medical services began returning to schools (IOM, 1997).

By the late 1860s New York City had instituted sanitary inspections of schools twice a year because of the poor sanitary conditions in schools (IOM, 1997). This practice of sanitary inspections of schools became the precursor of the healthy school environment component of Coordinated School Health. As environmental supports for addressing infectious diseases were initiated during the early and mid-20th century (e.g., potable water, sanitary latrines, and vaccinations), deaths from infectious diseases were dramatically reduced.

World War I marked a turning point in the history of two other components: health education and school physical education. Because of the poor physical condition of many draftees, almost every state between 1918 and 1921 enacted laws prescribing health education and physical education. Course work in health education expanded to include hygiene, nutrition, diseases, family health, sex education, and healthy habits as well as the consequences of alcohol and tobacco use. Physical training, which was also known as gymnastics, was introduced into most schools during the period following World War I, although Shattuck's 1850 report had also called for physical training as part of his plan for improving the public's health (IOM, 1997).

SECOND STAGE OF HEALTH PROMOTION: ADDRESSING INDIVIDUAL BEHAVIORS

By the 1960s mental, social, and emotional health problems of students became more important issues than infectious disease. Of particular concern was the increase in substance abuse, narcotic addiction, homicide, and suicide among adolescents. This shift in disease causation in youth corresponded in timing more or less with the second stage of health promotion, which began in 1970s with the release of the Lalonde report (1974). This report documented that a new perspective was needed to improve the health of the population. The root causes of disease and death could now be traced to four basic causes: biological factors, inadequacies in the health care system, environmental factors, and behavioral or lifestyle factors. This notion directly challenged the prevailing attitude that all improvements in health could be achieved by improving the health care system.

The U.S. Public Health Service (1979) used the Lalonde framework to analyze all deaths in the United States in 1976 (see figure 2.1). The Public Health Service found that the major cause of premature death (50 percent) was lifestyle factors. Biological factors (bacteria, viruses, genetics, and so on) contributed approximately 20 percent of the total of premature deaths, environmental factors (toxins, pollutants, safety issues, and so on) contributed another 20 percent, and health care (either lack of access to health care or mistakes by the health care professions) contributed 10 percent. The behaviors that people chose to adopt or not adopt contributed the most to chronic disease and injury—the leading causes of premature mortality and morbidity by the mid-20th century.

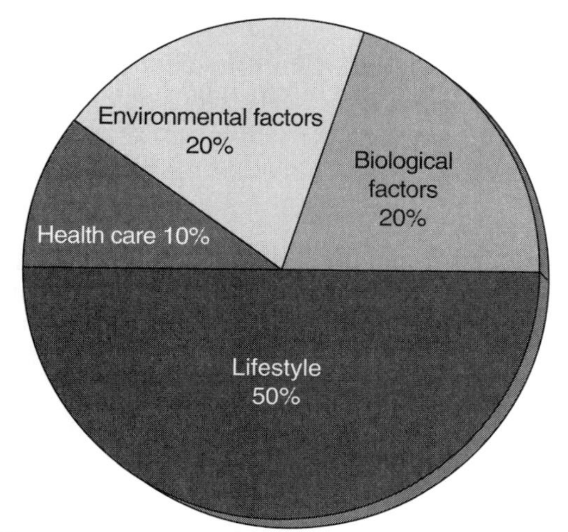

Figure 2.1 Root causes of premature deaths.
From U.S. Public Health Service, 1979.

Although the framework called attention to the continued need to ensure potable water; effective garbage and sewage disposal; and safe and unpolluted food, medicine, and air, it was the introduction of behavioral factors that shifted our understanding of disease causation. A person's health status became the responsibility of not only the physician, who promotes health with curative treatments, but also the individual, whose choice of lifestyle plays an important role in preventing or promoting disease and injury.

Substituting healthy behaviors for unhealthy behaviors, such as avoiding tobacco use, choosing a healthy diet, and engaging in regular physical activity, could prevent the development of various chronic diseases, including heart disease, diabetes, and cancer. By adopting many safety behaviors such as wearing seat belts, not riding with someone who has been drinking, and not engaging in fighting, a person could avoid unintentional and intentional injury.

Many students engaged in high-risk behaviors at this time. According to Dryfoos (1990), 10 percent of the 28 million students ages 10 through 17 engaged in a number of high-risk behaviors. Another 4 million students (15 percent) had excessively high prevalence rates for some but not all of the high-risk behaviors. These figures meant that the future of 7 million youth in this country was in jeopardy unless major and immediate changes were made in their lifestyle and their access to opportunities for healthy adolescent development. Another 25 percent of youth were at moderate risk, because of school problems, minor delinquencies, light substance abuse, and early intercourse. Only half the nation's youth (14 million) experienced few behavioral problems and were at low risk of negative consequences from their behavior. But even those students required general preventive services and health promotion programs. Because approximately 95 percent of students are enrolled in school, a quality school health program was seen as a social necessity for everyone.

To help students choose healthier behaviors, a number of curricula were developed, some with the assistance of federal funding for research and validation that the curricula were effective. Illustrious of curricula developed during the 1980s to encourage the adoption of healthy behaviors included Growing Healthy, Know Your Body, Teenage Health Teaching Modules, Go for Health, and Hearty Heart. Since then the number of evidenced-based programs has grown considerably, and they are now housed in several national and federal clearinghouses. (See "Resources" at the end of this chapter.)

Major political developments also contributed to changing the character of school programs. In 1965 a set of domestic programs, titled the Great Society, were enacted by Congress. Two main goals of the Great Society were the elimination of poverty and racial injustice. New spending programs that addressed education, medical care, urban problems, and nutrition were launched during this period. Although many of these programs focused on disadvantaged students and students with special needs, one direct effect was to triple the number of school nurses practicing in schools. Relevant legislation included Head Start, Medicaid, the Elementary and Secondary Education Act, the Education for All Handicapped Children Act, and the Child Nutrition Act (IOM, 1997).

The Child Nutrition Act of 1966 established the school breakfast program and permanently authorized reimbursements for school lunches served to needy students. Assistance in providing lunch to schoolchildren actually began by the United States Department of Agriculture in 1946 because of the poor nutrition of many of the draftees into World War II. The Education for All Handicapped Children Act (P.L. 94-142), enacted in 1975, required all public schools accepting federal funds to provide equal access to education and one free meal a day for children with physical and mental disabilities. Public schools were required to evaluate handicapped children and create an educational plan in conjunction with parental input that would prescribe as closely as possible the educational experience of nondisabled students. Before this law was enacted, many children with disabilities were denied access to education and opportunities to learn because many states had laws excluding children who were deaf, blind, emotionally disturbed, or mentally retarded.

Expansion of the School Health Model

During this stage of health promotion, the school health program also changed considerably. From the turn of the 20th century to the late 1980s, the three traditional components articulated for school health programs were health education, health services, and a healthy school environment. Kolbe (1986) suggested that an expanded school health model was a way that schools could help students live healthier, longer, more satisfying, and more productive lives. He suggested that if the three traditional components (health education, healthy school environment, and health services) were linked with physical education; counseling, psychology, and social services; school nutrition services; family and community involvement; and school site health promotion for faculty and staff that student health-related behaviors, health status, cognitive performance, and ultimately academic achievement would be enhanced.

Beyond the traditional three components that had composed the school health program, the other components were available at most schools. Counseling services began around the beginning of the 20th century, initially as vocational guidance, but by the 1930s school counseling started to address the personal, social, and emotional problems facing students. Although school psychologists have also been employed by some schools since the beginning of the 20th century to provide psychoeducational testing and services to address diagnosis and treatment of behavioral and learning problems in some schools, the passage of P.L. 94-142 quadrupled the number of school psychologists from 5,000 in 1970 to 20,000 by 1988 (Fagen, 1990). School site health promotion for faculty and staff was probably the one service that was the least developed in most schools. But it was recognized that schools are a work site for almost 10 million faculty and staff. Further, demonstration projects to engage faculty and staff in wellness activities had occurred in a number of schools with positive outcomes. Beyond the immediate health benefits that accrued to teachers, these programs also improved teacher morale and stimulated the teaching of more health to students.

Kolbe and Allensworth were in the American School Health Association's presidential rotation sequence when Kolbe's 1986 article, "Increasing the impact of school health programs: Engaging research perspective," was published. Allensworth suggested that a special issue of the association's *Journal of School Health* (*JOSH*) highlighting the roles and responsibilities of each component might help disseminate the model more quickly. After they both started working to secure authors for each component for the special issue, Kolbe's attention was redirected by a new threat to the nation's youth for which there was no cure and the only known treatment at the time was prevention—human immunodeficiency virus (HIV), which caused acquired immunodeficiency syndrome (AIDS). As the division director for the newly created Division of Adolescent and School Health within the Centers for Disease Control and Prevention (CDC), Kolbe had the responsibility of developing the national plan to reduce the spread of HIV among youth. Although he continued to assist with the development of the special issue, because of his limited involvement, he insisted that Allensworth become the lead author.

Originally, the model was named the Comprehensive School Health Program (CSHP) to identify the addition of five new components. The *JOSH* special issue focused more on describing quality programming in each component and less on how those eight components could be linked together in a process of continuous improvement. In later publications, Allensworth et al. (1994) articulated how the model could work at the school level. Strategies included

- coordinating the efforts of all faculty, staff, and administration by focusing on the priority behaviors interfering with learning and well-being;
- coordinating programming with interdisciplinary and interagency work teams, using the program planning process in a cycle of continuous improvement;
- replacing a health instruction model with a health promotion model using multiple strategies such as policy, environmental change, direct intervention (screening), role modeling, social support, and media as well as instruction;
- addressing structural and environmental changes as well as lifestyle changes;
- providing staff development to enhance professional skills;
- ensuring that all students have access to needed services; and
- viewing students as a resource by soliciting their active involvement in health promotion initiatives.

These strategies were updated in several publications (Resnicow & Allensworth, 1996; Allensworth, 1997). Allensworth later served on a CDC team that developed the roles and responsibilities for both local and state educational agencies to use in implementing a school health program (www.cdc.gov/healthyyouth/cshp/index.htm).

The new model for comprehensive school health was not without controversy. Physical educators often did not think of themselves as part of the school health program. And school nurses objected, in part because they were originally one-third of the school health program but now were reduced to being one-eighth of the program. But in spite of the objections from some professionals and some disciplines, the model has endured and has been found useful. The support and use of the model by the American School Health Association and the CDC facilitated dissemination of the model. The association published a number of articles in its journal focusing on the comprehensive school health model and developed a number of guides for schools explaining how to use the model. But the most dramatic and efficient dissemination occurred when Kolbe used the model at the Centers for Disease Control and Prevention (CDC) to address the prevention of HIV nationwide.

As the director of a new division at CDC, the Division of Adolescent and School Health, Kolbe took some bold actions that changed the way that CDC did its work. With the need to address the prevention of HIV among youth, Kolbe persuaded the agency to fund state departments of education because education was the only strategy available to prevent the spread of HIV. The CDC had only funded state departments of health before the HIV–AIDs epidemic. Kolbe also took the unique and novel position that HIV education should occur within a comprehensive school health model. This approach diffused resistance to HIV education as just a course in sex education and engaged physical educators, school nurses, counselors, and health teachers to work collaboratively as they helped school staff understand how to use universal precautions in cases of exposure to blood and body fluids in school and elsewhere and how to address the discrimination occurring with students or staff who were HIV positive.

When funding became available in the 1990s to fund chronic disease prevention, Kolbe required state departments of education and state departments of health to work collaboratively to address physical inactivity, poor nutrition, and tobacco use—the three major causes of chronic diseases. To receive the chronic disease funding, CDC required state departments of education and state departments of health to work collaboratively on school health issues as well as organize state coordinating councils that included other state agencies along with state professional and voluntary health and education organizations in a coordinated effort to plan school health programming. This innovative policy decision changed the way that states worked. Over the years, more than the original 20 states that received funding set up this collaborative planning.

The funding of **nongovernmental organizations (NGOs)** by CDC to work on school health concerns around HIV–AIDs also stimulated a variety of collaborative actions among health and

School Health *in Action*

The *Journal of School Health:* The Landmark CSH Issue

Many school health professionals and school administrators were first introduced to Coordinated School Health (CSH) through a landmark issue of the *Journal of School Health* in December 1987. The issue, funded by the Metropolitan Life Foundation, was titled "The Comprehensive School Program: Exploring an Expanded Concept." The introductory article, with the same title as the special issue of the journal, was authored by the original visionaries of what is now known as Coordinated School Health, Diane D. Allensworth and Lloyd J. Kolbe.

Two important concepts were stressed in the introductory article. The first concept was the importance of coordination among various school programs, the family, and the community. As Allensworth and Kolbe emphasized, "These eight components of a Comprehensive School Health Program, if coordinated to address a given health behavior or health problem, could have complementary if not synergistic effects" (p. 409). The second important concept was the connection of the health of students to academic success. In the Allensworth and Kolbe article, Michael McGinnis, at that time director, U.S. Office of Disease Prevention and Health Promotion, U.S. Department of Health and Human Services, noted:

> What is clear is that education and health are inextricably intertwined. A student who is not healthy, who suffers from an undetected vision or hearing defect, or who is hungry, or who is impaired by drugs or alcohol, is not a student who will profit from the educational process. Likewise, a person who has not been provided assistance in the shaping of healthy attitudes, beliefs, and habits early in life, will be more likely to suffer the consequences of reduced productivity in later years.

Besides the introductory article, the issue included one or two articles that addressed each of the eight components of comprehensive school health. The authors of these articles were asked to address the scope and parameters of the component; specific ways that the component influences the health and cognitive performance of students, faculty, and staff; results of research that describes the effectiveness of the component; and credentials required by and major national organizations for practitioners in the professions related to each component.

Allensworth and Kolbe hoped that the special issue would influence professionals to function together as a team to have a positive influence on the health and well-being of children and youth. The vision and leadership of Allensworth and Kolbe and the resources developed over the years after the publication of this landmark issue of the *Journal of School Health* have certainly made major contributions to maintaining and improving the health and academic achievement of school-age children and youth.

Reference

Allensworth & Kolbe. 1987. The Comprehensive School Health Program: Exploring an Expanded Concept. *Journal of School Health*, 57(10), 409–412.

education NGOs. One initiative that engaged five of the national agencies funded by CDC was the development of market research around the title of the Comprehensive School Health Program. Staff from the Council of Chief School Officers, the National Association of State Boards of Education, the National School Boards Association, the American Cancer Association, and the American School Health Association collaboratively found that the terminology "Comprehensive" School Health Programs (CSHP) caused much confusion because health education was often referred to as "comprehensive health education" and some people would say "comprehensive health education" when they were referring to the "Comprehensive School Health Program." Marketing research also discovered that school board members, superintendents, and principals thought that "comprehensive" sounded expensive and complicated. Two major publications of the era, *Health and Schools* and *Health Is Academic*, were published with the respective editors' full knowledge of the marketing research that had been completed by the five NGOs. The authors of both publications agreed to suggest to readers that using "coordinated" instead of "comprehensive" would be the best wording to use when referring to the school health program. CDC also began using this terminology. By 2006 most state departments of education had adopted the tenets of Coordinated School Health, but adoption at the school level was not as pervasive.

Additional Federal Support for Coordinated School Health Programs

Unlike other nations, the United States places the responsibility for education not at the federal level but at the state level. Therefore, any aspect of the curriculum, the amount of funding received per pupil, and the inclusion of any school health programming can vary considerably across states. But federal funding for specific programs such as the Child Nutrition Act and Title One of the Education for All Handicapped Children Act, which were implemented in all schools, provides a mechanism for some continuity in programming across the nation. Federal funding for demonstration projects as well as federal resources supporting the various components of school health can be found in most of the federal offices including the U.S. Departments of Education, Health and Human Services, Justice, and Agriculture. The resources and funding for demonstration projects over time can influence programming nationwide.

A major federal initiative promoting school health programming is the **Healthy People** program. The initiative, which began five years after the Lalonde report was issued, was released by the Office of Disease Prevention and Health Promotion in 1979. An updated Healthy People document has been published every 10 years (1980, 1990, 2000, and 2010). The document is a public–private national initiative that elicits input from a variety of stakeholders such as nongovernmental national organizations, state health agencies, professional associations, and universities as well as multiple federal agencies. This input provides direction for the identification of national priorities for health promotion at the beginning of each decade. The Healthy People goals and objectives guide and direct the health promotion actions of federal agencies, local and state health departments, health care practitioners, academicians, and health workers at all levels of government. The need to involve practitioners of school health became critical with the first update of new goals and objectives in 1989. Almost one-third of the objectives published in 1990 for achievement by 2000 could be attained only with the direct participation and support of the public schools.

THIRD STAGE OF HEALTH PROMOTION: ADDRESSING THE SOCIAL DETERMINANTS OF HEALTH

> That there should be a spread of life expectancy of 48 years among countries and 20 years or more within countries is not inevitable. A burgeoning volume of research identifies social factors at the root of much of these inequalities in health. Social determinants are relevant to communicable and noncommunicable disease alike.
>
> —Sir Michael Marmot, *Lancet*, 2005

By the beginning of the 21st century, it became apparent that just exhorting people to choose health-enhancing behaviors to improve health status was insufficient. Individual decisions about behaviors that people could adopt were rooted in the social environment in which they were born, lived, worked, and played. For example, many children lived where they could not play outside because of violence in their neighborhoods. Supermarkets that offered a variety of food and fresh produce were not located nearby. Toxic emissions from industry contaminated the air or water in the community, and access to medical care was limited. Schools in the community were often inferior, so these students received an inadequate education. The children (as well as the adults who cared for them) had little control over these various social situations that precluded their making healthy choices.

The social determinants of health include all societal conditions that affect health—poverty, the economic system, health care system including access, the educational system, housing, the transportation system, and the surrounding environment as well as the social relationships between community members, such as civic engagement or discrimination and racism. The root causes of premature illness and death have been updated to include the social determinants (see figure 2.2).

The World Health Organization, which has been at the forefront of describing the issues surrounding the social determinants of health, noted that these conditions existed not only in low-income countries but also in high-income countries that had provided universal health care for all their population. The United States, one of the richest

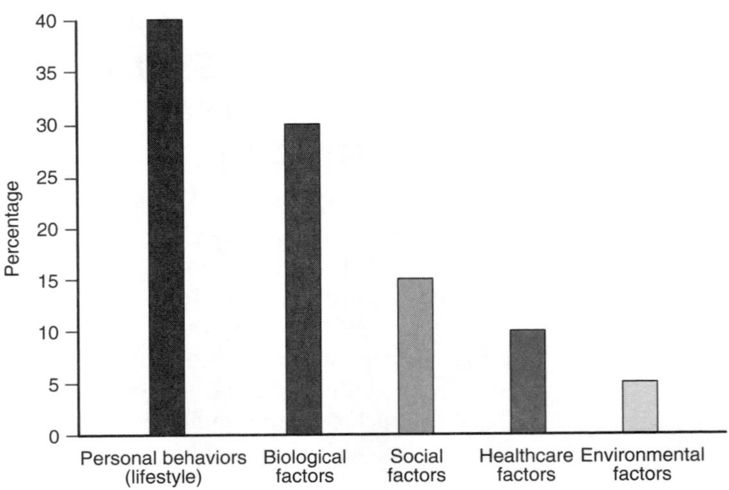

Figure 2.2 Contributing factors to premature death.
Data from Schroeder 2007.

countries in the world, also has one of the highest poverty rates for children of all developed countries. Children in poverty experience more of the negative social determinants. Currently, about 23 percent of students in the United States live in high-poverty families. These students are more likely to be exposed to toxins such as tobacco smoke and lead, experience food insecurity, have poorer health, and complete less schooling (Coley & Baker, 2013). Youth health disparities are evident in mortality rates, the incidence of chronic disease, and less access to general health care services and preventive services (Flores et al., 2010). The poor health of these students reduces not only their quality of life but also their educational attainment. The longer that children live in poverty, the slower their general maturation and the lower their educational achievement will be, not because of innate deficits, but because of the many poverty stressors including poor health care, food insecurity, inadequate housing, and inequitable educational opportunities (Richardson, 2007). Educational attainment is an acknowledged route out of poverty (Iton, 2006; Freudenberg & Ruglis, 2007). Yet for many poor students, inequitable educational opportunities and health problems will limit their achievement in school, which will also limit their productivity as adults. Students who have failed one or more courses are more likely to drop out of school (Allensworth & Easton, 2007) thus limiting career opportunities that could have helped them break the cycle of poverty.

Research that synthesized 10 years of progress within the Chicago Public School District on what is critical to improving student achievement found that five essential supports influenced student learning: school leadership, professional capacity of staff, an instructional guidance system that engages students, a student-centered learning climate that is safe and orderly, and parent and community support and linkages. *Community support and linkages* was the phrase that the authors used to describe how health needs were provided to students through linkages to community health and social services agencies. The researchers found that students in schools that assembled a first-rate social services support team and accessed external programs and services from community agencies to supplement the meager health and social services offered by the school system demonstrated improved reading and mathematics scores (Byrk et al., 2010).

In 2010 ASCD, a professional, educational membership organization with 165,000 members that was previously known as the Association for Supervision and Curriculum Development, and the Society for Public Health Education jointly convened an expert panel to explore the issues associated with health and education inequities in children and youth. The expert panel recommended:

- joint accountability for health and learning of students through cross-agency collaboration of the education and health sectors in every community,
- cross-agency collaboration using data to drive continuous improvement in programming,
- cross-agency collaboration ensuring health care access for all students,
- cross-agency collaboration ensuring a healthy and safe learning environment, and
- cross-agency collaboration ensuring health and physical education instruction so that all students could choose a healthy lifestyle (SOPHE, 2013).

Fact sheets describing each recommendation are available at www.sophe.org/SchoolHealth/Disparities.cfm.

The release of *Healthy People 2020* by the U.S. Department of Health and Human Services in 2010 included attention to the social determinants of health for the first time. The sentinel health indicator for all social determinant objectives is to increase the proportion of students who graduate with a regular diploma four years after starting ninth grade (HHS, 2010). This objective underscores the need for a link between the health and education sectors to ensure educational achievement and health for current students, the adults that they will become, and their future children (figure 2.3). Many students continue to have health problems that can reduce their achievement in course work by limiting their concentration or by increasing their absenteeism. Chronic student absenteeism is related to poor achievement and ultimately dropping out of school. Students who miss just two weeks of schooling each semester can be on a downward spiral of course failure and ultimately failure to graduate (Allensworth & Easton, 2007). The following list presents examples of student health problems that have the potential to negatively affect academic performance.

- Sixteen to 18 percent of students have a chronic health condition (Halfron & Newacheck, 2010).
- Approximately 20 percent of students have a diagnosable mental, emotional, or behavioral problem—mental health problems that often result in poor school performance, school dropout, or involvement with the child welfare or juvenile justice systems (Schwarz, 2009).
- Twenty-six percent of students living below 100 percent of poverty level and 18 percent of children living in families at 100 to 199 percent of poverty level have untreated dental caries (National Forum on Child Statistics, 2011). Each year more than 51 million school hours are lost to dental-related illness (Holt & Barzel, 2010).
- Eight percent of adolescents have a substance abuse or dependence disorder (Fox & McManus, 2009).

Besides diagnosed health problems, the health risk behaviors of students can impede learning, achievement, and high school graduation. Almost one-third of females who drop out of school cite pregnancy as the reason (Shuger, 2012). Substance abuse, unintended injury, and intentional injury (fighting, homicide, suicide) contribute to more immediate consequences. Among high school students, many are at risk because they engage in health-risk behaviors:

- Nearly 39 percent of teens had a drink of alcohol in the last 30 days, and 21.9 percent of students had engaged in binge drinking by having five or more drinks of alcohol in a row on at least one day during the 30 days before the survey;
- 33.7 percent of teens are sexually active, but only 9.5 percent used both a condom to protect against a sexually transmitted disease and a birth control method at their last sexual encounter;
- 71 percent of teens did not routinely engage in physical activity 60 minutes every day;

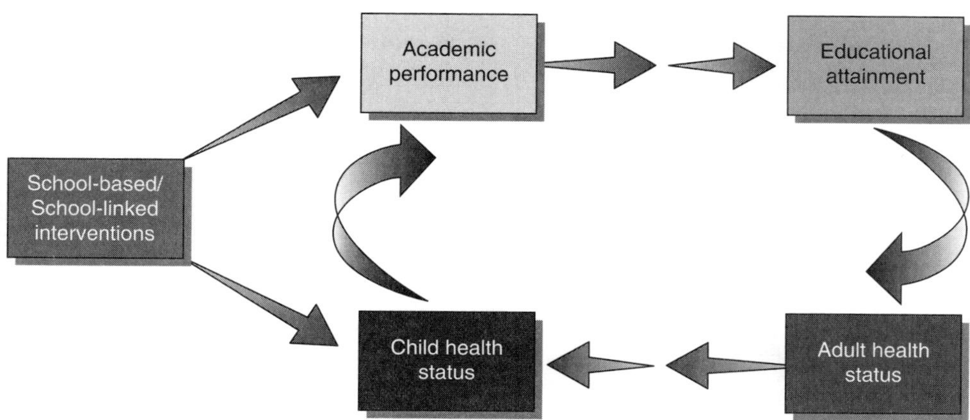

Figure 2.3 Education and health are interconnected.

Adapted, by permission, from N. Murray et al., 2006, Appendix E: *Education and health: A review and assessment. Code red: The critical condition of health in Texas* (Task Force on Access to Health Care in Texas). Available: http://www.coderedtexas.org/files/Appendix_E.pdf.

- 28 percent of teens ate vegetables two or more times per day; and
- 18.1 percent of teens smoked tobacco on at least one day 30 days before the survey (Eaton et al., 2012).

The prevalence of multiple health risk-taking behaviors is not uncommon. Fox and McManus (2009) found after reviewing adolescent engagement in 12 health risk behaviors that 52 percent of high school students reported engaging in two or more risk behaviors, 35 percent reported engaging in three or more, and 15 percent reported engaging in five or more. Students engaging in health risk behaviors threaten not only their health but also their academic achievement. Implementing a quality school health program that provides universal and targeted interventions can reduce health risk behaviors and improve chronic health conditions (figure 2.2).

A recent survey of teachers also underscores the health needs of students. A MetLife (2012) survey found that almost 50 percent of students do not arrive at school fit, healthy, rested, and alert (table 2.1). A majority of teachers (64 percent) in 2012 reported that during the past year the number of students and families who need health and social support services has increased. During the same period, 28 percent of teachers have seen reductions or eliminations of health or social services (MetLife, 2012).

A variety of structures and mechanisms currently exist to promote joint accountability between the education sector and health sector to improve the health status and the health behaviors of students by providing needed health care and social services. These mechanisms include coalitions promoting community schools, school-based health centers, school-linked health centers, children's cabinets, advisory committees, district and municipal coordinating committees, and school health councils and school health teams. Unfortunately, these infrastructures are not ubiquitous, nor are all functioning efficiently to link programming in a process of continuous improvement.

Two national organizations, the Coalition for Community Schools and Communities in Schools, have promoted the concept of community schools in which community agencies are solicited as partners to ensure that the physical, social, and emotional needs of students and families are being met. The Coalition of Community Schools has established five conditions to ensure that learning occurs:

- The school has a core instructional program with qualified teachers, a challenging curriculum, and high standards and expectations for students.
- Students are motivated and engaged in learning—both in school and in community settings, during and after school.
- The basic physical, mental, and emotional health needs of young people and their families are recognized and addressed.
- Mutual respect and effective collaboration occur among parents, families, and school staff.

Table 2.1 MetLife Survey of American Teachers

	Total (%)	Elementary school (%)	Middle school (%)	High school (%)
Teachers reporting that most/nearly all students...				
Arrive at school alert and rested	60	69	62	48
Are healthy and physically fit	56	61	56	51
Teachers strongly agree that the school provides support services ...				
Adequate health services to students	17	19	17	14
Adequate counseling and support for students	22	19	25	23
Healthy food choices for students	11	14	11	8

Based on MetLife 2012.

- Community engagement, together with school efforts, promotes a school climate that is safe, supportive, and respectful and that connects students to a broader learning community.

The Communities in Schools organization is based on five similar but unique strategies:

- A one-on-one relationship with a caring adult
- A safe place to learn and grow
- A healthy start and a healthy future (access to health and dental care, food programs, and counseling services)
- A marketable skill to use after graduation
- A chance to give back to peers and community

Both initiatives ensure that health services are provided to students, and both require active student participation in community service.

Evaluations from 20 community school initiatives have shown that 75 percent of these community schools improved academic achievement. More than half of the schools reported improvement in attendance, reduced behavior or discipline problems, greater compliance with school assignments, and more contact with supportive adults (Blank et al., 2004). A five-year evaluation of the Communities in Schools' dropout prevention program concluded that the program model resulted in the strongest reduction in dropout rates of any existing fully scaled dropout prevention program that has been evaluated by the U.S. Department of Education. The more fully and faithfully the model was implemented, the stronger the outcomes were (Communities in Schools, 2011).

BARRIERS TO UNIVERSAL ADOPTION OF CSH

Although most state education agencies have subscribed to a Coordinated School Health model, most local schools have not. One of the barriers to universal adoption of the Coordinated School Health model at the local school level has been the focus on achieving health goals. Although the original CSH model had identified improved cognitive performance as a short-term outcome and improved educational achievement as a long-term outcome, a document that compiled research on the value of each of the eight components in achieving educational goals lagged almost 15 years behind the initiation of the model. The publishing of *Making the Connection: Health and Student Achievement* in 2002 compiled the existing and emerging research on how each of the components contributed to various educational goals including reducing absenteeism, reducing tardiness, improving comportment, increasing school bonding, decreasing dropout rates, improving achievement, and increasing graduation rates. Only recently have leading educational researchers (Bryk et al., 2010) identified that a safe and nurturing learning environment, family involvement, and linkages with community agencies were among the five critical elements in organizing schools to improve achievement in elementary grades (but these researchers did not identify these elements as components of Coordinated School Health). Thus, the importance of school health programs to achievement of educational outcomes has not been a standard part of the preservice training of principals and superintendents whose support for the coordination of school health is critical at the local level.

Another barrier to universal adoption of the Coordinated School Health model was the lack of coordination among components and between the health and education sector. The launching of the special issue of the *Journal of School Health* in 1987 focused on exploring the status of the individual components but was not specific about how the coordination among the components should occur. As director of the Division of Adolescent and School Health, Kolbe identified how the school health program could be coordinated from the national level to the local level. Allensworth et al. (1994) first wrote about how local school coordination could be accomplished in *Healthy Students 2000* as well as in several other publications (Resnicow & Allensworth, 1996; Allensworth, 1997). But guidance on coordination from the CDC website was minimal until the mid-2000s when CDC identified roles, responsibilities, and coordination for both local and state school health programs (Allensworth et al., 2006). At the school level, a school health team composed of representatives of the eight components plus parents and community agency staff is recommended, and at the district level, a school health council composed of representatives from the school, community mental and physical health, public health, and civic and youth development agencies is recommended. An analysis by CDC of local school health teams found that the schools that have organized such structures have implemented more school health policies and programming (Brenner et al., 2004). The percentage of secondary schools that had one or more school health teams in 2010 ranged nationwide from 33.1 percent to 80.4 percent depending on the state (Brenner et al., 2011). Currently, the proportion of public health departments working with schools on the school health council ranges from 17.9 to 63.7 percent nationwide, again depending on the state (Brenner et al., 2011).

A final reason that the coordinated model seemed to be less accepted at the school level was that public health workers for the most part were focused on the achieving the health goals because they were responsible for those specific goals. Public health workers did not help school stakeholders understand how achieving health goals could at the same time achieve educational goals such as reduced absenteeism, reduced tardiness, improved comportment, improved time on task, and improved achievement.

A new model for promoting health and academic success was initiated by ASCD in 2007. The **Whole Child Initiative** focused on ways to ensure that young people's needs are met both at the higher levels of knowledge and achievement and at the most fundamental levels of health, safety, and belonging. The initiative challenged schools and communities to work together in new ways to develop "successful learners who are knowledgeable, emotionally and physically healthy, civically active, engaged, prepared for economic self-sufficiency, and ready for the world beyond formal schooling" (ASCD, 2007). ASCD's Commission on the Whole Child recommended that local schools work closely with the community to address the conditions that affect learning. Kolbe was a member of the ASCD's commission, an interdisciplinary panel that included public health, health care, and education leaders that identified the following five elements as necessary for learning:

- Each student enters school healthy and learns about and practices a healthy lifestyle.
- Each student learns in an intellectually challenging environment that is physically and emotionally safe for students and adults.
- Each student is actively engaged in learning and is connected to the school and broader community.
- Each student has access to personalized learning and to qualified and caring adults.
- Each graduate is prepared for success in college or further study and for employment in a global environment.

NEXT EVOLUTION FOR SCHOOL HEALTH

In 2014 ASCD and the Centers for Disease Control and Prevention merged their respective models into the Whole School, Whole Community, Whole Child (WSCC) model to ensure greater collaboration, integration, and alignment between the health and education sectors. Both Kolbe and Allensworth were among the subject matter experts in health and education who assisted with the development of the WSCC model.

The leadership and respect that these two organizations have in their respective sectors bodes well for encouraging both the education sector and the health sector to move simultaneously toward greater collaboration. Linking the Whole Child model with Coordinated School Health shifts the focus to students as opposed to the discipline or services. For the educational community, the model now will focus equally on educational outcomes and health outcomes. In addition, having the primary public health agency and its network of public health workers as community advocates can facilitate the collaboration needed at the community level.

The model expands the components by separating the healthy environment into the physical environment and the social and emotional climate. Family and community involvement has also been divided into two separate components to emphasize the role that community agencies, businesses, and organizations can play in support of both the health and learning of students. Further, the critical role of family engagement in improving health and learning outcomes of students is now highlighted. The key to moving from model to action requires collaborative development of policies, practices, and processes, resulting in complementary processes guiding each decision and action within both sectors in communities across the nation. Within the announcement of the merged model, ASCD is calling for more collaboration among sectors.

SUMMARY

Many children and youth face threats to their health and well-being. Because more than 95 percent of young people aged 5 to 17 years are enrolled in school, schools are in a unique position to improve both the education status and health status of young people throughout the nation. Although much progress has been made to improve school health programming during the last 25 years, much remains to be done. The quality of programming of most components in most schools nationwide needs to improve because they do not meet national standards. For example, instruction in neither health education (Kann, Telljohann, & Wooley, 2007; Brenner et al., 2011) nor physical education (CDC, 2013b; Demissie, et al., 2013) meets time requirements set by national standards. The services of a registered nurse are not available to all students, and when one is available the ratio of practitioner to students does not meet national standards (Brenner, Wheeler, et al. 2006). Nor are school counselors, psychologists, or social workers available for all students (Brenner, Weist, et al., 2007). Some schools that have adopted the goals of a "community school" have ensured linkages between schools and community agencies that provide physical and mental health services (Blank et al., 2004; Communities in Schools, 2011). But the coordination among schools, families, and community agencies could be improved in most communities. Children and youth make up one-fourth of our population and all of its future. Providing a quality school health program for each child ensures improved learning and achievement as well as a healthier and more productive future for our nation.

Glossary

community schools—A set of partnerships between school and community to ensure student access to health care as well as educational and other needed services.

Healthy People—A federal public–private partnership that began in 1980 and that at the beginning of every decade sets the public health goals and objectives for research and programming for the decade.

health promotion—A planned intervention to improve the health of a target population by changing lifestyle behaviors and environmental conditions through any combination of health education, organizational, economic, or environmental supports.

nongovernmental organization (NGO)—A nongovernmental agency that is nonprofit and organized at the local, state, national, or international level.

school health council—The term given to the team organized at the district level to facilitate continuous improvement in the school health program as well as collaboration between the school and the community. Ideally, the district school health council includes at least one district representative from each of the eight components, as well as school administrators, parents, students, and community representatives involved in the health and well-being of students, including a representative from the local health department and the school district's medical consultant.

school health team—The corollary of the school health council, the team that facilitates continuous improvement in the school health program at school site level. Ideally, the team includes an administrator, staff representing the eight components, parents, subject specialist, classroom teachers, students, and community members engaged in the health and well-being of students.

social determinants of health—The primary causes of premature illness and death, which are now recognized to be rooted in the social environment in which people are born, live, work, and play. The social determinants of health include all societal conditions that affect health—poverty, the economic system, the health care system including access, the educational system, housing, the transportation system, and the surrounding environment as well as the social relationships available between community members, such as civic engagement or discrimination and racism.

Whole Child—an initiative developed by ASCD in 2007 to improve the education and health outcomes of students by organizing school, families, and community agencies to ensure that all students are healthy, safe, engaged, supported, and challenged.

Application Activities

1. As a school health professional with a strong background in the Whole School, Whole Community, Whole Child (WSCC) approach, you have been invited by a school administrator to speak to teachers and school staff regarding this approach to school health. You will have 30 minutes for your presentation and 15 minutes for discussion and questions. You are asked to address the three stages of health promotion, the history of the CSH-WSCC approach, and the rationale for promoting school health. Develop a PowerPoint outline for your presentation and a list of questions that may be asked of you by teachers and staff members. Include your responses to the questions.
2. You are invited to write an opinion article (op-ed) for the local newspaper on WSCC. The purpose of your op-ed is to inform the local community of why promoting student health is important for the local district and why WSCC is a logical vehicle for advancing the health and wellness of those in the district. Your op-ed cannot be longer than 1,000 words.
3. You are a health educator with a youth health promotion organization that has worked with schools in coordinated school health (CSH). Your supervisor has asked you to draft an announcement, no longer than one page, that will be sent to other community organizations that have supported your organization's past CSH efforts. The purpose of the paper is to introduce the WSCC model to these organizations. You have been asked to present a comparison of WSCC to the CSH model in your paper and describe both the important elements of WSCC and the benefits of moving from CSH to WSCC. In developing your announcement, assume that readers will have limited background on the history of CSH and no background on WSCC.

Resources

Basch, Charles E. 2010. *Healthier Students Are Better Learners. A Research Initiative of the Campaign for Educational Equity.* Teachers College, Columbia University, Research Review No. 6. www.equitycampaign.org/i/a/document/12557_EquityMattersVol6_web03082010.pdf

City Connects: The Impact of City Connects: Progress Report 2012. 2012. Boston: City Connects, Boston College Center for Optimized Student Support. www.bc.edu/content/dam/files/schools/lsoe/cityconnects/pdf/CityConnects_ProgressReport_2012.pdf

Castrechini, Sebastian, & London, Rebecca A. 2012. *Positive Student Outcomes in Community Schools.* Center for American Progress. www.americanprogress.org/issues/2012/02/pdf/positive_student_outcomes.pdf

Coalition of Community Schools. 2013. *Rational and Results Framework.* Washington DC: Coalition of Community Schools. www.communityschools.org/results/overview.aspx

Communities in Schools. 2012. *Communities in Schools and the Five Basics. Fact Sheet.* Arlington, VA: Communities in Schools. www.communitiesinschools.org/media/uploads/attachments/Communities_In_Schools_and_the_Five_Basics_2.pdf

CDC. 2013. *Coordinated School Health.* Atlanta, GA: Centers for Disease Control and Prevention. www.cdc.gov/healthyyouth/cshp/index.htm

Federal Interagency Forum on Child and Family Statistics. 2013. *America's Children: Key National Indicators of Well-Being, 2013.* Washington, DC: U.S. Government Printing Office. www.childstats.gov/pdf/ac2013/ac_13.pdf

National Prevention Council, Office of the Surgeon General, U.S. Department of Health and Human Services. 2011. *National Prevention Strategy.* Washington, DC. www.surgeongeneral.gov/initiatives/prevention/strategy/report.pdf

Shirer, Karen, & Miller, Patricia P. 1998. *Promoting Healthy Students, Schools and Communities: A Guide to Community School Health Councils.* Atlanta, GA: American Cancer Society. www.cancer.org/healthymorewaysacshelpsyoustaywell/schoolhealth/schoolhealthcouncils/a-guide-to-community-school-health-councils

Registries of Effective and Evidenced-Based School Health Interventions

Child Trends "What Works" Listings: www.childtrends.org

SAMHSA's National Registry of Evidence-Based Programs and Practices: www.nrepp.samhsa.gov

Office of Juvenile Justice and Delinquency Prevention's Model Programs Guide: www.ojjdp.gov/mpg/

Institute of Education Sciences, What Works Clearinghouse: http://ies.ed.gov/ncee/wwc/

References

Allensworth, Diane, Symons, Cynthia, & Olds, R. Scott. 1994. *Healthy Students 2000: An Agenda for Continuous Improvement in America's Schools*. Kent, Ohio: American School Health Association.

Allensworth, Diane. 1997. Improving the Health of Youth Through a Coordinated School Health Programme. *Health Promotion & Education, 1*(4), 2–47.

Allensworth, Diane D., Fisher, C., & Hunt, P. 2006, October 12. An Expanded Understanding of Coordinated School Health Programs. American School Health Association Annual School Health Conference. St. Louis, MO.

Allensworth, Elaine, & Easton John Q. 2005. *The On-Track Indicator as a Predictor of High School Graduation*. Chicago: Consortium on Chicago School Research at the University of Chicago. http://ccsr.uchicago.edu/content/publications.php

Allensworth, Elaine, & Kolbe, Lloyd. 1987. The Comprehensive School Health Program: Exploring an Expanded Concept. *Journal of School Health*, 57(10), 409–412.

ASCD. 2007. *The Community Conversations Project: A Guide for Informal Discussion Groups*. Arlington, VA: ASCD.

ASCD. 2014. ASCD and CDC Announce Whole School, Whole Community, Whole Child Model. www.ascd.org/news-media/Press-Room/News-Releases/ASCD-and-CDC-announce-whole-child-model.aspx

Blank, Martin J., & Shah, Bela P. 2004. Educators and Community Sharing Responsibility for Student Learning. Info Brief. *Association for Supervision and Curriculum Development, 36*, 1–11.

Brenner, Nancy D., Kann, Laura, McManus, Tim, Stevenson, Beth, & Wooley Susan F. 2004. The Relationship Between School Health Councils and School Health Policies and Programs in U.S. Schools. *Journal of School Health, 74*(4), 130–135.

Brenner, Nancy D., Wheeler, Lani, Wolfe, Linda C., Vernon-Smiley, Mary, & Linda Caldart-Olsen. 2006. Health Services: Results from the School Health Policies and Programs Study, *Journal of School Health*, 77(8), 464–485.

Brenner, Nancy D., Weist, M., Adelman, H., Taylor L., & Vernon-Smiley, Mary. 2007. Mental Health Services: Results from the School Health Policies and Programs Study, 2006. *Journal of School Health*, 77(8), 486–499.

Brenner, Nancy D., Zewditu, Demissie, Foti, Kathryn, McManus. Tim, Shanklin, Shari L., Hawkins, Joseph, & Kann, Laura. 2011. *School Health Profiles 2010: Characteristics of health Programs Among Secondary Schools in Selected U.S. Sites*. Atlanta, GA: Centers for Disease Control and Prevention. www.cdc.gov/healthyyouth/profiles/2010/profiles_report.pdf

Byrk, Anthony S., Sebrig, Penny B., Allensworth, Elaine, Luppesca, Stuart, & Easton John Q. 2010. *Organizing Schools for Improvement. Lessons From Chicago*. Chicago: University of Chicago Press. http://ccsr.uchicago.edu/books/osfi/prologue.pdf

Centers for Disease Control and Prevention (CDC). 2013b. *Comprehensive School Physical Activity Programs: A Guide for Schools*. Atlanta, GA: U.S. Department of Health and Human Services.

Coley, Richard J., & Baker, Bruce. 2013. *Poverty and Education: Finding the Way Forward*. Princeton, NJ: Educational Testing Service. www.ets.org/s/research/pdf/poverty_and_education_report.pdf

Communities in Schools. 2011. *2009–2010 Results From the Communities in Schools Network*. Washington, DC: Communities in Schools. www.communitiesinschools.org/media/uploads/attachments/Network_Results_2009-2010.pdf

Demissie, Zewditu, Brener, Nancy D., McManus, Tim, Shanklin, Shari L., Hawkins, Joseph, & Kann, Laura. 2013. *School Health Profiles 2012: Characteristics of Health Programs Among Secondary Schools*. Atlanta, GA: Centers for Disease Control and Prevention. www.cdc.gov/healthyyouth/profiles/2012/profiles_report.pdf

Dryfoos, Joy G. 1990. *Adolescence at Risk: Prevalence and Prevention*. New York: Oxford Press.

Eaton, Danice K., Kann, Laura, Kinchen, Shari, Flint, Katherine, Hawkins, Joseph, Harris, William, Lowry, Richard, McManus, Tim, Chyen, David, Whittle, Lisa, Lim, Connie, & Wechsler Howell. 2012. Youth Risk Behavior Surveillance—United States. *MMWR, 61*(4), 1–162. www.cdc.gov/mmwr/pdf/ss/ss6104.pdf

Fagen, Thomas. 1990. A Brief History of School Psychology in the United States. In A. Thomas & J. Grimes (Eds.), *Best Practices in School Psychology*. Bethesda, MD: National Association of School Psychologists. www.nyasp.org/pdf/sp_timeline.pdf

Flores, Glenn, and the Committee on Pediatric Research. 2010. Racial and Ethnic Disparities in the Health and Health Care of Children. *Pediatrics, 125*(4), e979–e1020. http://pediatrics.aappublications.org/content/125/4/e979.full

Fox, Harriette B., & McManus, Margaret A. 2009, June. *Health Reform and Adolescents*. Issue Brief No. 3. National Alliance to Advance Adolescent Health. http://thenationalalliance.org/pdfs/Brief3.%20Health%20Reform%20and%20Adolescents.pdf

Freudenberg, Nicholas, & Ruglis, Jessica. 2007. Reframing School Dropout as a Public Health Issue. *Preventing Chronic Disease, 4* (4). www.cdc.gov/pcd/issues/2007/oct/07_0063.htm

Halfron, Neal, & Newacheck, Paul W. 2010. Evolving Notions of Childhood Chronic Illness. *JAMA, 303*(7), 665-666.

Holt, Katrina, & Barzel, Ruth. 2010. *Pain and Suffering Shouldn't Be an Option: School-Based and School-Linked Oral Health Services for Children and Adolescents.* Washington, DC: National Maternal and Child Oral Health Resource Center. www.mchoralhealth.org/PDFs/schoolhealthfactsheet.pdf

ICF International. 2010. *2010 Communities in Schools National Evaluation Five Year Summary* Report, Fairfax, VA: ICF International. www.communitiesinschools.org/media-center/resource/five-year-evaluation

Institute of Medicine (IOM). 1997. *Schools and Health: Our Nation's Investment—Final Report of the Committee on Comprehensive School Health Programs in Grades K–12.* Ed. Allensworth, Diane, Wyche, James, Lawson, Elaine, and Nicholson, Lois. Washington, DC: Institute of Medicine, National Academy of Science.

Iton, Anthony. 2006. Tackling the Root Causes of Health Disparities Through Community Capacity Building. In Richard Hofreichter (ed.), *Tackling Health Inequities Through Public Health Practice: A Handbook for Action* (pp. 115–136). Washington, DC: National Association of County and City Health Official. www.naccho.org/pubs/product1.cfm?Product_ID=11

Kickbush, Ilona, & Payne, Lea. 2003. Twenty-First Century Health Promotion: The Public Health Revolution Meets the Wellness Revolution. *Health Promotion International, 18*(4), 275–278.

Kann, Laura, Telljohann, Susan K., & Wooley, Susan F. 2006. Health Education: Results From the School Health Policies and Programs Study. *Journal of School Health, 77*(8), 408–434.

Kolbe, Lloyd J. 1986. Increasing the Impact of School Health Promotion Programs: Emerging Research Perspective. *Journal of Health Education, 17*(5), 47–52.

Lalonde, Marc. 1974. *A New Perspective on the Health of Canadians: A Working Document.* Ottawa, ON: Health and Welfare Canada.

Marmot, Michael. 2005. Social Determinants of Health Inequalities. *Lancet, 365,* 1099–104. www.who.int/social_determinants/strategy/Marmot-Social%20determinants%20of%20health%20inqualities.pdf

MetLife. 2012. *The MetLife Survey of American Teachers: Teachers, Parents and the Economy. A Survey of Teachers, Parents and Students.* www.metlife.com/assets/cao/contributions/foundation/american-teacher/MetLife-Teacher-Survey-2011.pdf

Murray, Nancy, Franzini, Luisa, Marko, Dritana, Lupo, Jr., Philip, Garza, Julie, & Linder, Stephen. 2006. *Education and Health: A Review and Assessment, Appendix E in Code Red: The Critical Condition of Health in Texas.* www.coderedtexas.org/files/Appendix_E.pdf

National Forum on Child Statistics. 2011. *America's Children: Key National Indicators of Well-Being, 2011.* Available at www.childstats.gov/pdf/ac2011/ac_11.pdf

Resnicow Ken, & Allensworth, Diane D. 1996. Conducting a Comprehensive School Health Program. *Journal of School Health,* 66(2), 59–63.

Richardson, Jeanita W. 2007. Building Bridges Between School-Based Health Clinics and Schools. *Journal of School Health, 77,* 337–343.

Schroeder, S.A. 2007. We Can Do Better—Improving the Health of the American People. *New England Journal of Medicine, 357,* 1221–8.

Schwarz, Susan W. 2009. *Adolescent Mental Health in the United States Facts for Policymakers.* New York: Columbia University, Mailman School of Public Health. www.nccp.org/publications/pdf/text_878.pdf

Shuger, Lisa. 2012. *Teen Pregnancy and High School Drop Outs.* Washington, DC: The National Campaign to Prevent Teen and Unplanned Pregnancy and America's Promise Alliance. www.thenationalcampaign.org/resources/pdf/teen-preg-hs-dropout.pdf

SOPHE/ASCD Expert Panel on Youth Health Disparities. 2013. *Reducing Youth Health Disparities Requires Cross-Agency Collaboration Between the Health and Education Sectors.* Washington DC: SOPHE, www.sophe.org/SchoolHealth/Disparities.cfm

U.S. Department of Health and Human Services. 2010. *Healthy People: Health Objectives for the Nation, 2020.* Washington, DC: U.S. Department of Health and Human Services. http://healthypeople.gov/2020/topicsobjectives2020/overview.aspx?topicid=33

U.S. Public Health Service. 1979. *Healthy People: The U.S. Surgeon General's Report on Health Promotion and Disease Prevention.* Washington, DC: U.S. Department of Health, Education and Welfare.

Walsh, Mary E. 2013. *City Connects: Optimized Student Supports.* www.socialimpactexchange.org/sites/www.socialimpactexchange.org/files/City%20Connects%20One%20Pager.pdf

Wong, Mitchell, Shapiro, Martin, Boscardin, John W., & Ettner, Susan L. 2002. Contribution of Major Diseases to Disparities in Mortality. *New England Journal of Medicine, 347,* 1585–1592.

3

Components of the WSCC Model

DAVID A. BIRCH • QSHEQUILLA P. MITCHELL • HANNAH M. PRIEST

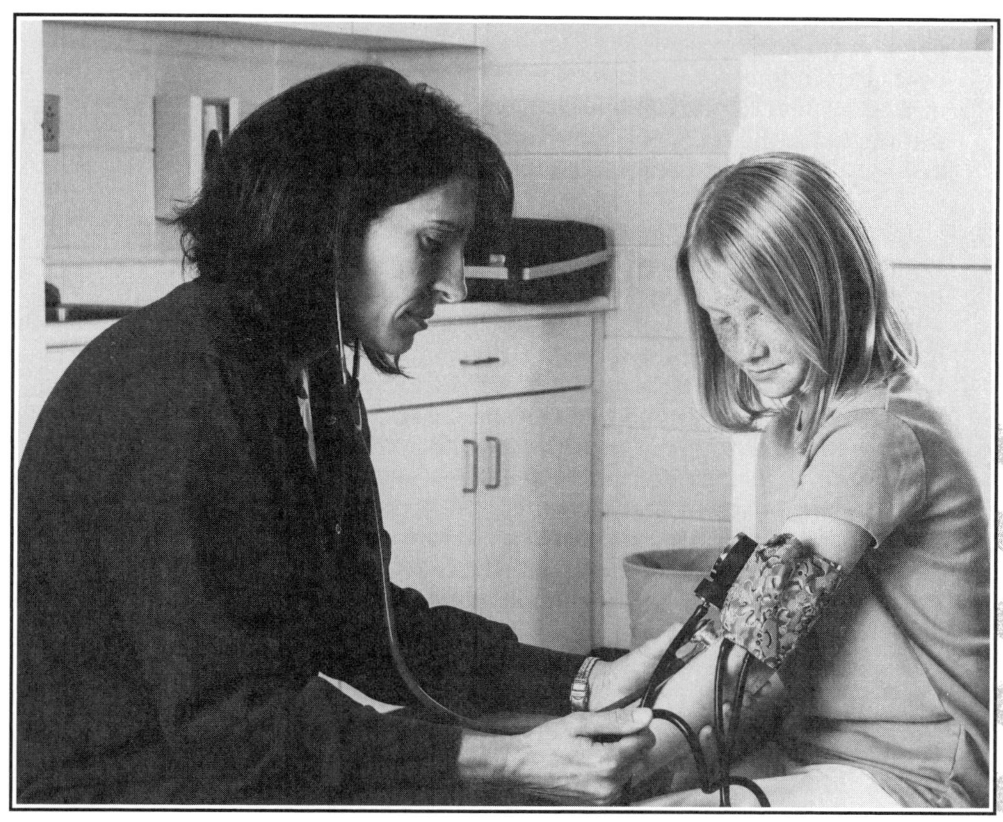

Many factors affect the health status of children and youth. To address the complexity of the health behaviors and health status of children and youth, a multicomponent approach to school health is needed. Since the early 1900s this approach has evolved from a three-component framework (health education, health services, school environment) to the eight-component Coordinated School Health (CSH) framework, and now to the recently developed 10-component Whole School, Whole Community, Whole Child (WSCC) approach. Coordination among components has been stressed as an essential aspect of both CSH and WSCC. Even with coordination, however, quality in each of the components is essential for maximum effect on both health and learning. Although these components often exist in schools, the presence of a program does not mean that it is implemented in a quality manner. As Allensworth stated in chapter 2, "The existence of a component within a school does not ensure that students receive the national standards established by that component."

The purpose of this chapter is to present background knowledge related to program quality in 9 of the 10 components of the WSCC approach. Because of its prominence in the WSCC model, the 10th component, community involvement is addressed in detail in chapter 7. Essential information related to program quality is presented for each component that is addressed in the chapter. This information includes appropriate national guidelines or standards, faculty or staff qualifications, and best practices related to implementation.

HEALTH EDUCATION

Comprehensive school health education is characterized by planned, sequential, developmentally appropriate, and culturally inclusive learning experiences taught by qualified trained teachers. The health education curriculum should be based on relevant health behavior theories; focus on the emotional, intellectual, physical, and social dimensions of health; provide students with exposure to diverse instructional techniques; and evaluate student achievement through a variety of assessment strategies (Joint Committee on National Health Education Standards [JCNHES], 2007). The learning experiences embedded within the curriculum should be designed to help students acquire functional health information; identify personal values that support healthy behaviors; recognize group norms that relate to a healthy lifestyle; and develop skills necessary to adopt, practice, and maintain health-enhancing behaviors (CDC, 2013a; JCNHES, 2007). Although many leaders in health and education suggest a linkage between quality health education and academic achievement, and some research verifies this linkage, many schools in the United States struggle to provide quality health education instruction (CDC, 2013b; JCNHES, 2007). Possible positive consequences of this linkage include a decrease in student absenteeism, higher academic achievement, and an increase in graduation rates (Allensworth, 2011; Basch, 2011a, 2011b; Freudenberg & Ruglis, 2007).

Healthy People 2020 includes an objective to increase the proportion of elementary, middle, and senior high schools that provide **comprehensive school health education** (USDHHS, 2013). Nationwide, 41.2 percent of elementary schools, 58.7 percent of middle schools, and 78.7 percent of high schools had specific time requirements for school health instruction (CDC, 2013b).

The second edition of **The National Health Education Standards** (figure 3.1) was released in 2007. The standards were developed by a panel of health education leaders with input from professionals in both health and education, as well as parents and community members. The standards are not federally mandated or designed to define a national curriculum. Instead, they are intended to provide a framework and resource for the development of state standards and health education curricula in local school districts (American Cancer Society, 2007). The standards include three distinct components: the individual health education standards, a rationale statement for each standard, and performance indicators linked to each standard for mastery by the completion of grades 4, 8, and 11 (American Cancer Society, 2007).

FIGURE 3.1

National Health Education Standards

Standard 1: Students will comprehend concepts related to health promotion and disease prevention to enhance health.

Standard 2: Students will analyze the influence of family, peers, culture, media, technology, and other factors on health behaviors.

Standard 3: Students will demonstrate the ability to access valid information, products, and services to enhance health.

Standard 4: Students will demonstrate the ability to use interpersonal communication skills to enhance health and avoid or reduce health risks.

Standard 5: Students will demonstrate the ability to use decision-making skills to enhance health.

Standard 6: Students will demonstrate the ability to use goal-setting skills to enhance health.

Standard 7: Students will demonstrate the ability to practice health-enhancing behaviors and avoid or reduce health risks.

Standard 8: Students will demonstrate the ability to advocate for personal, family, and community health.

Reprinted from Centers for Disease Control and Prevention, 2013. *National Health Education Standards for health education.* Available: http://www.cdc.gov/healthyyouth/sher/standards/

The standards can be applied to various health education content areas. The Centers for Disease Control and Prevention (CDC, 2011a) has identified six risk behaviors as being important focal points for instruction in school health education. These behaviors include alcohol and other drug use, physical inactivity, sexual behaviors that contribute to unintended pregnancy and sexually transmitted diseases, tobacco use, unhealthy dietary behaviors, and behaviors that contribute to unintentional injuries and violence. Other possible content areas for instruction include environmental health, human sexuality, and mental and emotional health (CDC, 2013a).

Beyond the National Health Education Standards, quality school health education should be based on quality health instruction. The following best practices have been identified by the CDC Division of Adolescent and School Health. They are based on reviews of effective programs and curricula and the positions of experts in the profession of health education (CDC, 2013d).

- Focus on clear health goals and related behavioral outcomes
- Are research-based and theory-driven
- Address individual values, attitudes, and beliefs
- Address individual and group norms that support health-enhancing behaviors
- Focus on reinforcing protective factors and increasing perceptions of personal risk and harmfulness of engaging in specific unhealthy practices and behaviors
- Address social pressures and influences
- Build personal competence, social competence, and self-efficacy by addressing skills
- Provide functional health knowledge that is basic, accurate, and directly contributes to health-promoting decisions and behaviors
- Use strategies designed to personalize information and engage students
- Provide age-appropriate and developmentally appropriate information, learning strategies, teaching methods, and materials
- Incorporate learning strategies, teaching methods, and materials that are culturally inclusive
- Provide adequate time for instruction and learning
- Provide opportunities to reinforce skills and positive health behaviors
- Provide opportunities to make positive connections with influential others
- Include teacher information and plans for professional development and training that enhance effectiveness of instruction and student learning

PARENT AND FAMILY ENGAGEMENT

Parents have a tremendous influence on their children's lives, including their education. The Department of Education and Human Services in Maine has described parents and family members as their children's chief educators because they provide the "primary cultural, linguistic, social, and economic learning environment" for them (State of Maine Department of Education and Department of Health and Human Services, 2002, G-6-7). The National Education Association's (NEA) President Dennis Van Roekel reinforced this role by stating, "Parents, families, educators and communities—there's no better partnership to assure that all students pre-K to high school—have the support and resources they need to succeed in school and in life" (NEA, 2008, 1). Family engagement in a child's education is supported by nongovernmental organizations such as the National Network of Partnership Schools (NNPS), Coalition for Community Schools (CCS), National Coalition for Parent Involvement in Education (NCPIE) (1995), National Parent Teacher Association (NPTA), and National Board for Professional Teaching Standards (NBPTS).

A substantial body of evidence demonstrates that parent, family, and community engagement in education is related to higher student achievement and school improvement. Specifically, students generally earn higher grades, attend school more regularly, remain in school longer, like school more, and enroll in higher-level programs when parents, families, schools, and communities work collaboratively to promote learning (Henderson & Mapp, 2002). Students with parents who are engaged in their schooling are less likely to smoke cigarettes, drink alcohol, become pregnant, or be physically inactive (CDC, 2012a).

Family and parent engagement uses an integrated school, community, and parent approach to improve the health and well-being of students (Jones, 2008). The terms *family(ies)* and *parent(s)* are used interchangeably throughout this book to mean the adult primary caregiver(s) of a child's basic needs. These words encompass biological parents and nonbiological parents, such as adoptive, foster, or stepparents, and other biological relatives such as aunts, uncles, grandparents, and siblings (CDC, 2012b).

Despite the support of several prominent organizations, schools may find it difficult to sustain family engagement, particularly as children mature into adolescence and progress to middle and high school. Engaging family members often involves challenges such as time conflicts with work and other responsibilities of family members; lack of transportation to school; and lack of comfort among family members in engaging in school activities, sometimes caused by a language barrier, feelings of inferiority when working with teachers and other school personnel, and unfamiliarity with the school culture. In addition, teachers and school staff may face challenges with adequate time and resources in working with families (CDC, 2013b).

Epstein et al. (2009) identified six types of involvement necessary for successful school, family, and community partnerships: (1) providing parenting support, (2) communicating with parents, (3) providing diverse volunteer opportunities, (4) supporting at-home learning, (5) encouraging parents to engage in decision-making opportunities in schools, and (6) collaborating with the community (CDC, 2012b, 12). Research has shown that implementing activities that incorporate all six types of involvement will increase the chances of engaging more families in the education and health of their children across all grades (Epstein et al., 2009; Simon, 2001). Strategies for the first five of Epstein's types of involvement are discussed here. Community collaboration is presented in detail in chapter 7.

1. **Providing parenting support**. The CDC (2012b) recommends offering parent education classes on a variety of topics and providing parents with information, seminars, and workshops on health topics that are directly related to content taught in health education and physical education classes. Additional parenting support strategies include developing a parent resource center that emphasizes child and adolescent health and other relevant family issues.
2. **Communicating with parents**. Schools can use a diverse array of communication methods such as flyers, memos, banners, signs, door hangers, postcards, newsletters, monthly calendars of events, report cards, progress reports, letters, websites and web boards, text messaging, and e-mail messages to increase parental awareness and involvement in school- and community-based health and safety programs (CDC, 2012c). Direct communication including phone calls, parent–teacher conferences, meetings, school events, radio station announcements, local access television, public service announcements, conversations at school, regular parent seminars, and automated phone system messages can also be used to communicate with parents. School staff can receive input from parents through parent surveys, parent–teacher focus groups, school-sponsored parent blogs, and on-site suggestion boxes. Schools also should be culturally sensitive and provide families with written and verbal information in their native language. In addition, schools should offer regular meetings with parents to discuss children's grades, behavior, and achievements, as well as school health issues. Meeting times should be flexible to accommodate parents' work schedules or other obligations.
3. **Providing diverse volunteer opportunities**. Parents should be encouraged to serve as monitors, chaperones, tutors, mentors, or coaching assistants for school health activities and events. School staff may invite parent volunteers to lead lunchtime walks, weekend games, or after-school exercise programs in dance, karate, aerobics, yoga, or other activities that demonstrate their talents and skills.
4. **Supporting at-home learning**. Teachers should use strategies designed to engage parents in discussions about health topics with their children. School staff can encourage parents to engage their children in specific health-related learning experiences that are designed to reinforce what is taught through the school health education curriculum. Students can

School Health *in Action*

CSH Success in Tennessee

In "Coordinated School Health: Getting It All Together," an article in *Educational Leadership*, Joyce Fetro, Connie Givens, and Kellie Carroll (2010) present an overview of how the state of Tennessee has moved forward in the statewide implementation of Coordinated School Health (CSH). The article describes how all school districts are moving toward compliance with Tennessee school health laws and Coordinated School Health standards and guidelines. Local districts are hiring full-time coordinators for the program; sending educators to mandatory professional development institutes; and establishing community school health advisory committees, district-level staff coordinating councils, and healthy school teams. In addition, the districts are developing action plans for improving school health programs and services.

The article also features the success experienced by the Gibson County Special School District in western Tennessee. The district has implemented numerous CSH activities including

- a comprehensive health education curriculum based on the Michigan Model curriculum;
- a health fair in each school;
- physical education for all students;
- an elementary-level walking program that requires all students to walk at least 5 minutes each school day for 12 weeks each semester;
- healthful food choices in the school cafeterias;
- nutrition newsletters for parents;
- numerous health screenings for students and staff; and
- programs conducted by counselors for students, staff and parents, and students.

Reference

Fetro, Joyce V., Givens, Connie, & Carroll, Kellie. 2010. Coordinated School Health: Getting It All Together. *Educational Leadership, 67*(4), 32–37.

engage their parents by teaching them about health based on what they learned in school.

5. **Encouraging parents to engage in decision-making opportunities in schools.** Parents can be involved through the parent teacher association (PTA) or parent teacher organization (PTO), school health council, school health teams, and other school committees charged with decision making.

PHYSICAL ENVIRONMENT

More than 53 million children and 6 million adults spend the majority of their day in over 120,000 public and private school buildings (United States Environmental Protection Agency, 2012). Many schools in the United States are in need of repair, and more than one-third of all students attend class in buildings that are in need of renovation or replacement (American Cancer Society, 2013). School leaders have a responsibility to provide a healthy and safe learning environment for students and staff and to implement and follow all appropriate accessibility, environmental, and safety policies and standards (National Association of Secondary School Principals, 2013). Protecting the health and safety of children and adolescents while in school is an essential part of any comprehensive education plan (Jones, 2008; Frumkin, Geller, & Nodvin, 2006; U.S. Department of Education, 2010). The physical environment of the school, along with the social and emotional climate, is essential to students' academic success and overall well-being.

Many factors influence the quality of a school's physical environment and student safety. These factors include the overall condition and safety of buildings, school grounds, playground equipment, and athletic fields. In addition, school property should be free from environmental hazards, tobacco, drugs, weapons, and violence and appropriately secure from unauthorized access

(ASCD, 2014; CDC, 2013a; Institute of Medicine [IOM], 1997).

Conditions within the school building can affect safety, teaching, learning, and overall satisfaction with the school experience for students, faculty, staff, and visitors. Factors for consideration inside the school include building design, adequate space for student traffic flow and learning, cleanliness, reasonable noise level, freedom from environmental hazards, adequate heating and cooling, appropriate ventilation, lighting, and well-maintained restrooms. All areas of the school should be accessible to people with disabilities. Like the environment outside the school, the school building should be free from tobacco, drugs, weapons, and violence (ASCD, 2014; Henderson & Rowe, 1998; IOM 1997).

One other important aspect of the school environment is linked to student transportation. Buses and other vehicles used for transportation must be maintained for safety and environmental regulations, and they should present an attractive and comfortable travel environment for passengers. In addition, pedestrian, bicycle, and motor vehicle traffic flow outside the school should be efficient and safe (ASCD, 2014).

Another important aspect of school safety is emergency preparedness. Schools should have emergency disaster plans in place that are understood by appropriate parties. Periodic emergency drills are a necessary component of emergency preparedness (IOM, 1997).

Learning is less likely to take place in an environment that is not enjoyable and not safe. The physical environment of a school is essential to promoting health and academic success.

SOCIAL AND EMOTIONAL CLIMATE

A comfortable, safe, and nurturing social and emotional climate is essential for maximizing health and academic achievement for students (JCNHES, 2007). Among the factors that should be present in a positive social and emotional climate are an attractive, comfortable physical environment; appreciation and respect for individual differences and cultural diversity; value placed on equity and social justice; high expectations and supportive actions for learning; size and structure of classes, organizations, and an overall school that promotes individual identity; and a general sense of comfort and safety for all who interact within the school environment (IOM, 1997).

A positive social and emotional climate contributes to a higher level of school connectedness. Basch (2011a; 2011b, 596) has described school connectedness as being "about interpersonal relationships, both with peers and school staff. It is the extent to which students perceive that adults and peers in the school community care about them as students and individuals." McNeely, Nonnemker, and Blum (2002, 20) present school connectedness as "the feeling of belonging and being cared for at school." Research supports the linkage between school connectedness and both academic success and health outcomes (Basch, 2011b).

All stakeholders in the school community should recognize and feel the message transmitted from a positive social climate. Specifically, that message should clearly indicate the following:

- We strongly believe that students, family members, staff and teachers, and community members are all important to the success and well-being of our school.
- We appreciate and celebrate the various cultures within our school community.
- We want students to have a healthy, safe, and enjoyable school experience.
- We expect students to be academically successful, and we will do whatever is necessary to promote success.
- We recognize that students learn differently and demonstrate their learning in diverse ways.
- We care.

To maintain an optimal physical environment and social and emotional climate, several specific actions are recommended for schools. A school environment committee should be formed that includes students, teachers, administrators, staff members, parents and family members, and community members. The composition of this committee should reflect the demographic composition of the school community. This group should oversee an ongoing assessment process that is designed to ascertain the quality and presence of all important elements of both the physical environment and the social climate. Based on the ongoing assessment, the committee should develop and implement an action plan. Progress on this plan should be reviewed on an ongoing basis. In addition, the plan should be communicated on a regular basis to all key stakeholders in the school community.

PHYSICAL EDUCATION AND PHYSICAL ACTIVITY

Physical education (PE) has been a fundamental part of the United States' public school curriculum for more than a century, first being offered in the early 1800s (National Association for Sport and Physical Education [NASPE], 2010a). After World War I, state education agencies began to issue mandates for physical education because many young males were deemed unfit for military service (NASPE 2010a). Traditionally physical education has taken a backseat to other subjects, namely math, science, history, and reading. For example, physical education was excluded as a core academic subject in the No Child Left Behind (NCLB) Act of 2001 and more recently in the reauthorization of the Individuals With Disabilities Education Act (IDEA), which was signed into law on December 3, 2004 (U.S. Department of Education, 2004; U.S. Department of Education, Office of Special Education Programs, 2007).

In recent years physical education has gained considerable attention and momentum. The primary reason for this paradigm shift is the overweight and obesity epidemic among American youth and the linkage to reduced physical activity levels. A significant body of research exists that supports the role of physical activity in health promotion and disease prevention. Substantial scientific evidence demonstrates a link between physical education and academic performance among school-aged youth (CDC, 2010). *Healthy People 2020* includes two primary goals related to physical education: (1) to increase the proportion of the nation's public and private schools that require daily physical education for all students and (2) to increase the proportion of adolescents who participate in daily school physical education (U.S. Department of Health and Human Services, 2013). The American Academy of Pediatrics, American Heart Association, CDC, NASPE, U.S Department of Education, U.S. Department of Health and Human Services, and the President's Council on Physical Fitness and Sport all support the need for high-quality physical education and physical activity (NASPE, 2010a). In May 2013 the Institute of Medicine (IOM) issued a report that recommended that the federal government designate physical education as a core subject because "it has commensurate values that are foundational for learning and therefore essential" (IOM, 2013, p. 3).

Physical education is defined as a planned, sequential K–12 course of study that provides cognitive content and learning experiences in a variety of activity areas (CDC, 2013a) that is "designed for students to gain the necessary skills and knowledge for lifelong participation in physical activity" (CDC, 2013a). NASPE describes the overarching goal of physical education as developing physically literate individuals who have the knowledge, skills and confidence to enjoy a lifetime of healthy physical activity. The **physically literate** person possesses the skills necessary to engage in a variety of physical activities; knows the implications of and the benefits from participation in various forms of physical activity; engages regularly in physical activity; is physically fit; and appreciates physical activity and its contributions to a healthy lifestyle (NASPE, 2013a). The national standards for K through 12 physical education provide a broad overview of the knowledge, skills, and attitudes that are essential for students to become physically literate individuals (figure 3.2).

High-quality physical education programs are paramount in developing physically literate people. NASPE (2010b) developed "opportunity to learn guidelines" that describe essential physical education program elements that provide effective learning foundations for students in grades K through 12. The following list is derived from the NASPE guidelines.

- Highly qualified physical education teachers
- A comprehensive, sequential, standards-based curriculum
- A healthy and safe learning environment for physical education
- Appropriate class size
- Quality facilities to promote learning, student participation, and safety
- Safe materials and equipment that maximize learning
- Appropriate time allocation for instruction
- Up-to-date instructional technology and related teacher training
- Formative and authentic summative assessment of student learning
- Annual program evaluation

Physical activity is defined as any type of body movement that requires energy expenditure (World Health Organization, 2013). For school-age children these activities may include walking, riding a bicycle, swinging, dancing,

FIGURE 3.2

National Standards for Physical Education

Standard 1: The physically literate individual demonstrates competency in a variety of motor skills and movement patterns.

Standard 2: The physically literate individual applies knowledge of concepts, principles, strategies, and tactics related to movement and performance.

Standard 3: The physical literate individual demonstrates the knowledge and skills to achieve and maintain a health-enhancing level of physical activity and fitness.

Standard 4: The physically literate individual exhibits responsible personal and social behavior that respects self and others.

Standard 5: The physically literate individual recognizes the value of physical activity for health, enjoyment, challenge, self-expression, and social interaction.

Reprinted from National Association for Sport and Physical Education, 2013, *National standards & grade level outcomes for K-12 physical education* (Champaign, IL: Human Kinetics). Available: http://www.aahperd.org/naspe/standards/nationalStandards/PEstandards.cfm

skipping, or flying a kite. A 2013 Institute of Medicine (IOM) report titled *Educating the Student Body: Taking Physical Activity and Physical Education to School* made several recommendations related to the schools' role in increasing physical activity. These suggestions included increasing the amount of time that youth spend in physical activity though brief classroom breaks, incorporating physical activity directly into academic sessions, offering intramural sports and physical activity clubs, providing access to school facilities during nonschool hours, and, when appropriate, providing active recess breaks throughout the school day (IOM, 2013). Providing inexpensive equipment for playground activities and training staff to organize and implement physical activity are important considerations related to recess (Robert Wood Johnson Foundation, 2012). Children and adolescents should engage in at least 60 minutes of physical activity each day (CDC, 2011b). Specifically, moderate-intensity aerobic activity (e.g., walking briskly) should compose the majority of this time. Vigorous-intensity aerobic activity should be incorporated on at least three days per week. Additionally, children and adolescents should engage in muscle-strengthening activities, such as push-ups, and bone-strengthening activities, such as running or jumping rope, at least three days per week.

COUNSELING, PSYCHOLOGICAL, AND SOCIAL SERVICES

Children and youth may be faced with a variety of difficult issues including abuse, suicide ideation, questioning sexuality, parental divorce, alcoholism, and drug addiction. Consequently, many students struggle with mental, emotional, and social problems that affect their ability to be successful in school. Counseling, psychological, and social services can provide important help in effectively identifying and addressing students' mental health issues.

Counseling, psychological, and social services are provided to improve students' mental, emotional, and social health and include individual and group assessments, interventions, and referrals (CDC, 2013a). Certified school counselors, school psychologists, and social workers typically provide these services (Jones, 2008).

School counselors promote student achievement through the design and delivery of comprehensive school counseling programs (American School Counselor Association [ASCA], 2012). Schools counselors spend their time, skills, and energy on providing direct and indirect services for students (ASCA, 2012). The American School Counselor Association (ASCA 2009, 2012) recommends a counselor-to-student ratio of 1:250 and an 80 percent or greater allocation of their time to direct and indirect services to students. **Direct services** involve face-to face communication between the school counselor and students and include individual student planning, the school counseling core curriculum, and responsive services. **Indirect services** are offered on behalf of students and result from the counselors' communication with others involving referrals for extended assistance or consultation and collaboration with parents, other educators, or community agencies. Guided by student data and academic, occupational, and personal or social development standards, comprehensive school counseling programs support and enhance the learning process for all students and are considered an essential part of the school's educational mission (ASCA, 2012).

ASCA (2009) recommends that school counselors have a minimum of a master's degree in school counseling and be certified or licensed educators. In addition, professional school counselors must meet state certification or licensure standards and adhere to all laws of the state in which they are employed.

School psychologists enable children and adolescents to thrive academically, behaviorally, socially, and emotionally. The school psychologist works with educators, parents, and other professionals to establish a supportive learning environment that is safe and healthy for all students and promotes connections between school, home, and the community (National Association of School Psychologists [NASP], n.d.). The National Association of School Psychologists model for comprehensive and integrated school psychological services (NASP practice model) is a guide for the organization and provision of comprehensive school psychological services across all levels (e.g., local, state, and federal) (NASP, 2010a) (figure 3.3). The NASP practice model clearly describes the services that school psychologists are expected to provide, within reason, and the overarching framework in which services should be delivered. As presented in the model, school psychologists provide services across 10 practice domains of school psychology.

The National Association of School Psychologists (NASP, 2010a) recommends that schools not exceed a school psychologist-to-student ratio of 1:1,000, but when school psychologists are responsible for providing comprehensive and preventive services such as evaluations, crisis response, behavioral interventions, and individual or group counseling, the ratio should not exceed one school psychologist per 500 to 700 students. NASP rec-

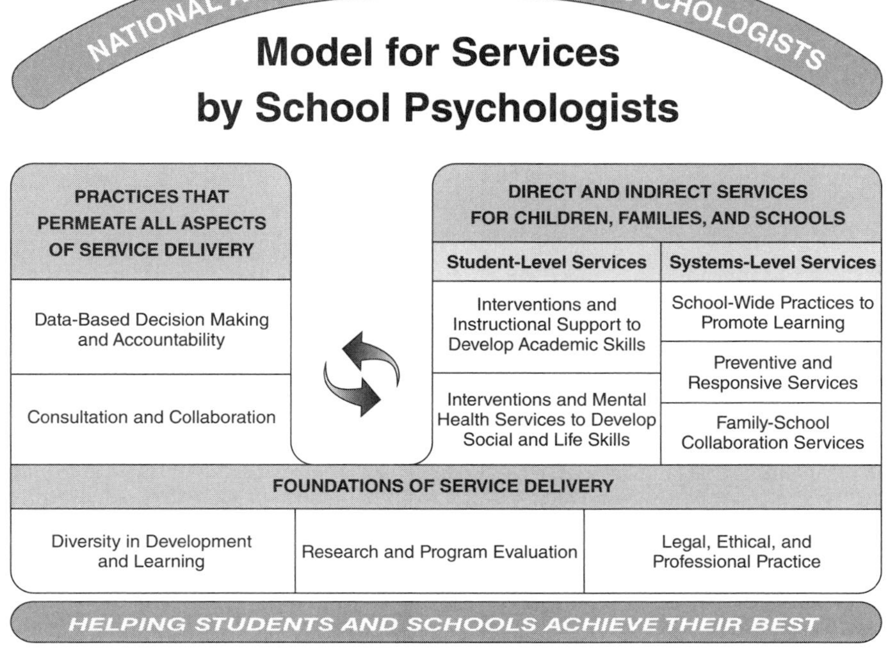

Figure 3.3 National Association of School Psychologists practice model.

ommends a lower ratio for school psychologists assigned to work with student populations that have intensive special needs (NASP, 2010a).

School social workers provide a critical link between the school, the home, and the community (School Social Work Association of America [SSWAA], 2003). School social workers provide direct services to students and their families (e.g., casework, group work, classroom presentations, crisis intervention, consultation, referrals to community agencies), engage in the assessment process for special education students, consult with teachers and administrators, and regularly serve on committees or teams within the school (SSWAA, 2003). These roles and responsibilities vary substantially, depending on the school, district, or state in which they are employed (Frey et al., 2013). SSWAA developed the school social work practice model (figure 3.4), which includes the following practices

- provide evidence-based education, behavior, and mental health services;
- promote a school climate and culture conductive to student learning and teaching excellence; and
- maximize access to school-based and community-based resources (Frey et al., 2013).

The model also proposes four key constructs that are integrated into each practice:

- Home-school-community linkages
- Ethical guidelines and educational policy
- Education rights and advocacy
- Data-based decision making

Additionally, the model stipulates that a full-time school social worker is required to implement the proposed practices and its key constructs. NASW (2012) recommends that school social workers have a graduate degree in social work from a program accredited by the Council on Social Work Education (CSWE). School social workers are required to obtain a license through the state boards of social work. When certification is available, school social workers should be certified by their respective state departments of education. An appropriate ratio of school social workers to students is 1:250 for a full-time social worker. This ratio may vary within school districts, depending

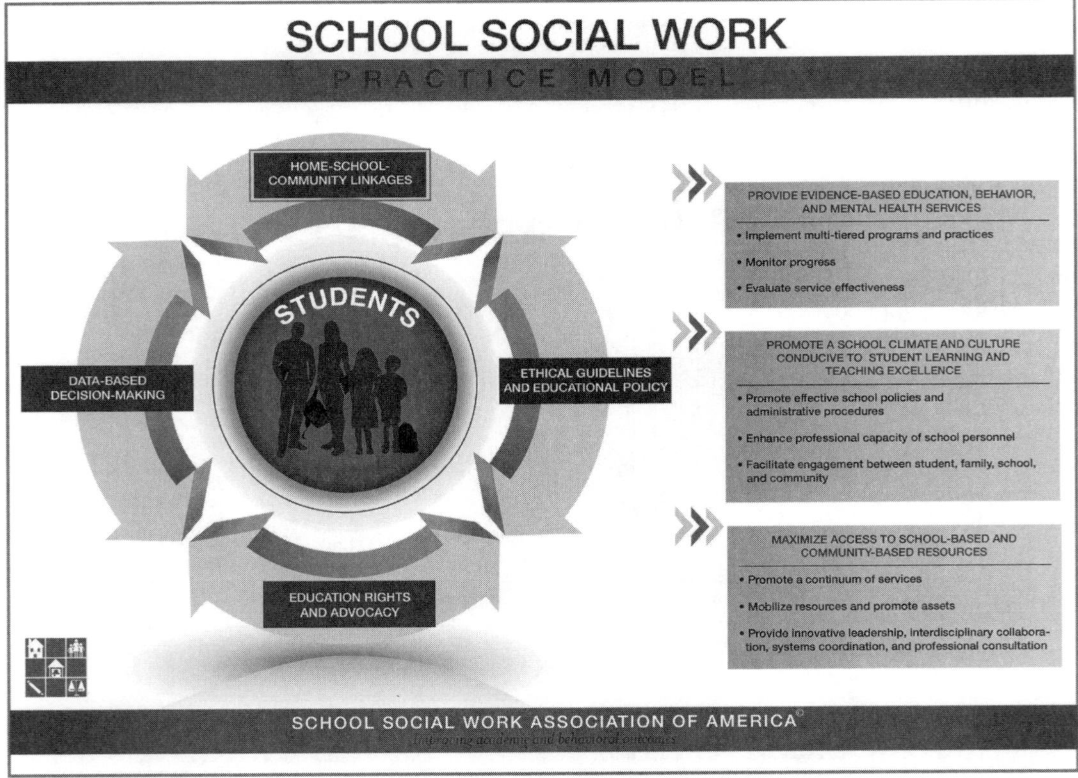

Figure 3.4 School social work practice model.

Reprinted, by permission, from School Social Work Association of America, 2013, *School social work practice model* (Summer, WA: SSWAA). Available: http://sswaa.org/associations/13190/files/SSWAA_Practice_Model%20Graphic.pdf

on factors such as the experience and expertise of the school social worker, percentage of high-risk students, and availability of other services within the school and around the community (Frey et al., 2013, p. 2).

HEALTH SERVICES

Health services are

> services designed to ensure access or referral to primary health care services or both, foster appropriate use of primary health care services, prevent and control communicable disease and other health problems, provide emergency care for illness or injury, promote and provide optimum sanitary conditions for a safe school facility and school environment and provide educational and counseling opportunities for promoting and maintaining individual, family, and community health. (CDC, 2013a, para. 3)

Professionals such as nurses, dentists, physicians, health educators, and other allied health personnel provide health services (CDC, 2013a).

The extent of school health services available within schools varies by school district. The American Academy of Pediatrics (AAP) recommends that the following minimum health services be offered in schools:

> (1) assessment of health complaints, medication administration, and care for students with special health care needs; (2) a system for managing emergencies and urgent situations; (3) mandated health screening programs, verification of immunizations, and infectious disease reporting; and (4) identification and management of students' chronic health care needs that affect educational achievement. (American Academy of Pediatrics Council on School Health, 2008, 1054)

The school nurse often functions as a "leader and coordinator of the school health services team," and is uniquely positioned to direct school health programs and policies and promote health education (NASN, 2010, p. 1; NASN, 2011). The American Academy of Pediatrics Council on School Health (2008) and National Association of School Nurses (2004) identified seven core roles for school nurses. These roles are administering direct care to students; demonstrating leadership for the provision of health services; offering screening and referral for health problems; fostering a healthy school environment; promoting health, functioning in a leadership position for health programs and policies; and serving as a liaison among school personnel, health professionals, family, and the community.

The National Association of School Nurses (NASN, 2010) asserts that schools should employ professionally prepared registered nurses (RNs) who are qualified to conduct and manage school health programs that address a variety of health issues faced by school-age children and youth. NASN also recommends that school nurses' academic preparation be at the baccalaureate level and that they should seek opportunities to participate in continuing nursing education and professional development. The American Academy of Pediatrics Council on School Health (2008) and NASN (2012) support national certification of school nurses by the National Board for Certification of School Nurses (NBCSN).

NASN (2010) recommends a formula-based approach with minimum nurses-to-student ratios based on the needs of the student populations: 1:750 for students in the general population, 1:225 for student populations that have complex health care needs, and 1:1 for individual students who require daily, ongoing professional nursing services. Additional factors should be considered in the formula-based approach, including average number of emergency services per year, number of students on free or reduced lunch, and number of students with a **medical home** (NASN, 2010). A medical home is a collaborative partnership between the patient, his or her family, the primary care provider, specialists, and the community (U.S. Department of Health and Human Services, n.d.).

The American Academy of Pediatrics Council on School Health (2013) recommends that every school district have a school physician. **School physicians** should possess expertise in pediatrics or be nationally board-certified pediatricians (American Academy of Pediatrics Council on School Health, 2013; American Medical Association [AMA] 2013). The responsibilities of the school physician can include administration and planning, liaison to community physicians, direct service, clinical consultation, policy consultation, health education, public relations, advocacy, and systems development consultation (Commonwealth of Massachusetts Executive Office of Health and Human Services, 2013).

School physicians are also responsible for reviewing guidelines, programs, and policies specific to health care that takes place in schools. School physicians should also work collaboratively with the school to make sure that patients' health plans are implemented effectively within the school setting. School physicians may also serve on a school wellness policy committee, school health advisory committee, emergency preparedness committee, and other school health decision-making teams.

School physicians can be assigned to a school district for a minimum of a few hours each year (e.g., part-time employee, independent contractor) or have full-time employee status. School physician assignments and responsibilities are dependent on the "social and medical needs or demands of the community, the school district's priorities, and state laws" (American Academy of Pediatrics Council on School Health, 2013, p. 180).

Health services are being expanded and increasingly provided through school-based, school-linked, and mobile programs. **School-based health centers** (SBHCs) are defined as "a health center located in a school or on school grounds that provides, at a minimum on-site primary and preventive health care, mental health counseling, health promotion referral and follow-up services for young people enrolled" (National Health and Education Consortium, 1995).

SBHCs typically use one of three types of service delivery models. In the **primary care model**, a nurse practitioner, physician assistant, or physician is on staff, but no mental health provider is present. SBHCs that use the primary care model usually have a health educator or an oral health provider on staff. The **primary care–mental health model** is composed of a primary care provider and a mental health professional, such as a licensed clinical psychologist, social worker, or substance abuse counselor. The **primary care–mental health plus model** is the most comprehensive in nature. This model involves collaboration and coordination between primary care, mental health providers, and other professionals such as health educators, social service case managers, oral health providers, and nutritionists (Lofink et al., 2013). SBHCs have improved availability and access to health care for traditionally underserved children and youth (Allison et al., 2007; Kisker & Brown, 1996; Mandel & Qazilbash, 2005; Shuler, 2000; Wood et al., 1990; Young, D'Angelo, & Davis, 2001).

School-linked health centers (SLHC) are generally coordinated at the school but do not provide clinical services on campus; SLHC recommend collaboration between hospitals, health agencies,

School Health *in Action*

A University–School Partnership for CSH

In 2004 Videto and Hodges, as part of a university–school partnership, conducted assessments with 25 central and upstate New York schools. The schools used the assessment data in the development of CSH action plans. Interviews were held in 2006 and 2007 with personnel from the schools to determine the current state of the CSH in those schools and to assess the level of institutionalization of the action plans.

The assessment appeared to result in positive outcomes such as providing a clear list of the strengths and weaknesses of health and safety policies and programs at the school; enabling the school to develop action plans that can be incorporated into a school improvement plan; and engaging administrators, teachers, and the community in conversations that can potentially result in promoting health-enhancing behaviors and ultimately better health. As a result of going through the assessment, many of the schools reported engaging in activities to maintain the established school teams and infrastructure and to improve their CSH in one or more areas.

The resulting data supported the continuation of the university–school partnership model for facilitating the assessment. Beyond the positive outcomes from the assessment, only moderate institutionalization of action plans for advancing the CSH framework was found in the investigation. The institutionalization efforts that did occur were mostly related to policy and school environmental changes. Findings indicated the need for health coordinators to take a strong role in the assessment, for developing administrative support, for expanding parent and community involvement, and for instituting a formal process evaluation monitoring system to increase accountability.

community-based clinics, or health professionals (Committee on School Health, 2001). SLHCs may use primary care only, primary care–mental health, and primary care–mental health plus models for staffing and service provision. **Mobile programs** lack a fixed site and "rotate a health care team through a number of schools" (Strozer, Juszczak, & Ammerman, 2010, p. 1). Mobile programs can use the primary care, primary care–mental health, or primary care–mental health plus service delivery and staffing models.

NUTRITION ENVIRONMENT AND SERVICES

According to the CDC (2013a), schools are responsible for providing students with meals that are both nutritious and appealing. More than 30 million children participate in the **National School Lunch Program** (NSLP), and approximately 11 million participate in the **School Breakfast Program** (SBP) (Let's Move Child Nutrition Program, 2014). "Comprehensive, integrated services in school, kindergarten through grade 12, are an essential component of coordinated health school health programs and will improve the nutritional status, health, and academic performance of our nation's children" (Briggs et al., 2003).

In the United States, school nutrition programs are based on the **U.S. dietary guidelines** to ensure nutritional value. The guidelines are based on three overarching goals: balance calories with physical activity for weight management; increase consumption of fruits, vegetables, whole grains, and fat-free and low-fat dairy products; and decrease consumption of salt, saturated fats, trans fat, cholesterol, added sugars, and refined grains (U.S. Government, 2010).

In 2010 the **Healthy, Hunger-Free Kids Act** was passed to authorize funding and set policies for the United States Department of Agriculture's (USDA) child nutrition program. The National School Lunch Program, the School Breakfast Program, the **Special Supplemental Nutrition Program for Women, Infants and Children** (**WIC**), the **Summer Food Service Program**, and the **Child and Adult Care Food Program** were all addressed under this legislation (United States Department of Agriculture Food and Nutrition Service, 2014). Since 2010 tremendous reform has occurred to improve the quality and accessibility of nutrition for children.

The American Academy of Family Physicians, American Academy of Pediatrics, American Dietetic Association, National Hispanic Medical Association, National Medical Association, and the USDA (n.d.) have proposed a call to action urging schools and communities to recognize the health and academic benefits of healthy eating and the importance of making nutrition services a priority in every school. This joint call to action outlined the following 10 keys to promote healthy eating in schools:

1. Engaging and collaborating with students, parents, and teachers to assess the eating environment of the school
2. Providing adequate funding at the local, state, and federal level to assist in the development of healthy eating patterns
3. Integrating behavior-focused nutrition education from pre-K through grade 12 and staff training for people who provide nutrition education
4. Providing school meals that meet the USDA nutrition standards of sufficient choices that include new foods and foods prepared in different ways to serve the taste preferences of diverse student populations
5. Providing sufficient time and designated lunch periods
6. Ensuring sufficient number of serving areas for student access to school to limit wait time
7. Allocating adequate space to accommodate all students and pleasant surroundings
8. Encouraging students, teachers, and community volunteers to practice healthy eating to serve as role models in the school dining areas
9. Ensuring that when foods are sold in addition to National School Lunch Program meals, the foods represent the five major food groups of the food guide pyramid
10. Making decisions that the sale of foods in addition to the National School Lunch Program meals are based on nutrition goals, not on profit making

The food services environment has the potential to influence a child's decisions and nutrition selections, thereby shaping nutritional habits into adulthood. The school cafeteria has been referred to as a learning laboratory aimed to reinforce student learning about food and nutrition that occurred in health education courses (Fetro, Givens, & Carroll, 2010). Providing adequate **nutrition education services** serves as a critical strategy to improve the health status of America's youth.

EMPLOYEE WELLNESS

U.S. school systems provide employment for more than 4.5 percent of the U.S. workforce, totaling more than 6.7 million people (Alliance for a Healthier Generation, 2013). Schools have the opportunity to provide the means to improve the health status of staff through a variety of activities. Opportunities for health assessments, health education, and health-related fitness activities are common approaches to health promotion for staff (CDC, 2013b). Common health promotion activities available to school staff include seminars and workshops related to stress, nutrition, first aid, CPR, and workplace safety (Fetro et al., 2010). Employee wellness programs can not only benefit the health of school employees but also promote the health and learning of students (Alliance for a Healthier Generation, 2013).

Unfortunately, many schools underemphasize the importance of employee wellness. The School Health Program and Policy Study (SHPPS) found that approximately 35 percent of all districts in the United States provided funding for an **employee assistance program** or offered this service to faculty and staff (CDC, 2013b). These data also indicated that 45.6 percent of districts provided funding for or offered at least one type of screening for faculty and staff, regardless of whether the employee had health insurance (CDC, 2013b). Ignoring the health of employees can negatively affect school systems (Alliance for a Healthier Generation, 2013). The CDC's Division of Adolescent Health developed *School Employee Wellness: A Guide for Protecting the Assets of Our Nation's Schools* in 2007. This guide provides practical tools and resources for the implementation and evaluation of school employee wellness programs (CDC, 2007).

Traditionally, the effect of health promotion among staff is assessed by an improvement of staff health status through health education, adequate nutrition, and physical activity opportunities available to staff. Another benefit is the potential for school staff to serve as role models for expediting the promotion of the health of the student body (Ruder, 2009). Schools can improve employee health and wellness in many ways.

The following suggestions for program implementation are adapted from actions presented in two documents—one from the Education Development Center (2001) (www2.edc.org/makinghealthacademic/concept/actions_staff.asp) and the second from National Association of State Boards of Education (www.nasbe.org/healthy_schools/hs/bytopics.php?topicid=2100&catExpand=acdnbtm_catB):

- School-site health promotion that extends beyond individual-level risk reduction
- Integration of evaluation methods to address the well-being of administrators, faculty, and school support staff
- Educational opportunities for staff on healthy eating, physical activity, injury prevention, and maintaining a healthy lifestyle
- Access to walking tracks, fitness equipment, and public and private recreation centers and incentives to encourage employee use
- Nutrition standards for food and beverages offered in vending machines
- School policies that prohibit tobacco products on school grounds
- Peer support groups for weight management, tobacco cessation, stress management, family guidance, and other identified needs
- Allowance of time for staff to participate in health-promoting activities
- Administration of staff health appraisals
- Health screening and immunizations offered at school
- Staff encouragement to keep medical appointments and participate in health screenings for cancer, heart disease, diabetes, and so forth
- Linkages to established employee assistance programs
- Ongoing evaluation and assessment

SUMMARY

Ensuring quality in the WSCC approach is essential for communities and schools to maximize health and academic success for students. Overall support and coordination among the various components of WSCC is essential, but the efficacy of support and coordination can be negated if there are issues related to the overall quality of the individual components of WSCC. Mediocrity should not be acceptable in school programs. Weakness in one or more of the individual components will chip away at the effect of the total WSCC approach.

Unfortunately, evidence and professional speculation indicate that quality in individual components is not always present. National studies, such as the CDC School Health Policies and Practice Study (SHPPS) (www.cdc.gov/healthyyouth/shpps/index.htm), have uncovered weaknesses in individual components. To move forward and address such gaps, communities and schools must make efforts to ensure that commitment, adherence to national guidelines and standards, strongly prepared professionals and staff, and best practices are in place for all components of the WSCC approach.

Glossary

advocacy—Actions taken individually or collectively to inform or provide support for maintaining or changing a law or policy.

assessment of student learning—An ongoing process aimed at understanding and improving student learning. It involves setting goals and standards for student learning and then gathering and analyzing evidence (data) to determine how well student performance matches expectations and standards. The two main goals in the assessment of student learning are (1) to document what learning is taking place and (2) to use the results of assessment activities to improve student learning.

Child and Adult Care Food Program—CACFP provides aid to child and adult care institutions and family or group day-care homes for the provision of nutritious foods that contribute to the wellness, healthy growth, and development of young children and the health and wellness of older adults and chronically impaired disabled persons (U.S. Department of Agriculture Food and Nutrition Service, 2014).

comprehensive school health education—Defined by CDC as a course of study for students in pre-K through grade 12 that addresses a variety of topics such as alcohol and other drug use and abuse, healthy eating and nutrition, mental and emotional health, personal health and wellness, physical activity, safety and injury prevention, sexual health, tobacco use, and violence prevention.

counseling, psychological, and social services—One of the components of CSH, described as services provided to improve students' mental, emotional, and social health and includes individual and group assessments, interventions, and referrals.

direct services—Involves face-to-face communication between the school counselor and students and includes individual student planning, the school counseling core curriculum, and responsive services.

goal setting—The identification of the attainment of a level of behavior, characteristic, or status. Goals are usually general achievements that are further defined by specific objectives.

employee assistance programs (EAPs)—Programs offered by employers intended to help employees deal with personal problems that might adversely affect their work performance, health, and well-being. EAPs generally include short-term counseling and referral services for employees and members of their household.

Healthy, Hunger-Free Kids Act—This legislation authorizes funding and sets policy for USDA's core child nutrition programs: the National School Lunch Program; the School Breakfast Program; the Special Supplemental Nutrition Program for Women, Infants and Children (WIC); the Summer Food Service Program; and the Child and Adult Care Food Program. The Healthy, Hunger-Free Kids Act allows USDA, for the first time in over 30 years, the opportunity to make real reforms to the school lunch and breakfast programs by improving the critical nutrition and hunger safety net for millions of children.

health literacy—Defined by the Institute of Medicine (IOM) as the degree to which individuals have the capacity to obtain, process, and understand basic health information and services needed to make appropriate health decisions.

health services—One of the components of CSH, health services are described by CDC as services designed to ensure access or referral to primary health care services or both; foster appropriate use of primary health care services; prevent and control communicable disease and other health problems; provide emergency care for illness or injury; promote and provide optimum sanitary conditions for a safe school facility and school environment; and provide educational and counseling opportunities for promoting and maintaining individual, family, and community health.

Healthy People 2020—In December 2010 the Department of Health and Human Services launched Healthy People 2020, which has four overarching goals: (1) attain high-quality, longer lives free of preventable disease, disability, injury, and premature death; (2) achieve health equity, eliminate disparities, and improve the health of all groups; (3) create social and physical environments that promote good health for all; and (4) promote quality of life, healthy development, and healthy behaviors across all life stages.

indirect services—Services offered on behalf of students and result from the counselors' communication with others involving referrals for extended assistance or consultation and collaboration with parents, other educators, or community agencies.

infants and children (WIC)—The **Special Supplemental Nutrition Program for Women, Infants and Children (WIC)** defines infants as individuals up to their first birthday and children as individuals up to their fifth birthday.

medical home—A home base for any child's medical and nonmedical care. Today's medical home is a cultivated partnership between the patient, family, and primary provider in cooperation with specialists and support from the community. The patient and family are the focal point of this model, and the medical home is built around this center.

mobile programs—The practice of health care or medical care not restricted by location; may refer to the practice itself being mobile, as in a dental clinic in a van that moves from school to school, or the use of electronic devices to provide diagnostic services and support.

National School Lunch Program (NSLP)—A federally assisted meal program operating in public and nonprofit private schools and residential child care institutions. It provides nutritionally balanced and low-cost or free lunches to children each school day. The program was established under the National School Lunch Act, signed by President Harry Truman in 1946.

National Health Education Standards—According to the CDC (2014), the National Health Education Standards (NHES) were developed to establish, promote, and support health-enhancing behaviors for students in all grade levels—from prekindergarten through grade 12. The NHES provide a framework for teachers, administrators, and policy makers in designing or selecting curricula, allocating instructional resources, and assessing student achievement and progress. The standards provide students, families, and communities with concrete expectations for health education.

nutrition education services—A component of the CSH framework as described by CDC. Ideal characteristics include access to a variety of nutritious and appealing meals that accommodate the health and nutrition needs of all students. School nutrition programs should reflect the U.S. dietary guidelines for Americans and other criteria to achieve nutrition integrity. School nutrition services should offer students a learning laboratory for classroom nutrition and health education and serve as a resource for linkages with nutrition-related community services. Qualified child nutrition professionals should provide these services.

physical activity—The World Health Organization (WHO) describes physical activity as any bodily movement produced by skeletal muscles that requires energy expenditure. For school-age children these activities may include walking, riding a bicycle, swinging, dancing, skipping, or flying a kite.

physical education—A component of the CSH framework the CDC describes physical education as a school-based instructional opportunity for students to gain the necessary skills and knowledge for lifelong participation in physical activity. Physical education is characterized by a planned, sequential K through 12 curriculum that provides cognitive content and learning experiences in a variety of activity areas. Quality physical education programs assist students in achieving the national standards for K through 12 physical education. The outcome of a quality physical education program is a physically educated person who has the knowledge, skills, and confidence to enjoy a lifetime of healthful physical activity.

physically literate—An individual who possesses the skills necessary to engage in a variety of physical activities; knows the implications of and the benefits from participation in various forms of physical activity; engages in regular physical activity; is physically fit; and appreciates the contributions of physical activity to a healthy lifestyle.

primary care model—Service delivery model that has a nurse practitioner, physician assistant, or physician on staff but no mental health provider. SBHCs that use the primary care model usually have a health educator or an oral health provider on staff.

primary care–mental health model—Service delivery model that includes a primary care provider and a mental health professional, such as a licensed clinical psychologist, social worker, or substance abuse counselor.

primary care–mental health plus model—The most comprehensive service delivery model, which involves collaboration and coordination between primary care, mental health providers, and other professionals like health educators, social service case managers, oral health providers, and nutritionists.

program evaluation—A systematic method for collecting, analyzing, and using information to answer questions about projects, policies, and programs. CDC describes effective program evaluation as a systematic way to improve and account for public health actions.

school-based health center (SBHC)—A health center located in a school or on school grounds that provides, at a minimum, on-site primary and preventive health care, mental health counseling, health promotion referral and follow-up services for young people enrolled.

School Breakfast Program (SBP)—Provides cash assistance to states to operate nonprofit breakfast programs in schools and residential child care institutions. The Food and Nutrition Service administers the SBP at the federal level. State education agencies administer the SBP at the state level, and local school food authorities operate the program in schools.

school psychologists—Psychologists who work with and or in the schools and generally specialize in issues related to school-aged youth. They function to enable children and adolescents to thrive academically, behaviorally, socially, and emotionally.

school physicians—A physician employed by or for a school district whose job it is to direct all health activities within that district. Specifically, school physicians are responsible for reviewing guidelines, programs, and policies specific to health care that takes place in schools.

school social workers—Social workers who work with and or in the schools and generally specialize in issues related to school-aged youth. School social workers provide direct services to students and their families (e.g., casework, group work, classroom presentations, crisis intervention, consultation, referrals to community agencies), engage in the assessment process for special education students, consult with teachers and administrators, and regularly serve on committees and teams within the school.

school-linked health centers (SLHCs)—Health centers that are generally coordinated at the school but do not provide clinical services on the school campus; involve collaboration between hospitals, health agencies, community-based clinics, or health professionals.

Special Supplemental Nutrition Program for Women, Infants and Children (WIC)—Provides federal grants to states for supplemental foods, health care referrals, and nutrition education for low-income, pregnant, breastfeeding, and nonbreastfeeding postpartum women and to infants and children up to age five who are found to be at nutritional risk.

Summer Food Service Program (SFSP)—Established to ensure that low-income children continue to receive nutritious meals when school is not in session. Free meals that meet federal nutrition guidelines are provided to all children 18 years old and under at approved SFSP sites in areas with significant concentrations of low-income children.

U.S. dietary guidelines—The dietary guidelines for Americans are the cornerstone of federal nutrition policy and nutrition education activities. The *2010 Dietary Guidelines for Americans* emphasize three major goals for Americans: (1) balance calories with physical activity to manage weight; (2) consume more of certain foods and nutrients such as fruits, vegetables, whole grains, fat-free and low-fat dairy products, and seafood: and (3) consume fewer foods with sodium, saturated fats, trans fats, cholesterol, added sugars, and refined grains.

Application Activities

1. You are invited by the local school district to serve as a consultant to assist them in improving their pre-K through grade 12 health and physical education program. They would like you to begin by presenting the rationale for why a comprehensive school health and physical education program is an important component of the overall school curriculum. Following the rationale you will highlight the best practices for a quality program. You will have 30 minutes for your presentation. The attendees at your presentation will consist of administrators, health education teachers, and the school wellness team, which includes teachers, administrators, parents, and community members. Develop an outline and related PowerPoint slides for the presentation. In addition, develop a list of questions that you anticipate might be asked of you during or after your presentation (and include your responses).
2. Choose one of the following activities:
   a. Interview at least five college students regarding their memories of their experiences related to seven of the WSCC components (include health education; physical education and physical activity; health services; nutrition environment and services; counseling, psychological, and social services; the physical environment; and the social and emotional climate). For the activity, develop a list of interview questions for the seven components. Then, following the interviews, develop a summary of the interviews and your written reflection of the interviews.
   b. Complete a similar interview with either a combination of five school administrators, teachers, and staff members or five parents of school-age children. For the school faculty and staff interview, focus on their perception of the current CSH–WSCC activities at their school and their perceptions of the viability of the model for their school. For the parents, focus your interview on their perceptions of WSCC for their children's schools, its importance, and their perceptions of the current program that exists in their schools.
3. Develop a five-minute video to introduce the WSCC approach to your viewers. Share the video with classmates and get their reaction on how well it would gain the attention of school personnel and how well it provides a visual understanding of the WSCC layout. If possible, have the video reviewed by school administrators, teachers, or parents for their response.

Resources

Counseling, Psychological, and Social Services

American School Counselor Association: www.schoolcounselor.org

National Association of School Psychologists: www.nasponline.org

School Social Work Association of America: www.sswaa.org

Family Engagement

Johns Hopkins' National Network of Partnership Schools: www.partnershipschools.org

Harvard Family Research Project: www.hfrp.org/family-involvement

Parental Information and Resource Centers: www.nationalpirc.org

Physical Education and Physical Activity

National Association for Sport and Physical Education: www.aahperd.org/naspe/

P.E. Central: www.pecentral.org

Physical Education Curriculum Analysis Tool (PECAT): www.cdc.gov/healthyyouth/pecat/

Health Services

National Association of School Nurses: www.nasn.org

School-Based Health Alliance: www.sbh4all.org

American Academy of Pediatrics: www.aap.org

Health Education

Health Education Curriculum Analysis Tool (HECAT): www.cdc.gov/healthyyouth/HECAT

Characteristics of Effective Health Education Curricula: www.cdc.gov/healthyyouth/SHER/characteristics/index.htm

Michigan Model for Health: www.emc.cmich.edu/mm

Physical Environment and Social and Emotional Climate

National School Climate Center: www.schoolclimate.org

HealthySEAT: www.epa.gov/schools/healthyseat/index.html

Sensible Steps to Healthier School Environments: www.aaees.org/downloadcenter/FutureEngineersandScientists-SensibleSteps.pdf

Employee Wellness

Employee Wellness: https://schools.healthiergeneration.org/wellness_categories/employee_wellness/why_employee_wellness

Health Promotion for Staff: www.cancer.org/healthy/morewaysacshelpsyoustaywell/schoolhealth/understandingthecoordinatedschoolhealthprogram/health-promotion-for-staff

Action Steps for Implementing Health Promotion for Faculty and Staff: www2.edc.org/MakingHealthAcademic/Concept/actions_staff.asp

Nutrition Environment and Services

USDA Nutrition Standards for School Meals: www.fns.usda.gov/school-meals/nutrition-standards-school-meals

Ten Keys to Promote Healthy Eating in Schools: www.fns.usda.gov/sites/default/files/CalltoAction.pdf

School Nutrition Association: www.schoolnutrition.org

References

Alliance for a Healthier Generation. 2013. *Facts on Employee Wellness*. https://schools.healthiergeneration.org/_asset/xd1mnq/08-734_EWFactSheet.pdf

Allison, Mandy A., Crane, Lori A., Beaty, Brenda L., Davidson, Arthur J., Melkinovich, P., & Kempe, Allison. 2007. School Based Health Centers: Improving Access and Quality of Care for Low Income Adolescents. *Pediatrics*, *120*, 511–518.

Allensworth, Diane. 2011. Addressing the Social Determinants of Health of Children and Youth: A Role for SOPHE Members. *Health Education & Behavior*, *38*(4), 331–338.

American Academy of Family Physicians, American Academy of Pediatrics, American Diabetes Association, National Hispanic Medical Association, National Medical Association, and the United States Department of Agriculture. n.d. *Healthy School Environments: Promoting Healthy Eating Behaviors*. http://teamnutrition.usda.gov/Resources/CalltoAction.pdf

American Academy of Pediatrics Council on School Health. 2008. Role of the School Nurse in Providing School Health Services. *Pediatrics*, *121*, 1052–1056.

American Academy of Pediatrics Council on School Health. 2013. Policy Statement: Role of the School Physician. *Pediatrics*, *131*, 178–182.

American Cancer Society. 2007. *National Health Education Standards: Achieving Excellence*. Atlanta, GA.

American Cancer Society. 2013. *Healthy School Environment*. www.cancer.org/healthy/morewaysacshelpsyoustaywell/schoolhealth/understandingthecoordinatedschoolhealthprogram/healthy-school-environment

American Medical Association. 2013. *Policy Statement H-60-991: Providing Medical Services Through School-Based Health Programs*. Chicago: American Medical Association. https://ssl3.ama-assn.org/apps/ecomm/PolicyFinderForm.pl?site=www.ama-assn.org&uri=%2fresources%2fdoc%2fPolicyFinder%2fpolicyfiles%2fHnE%2fH-60.991.HTM

American School Counselor Association. 2009. *The Role of the Professional School Counselor*. www.schoolcounselor.org/content.asp?contentid=240

American School Counselor Association. 2012. *Executive Summary: ASCA National Model—a Framework for School Counseling Programs* (3rd ed.). Alexandria, VA: Author.

ASCD. 2014. *The Whole Child Tenets*. www.ascd.org/whole-child.aspx

Basch, Charles E. 2011a. Healthier Students are Better Learners: A Missing Link in School Reforms to Close the Achievement Gap. *Journal of School Health, 8(10)1*, 593–598.

Basch, Charles E. 2011b. Executive Summary: Healthier Students Are Better Learners. *Journal of School Health, 81*(10), 591–592.

Briggs, Marilyn, Safaii, SeAnne, & Beall, Deborah Lane; American Dietetic Association; Society for Nutrition Education; American School Food Service Association. 2003. Position of the American Dietetic Association, Society for Nutrition Education, and American School Food Service Association-Nutrition Services: An Essential Component of Comprehensive School Health Programs. *Journal of Nutrition Education & Behavior, 35*, 57–67.

Centers for Disease Control. 2007. *School Employee Wellness: A Guide for Protecting the Assets of our Nation's Schools*. www.healthyschoolsms.org/staff_health/documents/EntireGuide.pdf

Centers for Disease Control and Prevention. 2010. *The Association Between School Based Physical Activity, Including Physical Education, and Academic Performance*. Atlanta: U.S. Department of Health and Human Services.

Centers for Disease Control and Prevention. 2011a. *School Health Programs—Improving the Health of Our Nation's Youth*. www.cdc.gov/chronicdisease/resources/publications/aag/dash.htm

Centers for Disease Control and Prevention. 2011b. *How Much Physical Activity Do Children Need?* www.cdc.gov/physicalactivity/everyone/guidelines/children.html

Centers for Disease Control and Prevention. 2012a. *Engaged Parents Have Healthier Adolescents*. www.cdc.gov/Features/parentengagement/

Centers for Disease Control and Prevention. 2012b. *Parent Engagement: Strategies for Involving Parents in School Health*. Atlanta, GA: U.S. Department of Health and Human Services.

Centers for Disease Control and Prevention. 2012c. *School Health Index: Self-Assessment and Planning Guide. Middle School/High School Version*. Atlanta, GA: U.S. Department of Health and Human Services.

Centers for Disease Control and Prevention. 2013a. *Components of Coordinated School Health*. www.cdc.gov/healthyyouth/cshp/components.htm

Centers for Disease Control and Prevention. 2013b. *Results From the School Health Policy and Practices Study*. www.cdc.gov/healthyyouth/shpps/2012/pdf/shpps-results_2012.pdf

Centers for Disease Control and Prevention. 2013c. *National Health Education Standards for Health Education*. www.cdc.gov/healthyyouth/sher/standards/

Centers for Disease Control and Prevention. 2013d. *Characteristics of an Effective Health Education Curriculum*. www.cdc.gov/HealthyYouth/SHER/characteristics/

Commonwealth of Massachusetts Executive Office of Health and Human Services. 2013. *Template for Massachusetts School Physician/Medical Consultant Role*. www.mass.gov/eohhs/gov/departments/dph/programs/community-health/primarycare-healthaccess/school-health/publications/template-for-school-physician medical-consultant.html

Committee on School Health. 2001. School Health Centers and Other Integrated School Health Services. *Pediatrics, 107*(1), 198–201.

Education Development Center. 2001. Action Steps for Implementing a Healthy School Environment. www2.edc.org/makinghealthacademic/concept/actions_environment.asp

Epstein, Joyce L., Sanders, Mavis G., Sheldon, Steven B., Simon, Beth S., Salinas, Karen C., Jansorn, Natalie R., Van Vooris, Frances L., Martin, Cecelia S., Thomas, Brenda G., Greenfield, Marsha D., Hutchins, Darcy J., & Williams Kenyatta J. 2009. *School, Family, and Community Partnerships: Your Handbook for Action* (3rd ed.). Thousand Oaks, CA: Corwin Press.

Fetro, Joyce, Givens, Connie, & Carroll, Kellie. 2010. Coordinated School Health: Getting It All Together. *Educational Leadership, 67*(4), 32–37.

Freudenberg, Nicholas, & Ruglis, Jessica. 2007. Peer Reviewed: Reframing School Dropout as a Public Health Issue. *Preventing Chronic Disease, 4*(4).

Frey, Andy J., Alvarez, Michelle E., Dupper, David R., Sabatino, Christine A., Lindsey, Brenda C., Raines, James C., Streeck, Frederick, McInerney, Anne, & Norris Molly, A. 2013. *School Social Work Practice Model Overview. Improving Academic and Behavioral Outcomes*. http://sswaa.org/displaycommon.cfm?an=1&subarticlenbr=459

Frumkin, Howard, Geller, Robert J., & Nodvin, Janice. 2006. *Safe and Healthy School Environments*. New York: Oxford University Press.

Henderson, Anne T., & Mapp, Karen L. 2002. *A New Wave of Evidence: The Impact of School, Family, and Community Connections on Student Achievement—Annual Synthesis 2002*. Austin, TX: Center for Family and Community

Connections with Schools, Southwest Educational Development Laboratory.

Henderson, Alan, & Rowe, Daryle E. 1998. A Healthy School Environment. In Eva Marx & Susan Frelick Wooley (Eds.), *Health Is Academic: A Guide to Coordinated School Health Programs*. New York: Teachers College Press.

Institute of Medicine. 1997. *Schools and Health: Our Nation's Investment*. Diane Allensworth, Elaine Lawson, Lois Nicholson, & James Wyche (Eds.). Washington, DC: National Academy Press.

Institute of Medicine. 2013. *Educating the Student Body: Taking Physical Activity and Physical Education to School. Report Brief.*

Joint Committee on National Health Education Standards. 2007. *National Health Education Standards: Achieving Excellence* (2nd ed.). American Cancer Society.

Jones, Sherry E. 2008. Executive Summary. *Journal of School Health*, *78*(2), 69–117.

Kisker, Ellen E., & Brown, Randall S. 1996. Do School Based Health Centers Improve Adolescents' Access to Health Care, Health Status, and Risk Taking Behavior? *Journal of Adolescent Health*, *18*, 335-343.

Let's Move Child Nutrition Program. 2014. *Child Nutrition Programs*. www.letsmove.gov/child-nutrition-programs

Lofink, Haley, Kuebler, Joanna, Juszczak, Linda, Schlitt, John, Even, Matt, Rosenberg, Jessica, & White, Iliana. 2013. *2010-2011 School-Based Health Alliance Census Report*. Washington, DC: School-Based Health Alliance.

Mandel, Leslie A., & Qazilbash, Jasmine. 2005. Youth Voices as Change Agents: Moving Beyond the Medical Model in School-Based Health Center Practice. *Journal of School Health*, *75*, 239–242.

McNeely, Clea A., Nonnemker, James M., & Blum, Robert W. 2002. Promoting School Connectedness: Evidence from the National Longitudinal Study of Adolescent Health. *Journal of School Health*, *72*(4), 138–146.

National Association for Sport and Physical Education. 2010a. *Physical Education Is an Academic Subject*. Reston, VA: Author.

National Association for Sport and Physical Education. 2010b. *Opportunity to Learn Guidelines for Elementary, Middle, & High School Physical Education: A Side-by-Side Comparison*. Reston, VA: Author.

National Association for Sport and Physical Education. 2013a. *Why Children Need Physical Education*. www.aahperd.org/naspe/publications/teachingTools/whyPE.cfm

National Association for Sport and Physical Education. 2013b. *National Standards and Grade-Level Outcomes for K–12 Physical Education*. www.shapeamerica.org/standards/upload/Grade-Level-Outcomes-for-K-12-Physical-Education.pdf

National Association of School Nurses. 2004. *School Health Nursing Service Role in Health Care: Health Promotion and Disease Prevention Issue Brief.* Silver Spring, MD: Author.

National Association of School Nurses. 2010. *Caseload Assignments* [Position Statement]. Silver Spring, MD: Author.

National Association of School Nurses. 2011. *Role of the School Nurse* [Position Statement]. Silver Spring, MD: Author

National Association of School Nurses. 2012. *Education, Licensure, and Certification of School Nurses* [Position Statement]. Silver Spring, MD: Author.

National Association of School Psychologists. n.d. *What Is a School Psychologist?* Bethesda, MD: Author.

National Association of School Psychologists. 2010a. National Association of School Psychologists Model for Comprehensive and Integrated School Psychological Services. *School Psychology Review*, *39*(2), 320–333.

National Association of School Psychologists. 2012. *NASP Practice Model: Improving Outcomes for Students and Schools*. www.nasponline.org/standards/practice-model/

National Association of School Psychologists. 2013 *NASP Recommendations for Comprehensive School Safety Policies*. http://www.nasponline.org/communications/press-release/NASP_School_Safety_Recommendations_January%20 2013.pdf

National Association of Secondary School Principals. 2013. *Safe Schools*. www.nassp.org/Content.aspx?topic=47111

National Association of Social Workers. 2012. *NASW Standards for School Social Work Services*. Washington, DC: Author.

National Coalition for Parent Involvement in Education. 1995. *Developing Family/School Partnerships: Guide for Schools and School Districts*. Washington, DC: Author.

National Education Association Education Policy and Practice Department. 2008. *Parent, Family, Community Involvement in Education: An NEA Policy Brief. PB 11*. Washington: Author.

National Health and Education Consortium. 1995. *Starting Young: School-Based Health Care Census*. Washington, DC: Author.

Robert Wood Johnson Foundation. 2012. *Increasing Physical Activity Through Recess—Research Brief.* http://activelivingresearch.org/files/ALR_Brief_Recess.pdf

Ruder, Robert. 2009. Healthier Students Through Positive Role Modeling. *PSAHPERD, Spring/ Summer, 9,* 15.

School Social Work Association of America. 2003. *School Social Work as a Career*. http://sswaa.org/ displaycommon.cfm?an=1&subarticlenbr=99

School Social Work Association of America. 2013. *School Social Work Practice Model*. http://sswaa. org/associations/13190/files/SSWAA_Practice_ Model%20Graphic.pdf

Shuler, Pamela A. 2000. Evaluating Student Services Provided by School-Based Health Centers: Applying the Shuler Nurse Practitioner Practice Model. *Journal of School Health*, *70*, 348–352.

Simon, Beth S. 2001. Family Involvement in High School: Predictors and Effects. *NASSP Bulletin*, *85*(627), 9–19.

State of Maine Department of Education and Department of Health and Human Services. 2002. *Youth, Parent, Family, and Community Involvement: Coordinating School Health Programs*. www.maine.gov/education/ mainecshp/GuideLine_PDF/Cover&Disc.pdf

Strozer, Jan, Juszczak, Linda, & Ammerman, Adrienne. 2010. *2007–2008 National School-Based Health Care Census*. Washington, DC: National Assembly on School-Based Health Care.

U.S. Department of Agriculture Food and Nutrition Service. 2014. *School Meals*. www.fns.usda.gov/ school-meals/healthy-hunger-free-kids-actaf

U.S. Department of Education. 2004. "Elementary and Secondary Education Act – Title IX – General Provisions – Section 9101 – No. 11." Last modified September 15, 2004. www2.ed.gov/ policy/elsec/leg/esea02/pg107.html

U.S. Department of Education, Office of Special Education Programs. 2007. "IDEA Regulations: Alignment With the No Child Left Behind (NCLB) Act." http://idea.ed.gov/explore/view/p/. root.dynamic.TopicalBrief.3.

U.S. Department of Education. 2010. *Indicators of School Crime and School Safety: 2010*. http:// nces.ed.gov/pubs2011/2011002.pdf

U.S. Department of Health and Human Services, Office of Disease Prevention and Health Promotion. 2013. *Healthy People 2020*. Washington, DC. http://healthypeople.gov/2020/ topicsobjectives2020/default.aspx

U.S. Department of Health and Human Services. n.d. *What Is a Medical Home? Why Is It Important?* www.hrsa.gov/healthit/toolbox/ Childrenstool box/BuildingMedicalHome/whyimportant.html

U.S. Environmental Protection Agency. 2012. *Sensible Steps to Healthier School Environment*. www.aaees.org/downloadcenter/ FutureEngineersand Scientists-SensibleSteps.pdf

U.S. Government. 2010. *2010 Dietary Guidelines for Americans*. www.health.gov/dietaryguide lines/2010.asp

Videto, Donna M., & Hodges, Bonni C. 2009. Use of University/School Partnerships for the Institutionalization of the Coordinated School Health Program. *American Journal of Health Education*, *40*(4), 216–219.

Wood, David L., Hayward, Rodney A., Corey, Christopher R., Freeman, Howard E., & Shapiro, Martin F. 1990. Access to Medical Health Care for Children and Adolescents in the United States. *Pediatrics*, *86*, 666–673.

World Health Organization. 2013. *WHO: Physical Activity*. www.who.int/dietphysicalactivity/pa/ en/index.html

Young, Thomas L., D'Angelo, Sandra L., & Davis, James. 2001. Impact of a School-Based Health Center on Emergency Department Use by Elementary School Students. *Journal of School Health*, *71*, 196–198.

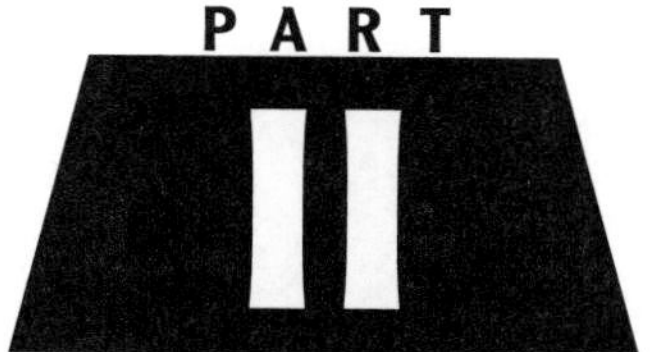

PART II

Putting the Focus on the Child

4

The Whole Child Initiative

SEAN SLADE

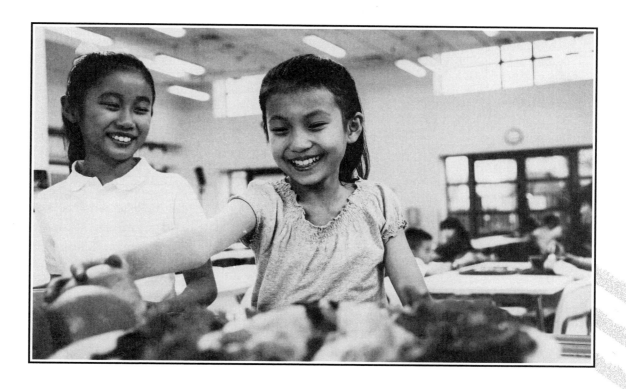

Schools that focus on establishing safe and secure environments, building connections, and developing relationships between students, staff, families, and community find reduced levels of substance abuse, reduced levels of anxiety and stress, and increased attendance and academic scores. Schools that take this role can build a culture of support to promote excellence for all students.

The relationship between health, healthful and safe school environments, and the educational success of students goes both ways. Just as education can benefit from improved health, health is improved through education. Education has been shown to improve health, health outcomes, and longevity. Education is the one social factor that is consistently linked to longer lives in every country where it has been studied (A Surprising Secret, 2007).

This chapter examines the health and academic success connection through the framework of ASCD's Whole Child Initiative. The five tenets of this initiative are presented with specific attention to the healthy tenet, including its 10 indicators. Besides an overview of the healthy tenet, nine levers of change for school health initiatives are included in the chapter. Going beyond change, the importance of sustainability is also addressed in this chapter.

WHOLE CHILD TENETS

In 2006 ASCD convened the Commission on the Whole Child (ASCD, 2007). This commission was composed of leading thinkers, researchers, and practitioners, all drawn from a variety of sectors. The commission was charged with recasting the definition of a successful learner from one whose achievement is measured solely by academic tests to one who is knowledgeable, emotionally and physically healthy, civically inspired, engaged in the arts, prepared for work and economic self-sufficiency, and ready for the world beyond formal schooling. The commission was convened to start a dialogue to change what is meant by a successful school, a successful education, and ultimately a successful student. The discussion was aimed directly at the educational landscape of 2007, which was dominated by the **No Child Left Behind Act** (NCLB) of 2001. NCLB clearly emphasized a greater focus on an academics-above-all-else educational system, further shifting the focus away from seeing the student holistically.

The commission began with a discussion of what an ideal education—one that places the child at the center—would look like. It asked how resources, both personnel and facilities, would be arranged if the child was key in the equation.

From this discussion, the ASCD **Whole Child Initiative** was launched in 2007. The initiative is a long-term effort to change the conversation about education from a focus on narrowly defined academic achievement to one that promotes the long-term development and success of children. The initiative established five tenets:

- **Healthy**—Each student enters school healthy and learns about and practices a healthy lifestyle.
- **Safe**—Each student learns in an environment that is physically and emotionally safe for students and adults.
- **Engaged**—Each student is actively engaged in learning and is connected to the school and broader community.
- **Supported**—Each student has access to personalized learning and is supported by qualified, caring adults.
- **Challenged**—Each student is challenged academically and prepared for success in college or further study and for employment and participation in a global environment.

These tenets provide the framework for the Whole Child Initiative. This initiative provides the direction for a well-rounded, holistic, and effective education and ensures that each child in each school and in each community is healthy, safe, engaged, supported, and challenged. The Whole Child Initiative is based on the understanding that students cannot learn if they are not healthy or safe. Subsequently, they won't learn unless they are engaged, supported, and challenged. The initiative has moved to align the fields of health and education in achieving healthy and safe environments and has propagated the idea that such an alignment is required for educational success.

When students' basic physiological and psychological needs—including being physically healthy, socially and emotionally safe, connected, and secure—are satisfied, they are more likely to

- become engaged in school,
- act in accord with school goals and values,
- develop social skills and understanding,
- contribute to the school and community, and
- achieve academically.

Further, when schools fail to meet those needs, students are more likely to become less motivated, more alienated, and poorer academic performers. The tenets refer directly back to Abraham Maslow's **hierarchy of needs**, which was set out in the 1943 paper "A Theory of Human Motivation" (Maslow, 1943). The original hierarchy established the foundational needs (physiological) at the base of a pyramid, followed subsequently by safety, belongingness, esteem, and self-actualization. By its pyramid structure, the hierarchy demonstrated the understanding that certain needs were possible only after others had been established.

Following on this structure the Whole Child tenets were arranged to demonstrate that health and then safety were fundamental in establishing environments in which students could then be engaged, supported, and ultimately challenged (figure 4.1).

LINKS BETWEEN HEALTH AND EDUCATION

The many links between health and education are well documented. A 2005 California Department of Education report outlined some of the links

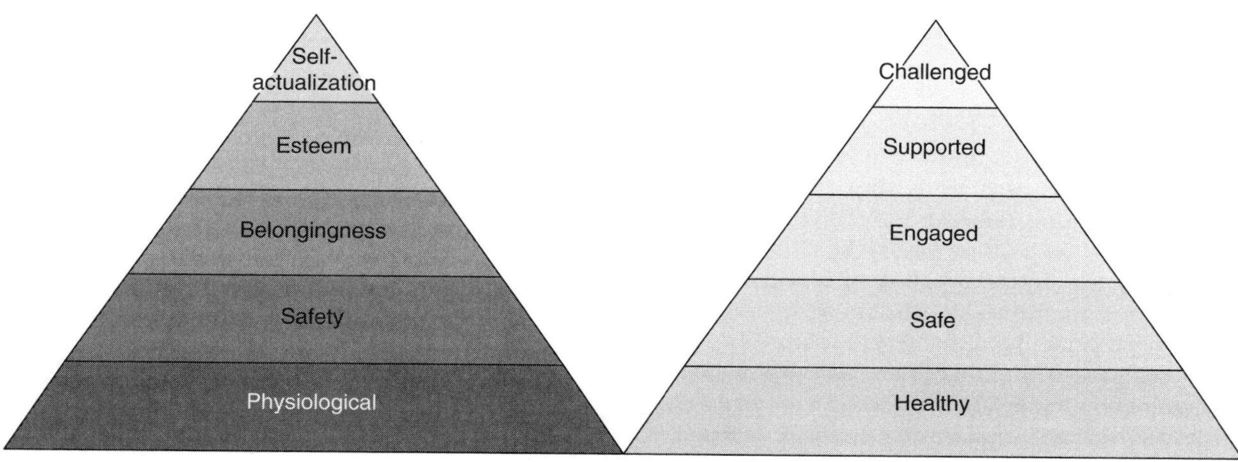

Figure 4.1 Maslow's hierarchy of needs (left) and the five Whole Child tenets (right) are both built on a structure that presumes that the body's physiological needs must be met before other human needs (such as emotional and social needs) may be addressed.

between health and education and the symbiotic role and effect of both.

- When health needs are met, students earn better grades.
- Investing in children's physical health needs promotes learning over the school years and has profound effects on school readiness and early learning.
- Increases in the amount and quality of physical education time have a favorable effect on academic achievement, even when time devoted to academic instruction has been reduced.
- Schools that are able to provide in-house or in-community health service connections see an increase in attendance, a decrease in the dropout rate, and improved gains in students' attitudes about learning.
- Substance abuse, hunger, lack of breakfast, and a perceived lack of safety at school have particularly strong relationships to students' poorer school performance.

The results suggest that addressing the health and developmental needs of youth is a critical component of a comprehensive strategy for meeting the accountability demands for improved academic performance.

Charles Basch (2010) identified seven educationally relevant health disparities problems based on prevalence within a low-income urban minority youth population. He also identified the causal effects on achievement of these health concerns and the feasibility of school systems to ameliorate at the school site. The seven educationally relevant health-related disparities were vision, asthma, teen pregnancy, aggression and violence, physical activity, breakfast, and inattention and hyperactivity.

Pertaining to the role of health status in relationship to educational success and quality of life, Basch states, "Health-related problems play a major role in limiting the motivation and ability to learn of urban minority youth, and interventions to address those problems can improve educational as well as health outcomes. Healthier students are better learners" (Basch, 2010, p. 4). Even if health factors had no effect on educational outcomes, they clearly influence the quality of life for youth and their ability to contribute and live productively in a democratic society. Improving the health of youth is a worthy goal for elementary and secondary education. Indeed, pursuing this goal is a moral imperative (Basch, 2010).

Beyond physical health, children who are anxious, fearful, or depressed cannot concentrate on the task at hand. Even if we employ the best teaching techniques and pedagogy, none will work if children do not feel safe. How can students collaborate, problem solve, or think critically if

School Health *in Action*

City Connects: Revitalizing Student Support

City Connects is an innovative school-based system that revitalizes support for students in urban schools and currently runs programs in Boston and Springfield, Massachusetts, and New York City. City Connects collaborates with teachers and school staff to identify the strengths and needs of every child in the elementary school setting. They then create a tailored set of intervention, prevention, and enrichment services located in the school and community designed to help each student learn and thrive. By addressing the in- and out-of-school factors that affect children, City Connects is able to help students succeed in school. City Connects is focused on helping students come to school ready to engage and learn. The theory behind this program is that each student's ability to thrive in the classroom depends on a unique set of academic, social-emotional, health, and family-related factors. The program is designed to address each child's strengths and needs across these four dimensions.

City Connects uses the existing structures of public schools and the resources of community agencies to deliver tailored supports and enrichment opportunities for students. In 2012-13, across all City Connects sites, 15,100 students were linked to more than 57,300 services and enrichment opportunities, ranging from tutoring to athletics programs. The City Connects *Progress Report 2012* (2012) shows strong evidence of the positive effects of the program. For students, new analyses show improvements in middle school report card scores, reduced chronic absenteeism, and lower probability of dropping out of school.

Based on City Connects. Available: http://www.bc.edu/schools/lsoe/cityconnects/

they are concerned about their personal safety? How can children dream new dreams, create new ideas, or form new concepts if they are suffering from depression, anxious about their home life, or stressed by what they experience after they leave the school building?

Graduation from high school has been associated with not only reduced bouts of illness but also less harmful illness. Ultimately, graduation has been shown to increase the average lifespan by six to nine years (Allensworth et al., 2011). Failure to graduate from high school too often commits people to a likelihood of both health issues and educational failure. Likewise, graduation can promote success.

Some groups are disproportionately affected by issues of health, poverty, and educational success. The struggles of youth are often directly related to issues in their environment such as malnutrition, mental health issues, substance abuse, and limited access to services and resources. These challenges often occur within the context of struggling schools, which are a reflection of the poorly resourced communities in which they live. But the environment of a school has the potential to change this trajectory. By environment, we are talking of both the physical and psychosocial environment, in other words, the climate and culture of the school.

A recent Chicago study (Steinberg, et al, 2011) outlined the elements that played a direct role in determining whether an environment was safe, supportive, and conducive to learning. The following four elements explained 80 percent of the differences in school safety across a major urban school district:

- **School–family interactions**: Schools in which teachers reported the highest levels of parent involvement were also the safest. Additionally, strong parental involvement with the school was seen as even a stronger indicator of school safety than was student achievement.
- **Student–teacher interactions**: Schools that served the most disadvantaged students but had documented high-quality student–teacher interactions were perceived as safer than those schools that served more advantaged students but had a poorer record of quality student–teacher interactions.
- **Teacher collaboration and support**: School environments were perceived as safer when the school staff took deliberate actions and collective responsibility toward ensuring it.

- **School leadership**: Strong connections exist between developing and sustaining a positive school climate and the principal's efforts in leading the initiative.

Schools that were perceived as safer tended to have higher achieving students and vice versa. Schools are able to play an active role in developing a climate and culture that is not only conducive to learning but also perceived as safer, more supportive, and more connected. The same Chicago study also highlighted how a school is able, by boosting the four elements, to provide safety and support even if that school sits inside an unsafe local environment (Steinberg et al., 2011).

"HEALTHY" AS A KEY TENET OF THE WHOLE CHILD INITIATIVE

By identifying "healthy" as a tenet in the Whole Child Initiative, attention was focused on the role of school health programs and services in the school and community. Healthy also focused a light on the need for schools to consider not just the academic outcomes of the students but also the health and well-being of students as a strategy to improve educational outcomes and address their holistic development. Putting a focus on being healthy proposed that schools and districts place additional attention on the environment in which learning takes place before embarking directly upon that learning. This approach was borne out of an understanding that students cannot learn if they are not healthy and safe. Subsequently, students won't learn unless they are also engaged, supported, and challenged.

The healthy tenet went beyond concentrating only on physical health. Healthy referred not only to physical health but also to social, emotional, and mental health. Schools should not be content with focusing only on physical activity and nutrition. They should also focus on the social and emotional development, along with the development of safe, supportive environments and access to mental health services, counseling, and social workers.

The **tenets**, including healthy, provide a framework for schools, but at its beginning the use of tenets provided but a bare framework. For many school-based administrators and personnel it sufficed well as a philosophy but fell short as a tool to affect school improvement and adjust school policies. In 2010 the Whole Child Initiative expanded the scaffold and included 10 **indicators** under each tenet to show and outline what each tenet looked like. The 10 indicators for the healthy tenet are the following:

1. Our school culture supports and reinforces the health and well-being of each student.
2. Our school health education curriculum and instruction support and reinforce the health and well-being of each student by addressing the physical, mental, emotional, and social dimensions of health.
3. Our school physical education schedule, curriculum, and instruction support and reinforce the health and well-being of each student by addressing lifetime fitness knowledge, attitudes, behaviors, and skills.
4. Our school facility and environment support and reinforce the health and well-being of each student and staff member.
5. Our school addresses the health and well-being of each staff member.
6. Our school collaborates with parents and the local community to promote the health and well-being of each student.
7. Our school integrates health and well-being into the school's ongoing activities, professional development, curriculum, and assessment practices.
8. Our school sets realistic goals for student and staff health that are built on accurate data and sound science.
9. Our school facilitates student and staff access to health, mental health, and dental services.
10. Our school supports, promotes, and reinforces healthy eating patterns and food safety in routine food services and special programming and events for students and staff.

The development of these indicators enables schools and districts to conduct needs assessments, analyze assets, and plan for improved health and education alignment. This was done through a focus on alignment from an educational perspective and outlook.

School Health *in Action*

Chicago Healthy Schools Campaign: Change for Good

In 2009 the Healthy Schools Campaign, Chicago Public Schools, and their partners came together to support schools in promoting healthy eating, nutrition education, and physical activity. Over 200 schools have made significant changes that have affected more than 90,000 students. In addition, all students are benefiting from major improvements to district health and wellness policies. This successful work has laid the foundation for even more significant and lasting change. HSC has an ambitious new plan to transform schools, communities, and the entire city and support the long-term health and success of all Chicago students. The new plan, called Change for Good, will engage Chicago Public Schools, parents, teachers, principals, school nurses, students, and partners at the local, state, and national levels. HSC's new initiative is intended to make permanent and lasting change that will have a significant positive effect on the long-term health and success of all Chicago children and will benefit the entire city. Change for Good includes four key areas: healthy food, physical activity, healthy classrooms, and green schoolyards. Change for Good is focused on the goals that align with the following four key areas:

- Working with Chicago Public Schools to make more improvements to the school food program and expand the district's farm-to-school program
- Improving physical education and supporting the district's longer-term goal of bringing daily physical education to all schools
- Providing leadership and skills training to principals, teachers, parents, and school nurses and supporting the district's increased focus on professional development
- Working to bring green schoolyards that support play, outdoor education, and community engagement to every corner of the city

Healthy Schools Campaign president and CEO Rochelle Davis stated in 2012,

> Despite this significant progress, our work is not done. Our work will not be finished until all children are offered, and actually eat and enjoy, a fresh and healthy school breakfast and lunch, have daily physical education that allows them to focus and learn, have the opportunity for active play and outdoor learning in schoolyards that are centers of community activity, and learn in a school with principals, teachers, school nurses, and parents who care about and promote student health and wellness. (Healthy School Campaign, n.d.)

Based on Health Schools Campaign. Available: http://healthschoolscampaign.typepad.com/healthy_schools_campaign/chicago_public_schools/

GAINING SUPPORT FOR THE WHOLE CHILD INITIATIVE

Through an earlier initiative, Healthy School Communities and a pilot study of the HSC initiative in 2007-09, ASCD gained a greater understanding of the importance of getting educational buy-in for initiatives that may have a strong health focus. Educators appear to be reluctant to view health-focused initiatives as anything more than health initiatives. Outlining the benefits of health was not enough; the benefits needed to be highlighted as educational benefits to gain support from those outside the health education sector.

The 2010 ASCD publication, *The Healthy School Communities Model: Aligning Health and Education in the School Setting*, surmised it this way.

> What is required is a change in how we view health and education; changes in how the two operate, align, and integrate in the school and community setting. Moreover, the biggest change must be in how education views health. The conversation needs to be directed not toward health professionals but toward education professionals. We must outline and define the education benefits of healthy students; healthy staff; and a healthy, effective school—for education's sake. (p. 4)

To better align, coordinate, and link health and education in the school setting, we must expand the conversation to include educators—teachers, school staff, and administrators. That is the premise of this publication. It takes the concept of health, combines it with education in the school setting and—most important for its implementation and sustainability—outlines for school personnel action steps and their benefits for the education process. (p. 5)

NINE LEVERS FOR CULTURAL CHANGE

Based on the 2007-09 pilot study, several elements or processes typically used for implementing a health initiative were identified as counterproductive. The pilot study indicated that health initiatives had to be introduced, implemented, and overseen as educational initiatives if they were to succeed in the school setting. Overall, the ASCD team of evaluators found a series of nine levers that catalyzed significant change in the culture of the participating school communities toward achieving success:

- The principal as leader
- Active and engaged leadership
- Distributive leadership
- Integration with the school improvement plan
- Effective use of data for continuous school improvement
- Ongoing and embedded professional development
- Authentic and mutually beneficial community collaborations
- Stakeholder support of the local efforts
- The creation or modification of school policy related to the process

The team's assessment of each site suggests that these levers work in concert to support the implementation and sustainability of the HSC concept as part of school improvement. Although all nine levers are important, several levers were determined to be pivotal. The most important was the first, the principal as leader. The evaluation team deemed the role of the principal the most critical piece of the process in implementing meaningful school change and school improvement. Without principal leadership, which is distinct from principal support, the process was likely to stagnate; with principal leadership, it thrived.

Consistent with the importance of principal leadership rather than support, Hoyle, Bartee, and Allensworth (2010) stressed that rather than attempting to gain support under the health banner, advocates should attempt to position CSH as part of school improvement plans. Kolbe (2002) summarized this thinking by stating,

> In sum, if American schools do not coordinate and modernize their school health programs as a critical part of educational reform, our children will continue to benefit at the margins from a wide disarray of otherwise unrelated, if not underdeveloped, efforts to improve interdependent education, health, and social outcomes. And, we will forfeit one of the most appropriate and powerfu l means available to improve student performance. (p. 10)

SUSTAINABILITY

Using the key findings of the HSC study, ASCD understood that for any initiative to be successful and sustainable, it has to be both viewed as educationally beneficial and linked to the overall school improvement process. In 2012 the initiative took two more steps to integrate the tenets and indicators approach into the school improvement process.

The first step toward integration was to develop an additional topic, **sustainability**, aligned to the tenets and 10 corresponding indicators (figure 4.2). These indicators are intended to increase the likelihood of sustainability of a school health initiative.

The second step toward integration was to take all 50 indicators for the Whole Child tenets, as well as the 10 additional indicators created under the topic of sustainability, and cross-link them to the six components of effective **school improvement**. The six components of school improvement are as follows:

- **School climate and culture:** Students entering school feel safe, engaged, and connected and see school as a place where they can learn and contribute to the world around them. They receive coordinated and continuous support to strengthen their social and emotional skills and enhance positive character traits.
- **Curriculum and instruction:** Students develop critical-thinking and reasoning

FIGURE 4.2
Indicators of Sustainability

Implementation of a Whole Child approach to education is a cornerstone of our school improvement plan and is included in our data collection.

Our professional development plan reflects emphasis on and implementation of a Whole Child approach to education, is individualized to meet staff needs, and is coordinated with an ongoing school improvement efforts and analysis process.

Our school regularly reviews the alignment of our policies and practices to ensure the health, safety, engagement, support, and challenge of our students.

Our school uses a balanced approach to formative and summative assessments that provide reliable, developmentally appropriate information about student learning.

Our professional evaluation process emphasizes meeting the needs of the whole child and provides opportunities for individualized professional growth.

Our school identifies and collaborates with community agencies, service providers, and organizations to meet specific goals for students.

Our school implements a proactive approach to identifying students' social, emotional, physical, and academic needs and designs coordinated interventions among all service providers.

Our school leaders implement a distributed leadership plan to ensure progress.

Our school staff, community-based service providers, families, and other adult stakeholders share research, appropriate data, idea generation, and resources to provide a coordinated, Whole Child approach for each student.

Our school and all our partners consistently assess and monitor our progress on all indicators of student success to ensure progress and make necessary changes in a timely manner.

Reprinted from ASCD, 2014, *The Whole Child initiative: Sustainable* (Alexandria, VA: ASCD). Available: http://www.ascd.org/programs/The-Whole-Child/Sustainable.aspx

skills, problem-solving competencies, technology proficiency, and content knowledge through evidence-based, relevant, differentiated instructional pedagogy and comprehensive curriculum.

- **Community and family:** Families, community members and organizations, and educators collaborate on shared decisions, actions, and outcomes for children.
- **Leadership**. Leaders act as visionaries, influencers, learners, and instructional guides to ensure that school policies and practices support a Whole Child approach.
- **Professional development and capacity:** Staff demonstrate the knowledge, skills, and dispositions necessary to ensure that each child is prepared for long-term success. They are supported by differentiated, job-embedded professional development.
- **Assessment:** Assessment is varied and timely, conducted to adjust teaching and learning activities to maximize student progress in all areas, and generates meaningful, useful data for decision making.

By doing this, the Whole Child Initiative formally linked the tenets, including healthy, and the indicators to the school improvement process, not as an extra or an altruistic add-on but as a fundamental part of the annual planning for the school and its community.

RELEVANCE FOR WHOLE SCHOOL, WHOLE COMMUNITY, WHOLE CHILD

Many lessons have been learned from the history of Coordinated School Health (CSH). CSH and the original eight-component model has undoubtedly been a well-planned and easily understood initiative, but it has not had the effect for which it was intended or designed. In 1998 Eva Marx, Susan Wooley, and Daphne Northrop wrote in the landmark publication *Health Is Academic*, "The promise of a Coordinated School Health program thus far outshines its practice" (p. 10).

Little has changed in the years since that statement was written to alter that viewpoint. Schools are the domain of education, so any initiative to be implemented in the schools must have educational benefit and be in alignment with the existing educational setting.

Although the appreciation of what constitutes an effective education is changing and has changed since the introduction of No Child Left Behind (ESEA) in 2001 and, somewhat coincidentally, since the introduction of the Whole Child Initiative, any new initiative must be linked back to the processes and functions of the school and its educational outcomes, whether these are academic, cognitive, or developmental.

For initiatives, and especially initiatives that may at first glance be viewed as superfluous to the school's primary mission, the following recommendations are key to successful implementation and sustained success.

Initiatives need to be

- adapted and subsequently adopted into the school as educationally beneficial initiatives,
- aligned or integrated into the school improvement process,
- aligned and written into school policies, and
- include the support and leadership of the school administration.

It was with this understanding and basis that ASCD and the U.S. Centers for Disease Control and Prevention, along with a select group of education, public health, and school health experts, undertook a revision and update of the traditional Coordinated School Health model.

The Whole School, Whole Community, Whole Child collaborative approach to learning and health model combines and builds on elements of the traditional Coordinated School Health (CSH) model and the Whole Child tenets. This new combined model responds to the call for greater alignment, integration, and collaboration between health and education to improve each child's cognitive, physical, social, and emotional development.

The fact is that health and education affect individuals, society, and the economy. They must work together whenever possible, and the schools represent a perfect setting for this collaboration. Schools are one of the most efficient systems for reaching children and youth to provide health services and programs, and approximately 95 percent of all U.S. children and youth attend school. At the same time, integrating health programs and services more deeply into the day-to-day life of schools and students represents an untapped tool for raising academic achievement.

SUMMARY

The Whole Child Initiative has made great strides in both moving the conversation about what constitutes an effective education and aligning the health and education sectors in the school setting. It has readjusted what many schools see as their core mission and has enabled schools to focus attention to elements that support the development of effective teaching and learning environments.

Health and well-being play a big role in supporting the mission of schools, but the health sector has promoted itself and its programs, including Coordinated School Health, as superfluous and adjacent to education rather than foundational to the educational process. To ensure consideration and implementation, WSCC must be presented as being crucial and beneficial to the educational process, be aligned with school improvement, and recognize that environments that promote health and well-being are the same environments that are conducive to effective teaching and learning.

Glossary

hierarchy of needs—Abraham Maslow's presentation of the needs for human development. Frequently displayed as a pyramid starting with the foundational need at the base and self-actualization at the top.

No Child Left Behind (NCLB) Act—Name provided in the Elementary and Secondary Education Act (ESEA) in 2001. The act supports standards-based educational reform and has been responsible for increased focus on setting high standards and establishing measurable goals to improve individual outcomes in education. Critics believe that NCLB has diverted needed resources away from a well-rounded education and instead focused attention on just two subject areas, language arts and math.

school improvement—The planning and process that all schools in the United States undertake to improve their schools. The majority of schools have school improvement teams, plans, and metrics that are analyzed annually. The school improvement plan is generally a comprehensive plan that identifies long-range improvement goals for the school to improve academic performance, school facilities, and professional development.

sustainability—The ability of a school to maintain an initiative or program long term beyond implementation or the initial phase that was funded or supported by an outside agency.

tenets and indicators—Key principles that provide the framework for the Whole Child Initiative. Each tenet—healthy, safe, engaged, supported, and challenged—is supported by 10 indicators provided by ASCD.

Whole Child Initiative—The initiative started in 2007 by ASCD that aims to focus greater attention on a holistic, well-rounded education that caters to each child's social, emotional, mental, physical, and cognitive development.

Application Activities

1. Conduct an interview with a school administrator. At the beginning of the interview, present a brief overview of the WSCC approach either verbally or in a written summary. During the interview, inquire about the administrator's perception of the school and school district's current efforts related to WSCC, the 9 levers for change, and the 10 indicators for sustainability. Write a summary of the interview and your perceptions of the district's status related to the Whole Child concept following the interview.
2. Choose either of the following two activities.
   a. Think back to your time as a student in elementary school. What was your experience as a student relative to your school's support of the five Whole Child tenets? Develop a reflection paper that describes your experiences related to the tenets, both positive and negative, and recommendations for improvement. Write the paper as if you would be providing it to an administrator at your former school.
   b. If you are currently working in a school, review how your school emphasizes the five Whole Child tenets. Develop a reflection paper that describes your perception of the school's emphasis on the tenets, both positive and negative, and your recommendations for improvement. Write the paper as if you would be providing it to an administrator or colleagues at the school.
3. Review the Healthy School Communities and the Whole Child information on the ASCD website at www.ascd.org/wholechild.aspx. After you have reviewed the information, create a professional development presentation targeted at colleagues in the school district in which you work (real or imagined). Present an understanding of the role of the Whole Child Initiative in advancing the academic success of students at your school. Develop a PowerPoint presentation that will highlight the key points of your report.

Resources

ASCD: www.ascd.org

Whole Child education: www.wholechildeducation.org

Whole Child tenets and indicators: www.wholechildeducation.org/assets/content/mx-resources/wholechildindicators-all.pdf

ASCD School Improvement Tool: http://sitool.ascd.org

Healthy School Communities: www.ascd.org/programs/healthy-school-communities.aspx

Healthy School Communities Model, Aligning Health and Education in the School Setting: www.ascd.org/ASCD/pdf/siteASCD/publications/Aligning-Health-Education.pdf

Healthier Students Are Better Learners, A Missing Link in School Reforms to Close the Achievement Gap, Equity Matters: www.equitycampaign.org/i/a/document/12557_equitymattersvol6_web03082010.pdf

Ensuring That No Child Is Left Behind; How Are Student Health Risks and Resilience Related to the Academic Progress of Schools? http://chks.wested.org/resources/EnsuringNCLB.pdf

References

A Surprising Secret to a Long Life: Stay in School. 2007, January 3. *New York Times*. www.nytimes.com/2007/01/03/health/03aging.html

ASCD. 2007. *The Learning Compact Redefined: A Call to Action. A Report of the Commission on the Whole Child*. Alexandria, VA: ASCD.

Allensworth, Diane, Lewallen, Theresa C., Stevenson, Beth, & Katz, Susan. 2011. Addressing the Needs of the Whole Child: What Public Health Can Do to Answer the Education Sector's Call for a Stronger Partnership. *Preventing Chronic Disease*, *8*(2), A44. www.cdc.gov/pcd/issues/2011/mar/10_0014.htm

Basch, E. Charles. 2010. Healthier Students Are Better Learners: A Missing Link in School Reforms to Close the Achievement Gap. *Equity Matters: Research Review*, No. 6.

California Department of Education. 2005. *Getting Results: Update 5—Student Health, Supportive Schools, and Academic Success*. Sacramento, CA: CDE Press.

City Connects. 2012. *The Impact of City Connects. Progress Report 2012*. www.bc.edu/content/dam/files/schools/lsoe/cityconnects/pdf/CityConnects_ProgressReport_2012.pdf

Healthy School Campaign. n.d. http://healthyschoolscampaign.typepad.com/healthy_schools_campaign/chicago_public_schools/

Hoyle, Tena B., Bartee, Todd R., & Allensworth, Diane D. 2010. Applying the Process of Health Promotion in Schools: A Commentary. *Journal of School Health*, *80*(4), 163–166.

Kolbe, Lloyd J. 2002. Education Reform and the Goals of Modern School Health Programs: How School Health Programs Can Help Students Achieve Success. *State Education Standard*, *3*(4), 4–11.

Maslow, Abraham H. 1943. A Theory of Human Motivation. *Psychological Review*, *50*(4), 370–96. http://psychclassics.yorku.ca/Maslow/motivation.htm

No Child Left Behind (NCLB) Act of 2001, Pub. L. No. 107-110, § 115, Stat. 1425, 2002.

Marx, Eva, Wooley, Susan, & Northrop, Daphne (Eds.). 1998. Health Is Academic: A Guide to Coordinated School Health Programs. New York: Teachers College Press.

Steinberg, Matthew P., Allensworth, Elaine M., and Johnson, David W. 2011. *Student and Teacher Safety in Chicago Public Schools: The Roles of Community Context and School Social Organization*. Chicago: Consortium on Chicago School Research.

5

Linking Health and Academic Success

MICHELE WALLEN

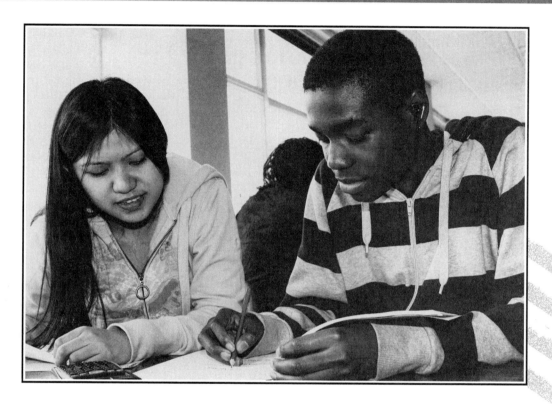

Education is a strong predictor of health and health outcomes (Woolf et al., 2007). People who did not graduate from high school are more likely to be in poor or fair health when compared with college graduates. The age-adjusted mortality rate of high school dropouts (ages 25 to 64) is twice that of adults who have some college education. People who do not complete high school are more likely to suffer from acute and chronic illnesses and conditions such as heart disease, hypertension, stroke, high cholesterol, emphysema, diabetes, asthma attacks, and ulcers. College graduates live, on average, five years longer when compared with those who do not complete high school (United Health Foundation, 2013; Arendt, 2005).

Health has great influence on academic achievement and education outcomes. Clearly, the health of students and academic success are inextricably linked. Statistical analyses reflect a negative association between high schools students' health-risk behaviors and their academic performance (CDC, 2009). Students who engage in health-risk behaviors are more likely to have lower grades than those who do not engage in health-risk behaviors. Health assets that students develop when transitioning from childhood to adolescence (for example, coping skills that reduce levels of anxiety and stress, physical activity habits, healthy dietary habits, sense of self-worth, and positive body image) may buffer them from the negative effects on academic performance that are often linked to the social and emotional challenges associated with puberty and transitions from elementary to middle and middle to high school settings (Forrest, 2013). Improvement in even one risk factor may help improve academic achievement.

In this chapter we explore the relationship between health and academic achievement in schools and examine strategies for advancement of these important outcomes. Examples of Whole School, Whole Community, Whole Child strategies are provided throughout the chapter. Success stories are highlighted, as are the benefits of this approach to address the multifaceted goals and responsibilities of schools today.

HEALTH AND EDUCATION IN EARLY CHILDHOOD

High-quality early childhood education can increase parental involvement, identify and use resources to address learning delays in children, contribute to improved education outcomes, increase future earning potential, and lead to healthier and longer lives. The National Education Goals Panel, a bipartisan intergovernmental body of federal and state government officials created to assess and report progress toward national education goals, identified five distinct yet connected domains of school readiness. These domains are developmental building blocks and currently at the center of the Head Start child development and early learning framework:

- Language and literacy
- Approaches to learning
- Cognitive and general knowledge
- Physical development and health
- Social and emotional development

Note that two of the five domains for early learning can be specifically addressed with the Whole School, Whole Community, Whole Child (WSCC) approach. When considering the critical role that health and physical development play in early learning and school readiness, it is understandable that children who experience poor health at a young age have lower academic achievement, experience poorer health as they age, and have lower socioeconomic status as adults. Longitudinal findings quantified the effects of childhood health and economic circumstances on adult health, employment, and socioeconomic status. Children who experience poor health have significantly lower educational attainment, lower social status, and poorer health as adults when controlling for parental income, education, and social class (Case et al., 2005).

Researchers investigated the relationship between child health and academic achievement during the formative years by using a large database of former Head Start children. Child health status was found to be an independent risk factor for lower academic achievement. Longitudinal analyses showed that poor general health status in kindergarten independently predicted lower reading and math scores in third grade (Spernak, Schottenbauer, Ramey, & Ramey, 2006, 1258). National early childhood education programs such as Head Start place a concurrent emphasis on the health and educational needs of children and demonstrate long-term benefits such as school achievement, increased graduation rates, and active participation in the work force (Novello, DeGraw, & Kleinman, 1992). Health and educational priorities do not recede after kindergarten for children and should therefore be a central focus of policy makers and educators. Resources and priority should be given to both educational and health outcomes through all grade spans because students' engagement in health risks increases with age (CDC, 2012).

HEALTH-RISK BEHAVIORS AND ACADEMIC ACHIEVEMENT

The Centers for Disease Control and Prevention (CDC) oversees data collection from middle school and high school students every other year with the Youth Risk Behavior Survey (YRBS). This surveillance effort allows researchers to follow trends and identify relationships associated with adolescent health-risk behaviors. One relationship important to educators and health professionals is the link between academic performance and engagement in health-risk behaviors. Researchers investigating the correlation between health and academics use measures such as grade point average (GPA) and standardized test scores to quantify academic performance. After controlling for sex, race and ethnicity, and grade level, the 2009 YRBS high school data suggest a negative association between health-risk behaviors and academic achievement. Students with lower grades are more likely to participate in risky health behaviors, and students earning higher grades are less likely to engage in risky health behaviors (CDC, 2009). The data presented in figure 5.1 represent questions asked of high school students regarding their participation in health-risk behaviors that are considered the leading causes of morbidity and mortality for their age group and their grade average.

MAKING A DIFFERENCE THROUGH THE WSCC APPROACH

Public health and education can work together to implement effective and efficient school health programs and policies to improve each student's cognitive, physical, social, and emotional development. Through the coordination and planning of policies, programs, and services, schools can reduce violence and aggression, address mental health problems, serve as providers of health services and school-based health centers, promote family and community involvement and parental engagement, provide a healthy breakfast and promote balanced nutritional services, and provide quality physical education and additional opportunities for physical activity. All these efforts will be addressed in following subsections. Focused efforts to promote WSCC will provide students with a healthy, safe, engaging, supportive, and challenging environment and improve school connectedness.

Create School Connectedness

Studies show that students who experience positive **school connectedness** are less likely to experience mental health problems, less likely to engage in health-risk behaviors, and more likely to have good educational outcomes (Catalano et al., 2004; Klem & Connell, 2004; Bond et al., 2007; Forrest et al., 2013). School connectedness emerges when students feel as though they are a part of the school and perceive an attachment between themselves and the adults and other students at school. Connectedness occurs when students feel as though adults care about their success in learning and their well-being as people. Researchers, educators, and health professionals attended the 2004 Wingspread Conference to review and discuss current findings related to school connectedness and its effects on education outcomes and health. As a result of the 2004 conference, the "Wingspread Declaration on School Connections" was written based on detailed research reviews and discussions among an interdisciplinary group of leaders in education. These discussions distilled key factors for school connectedness (Blum & Libbey, 2004; Wingspread, 2004). The core elements of this statement include the following.

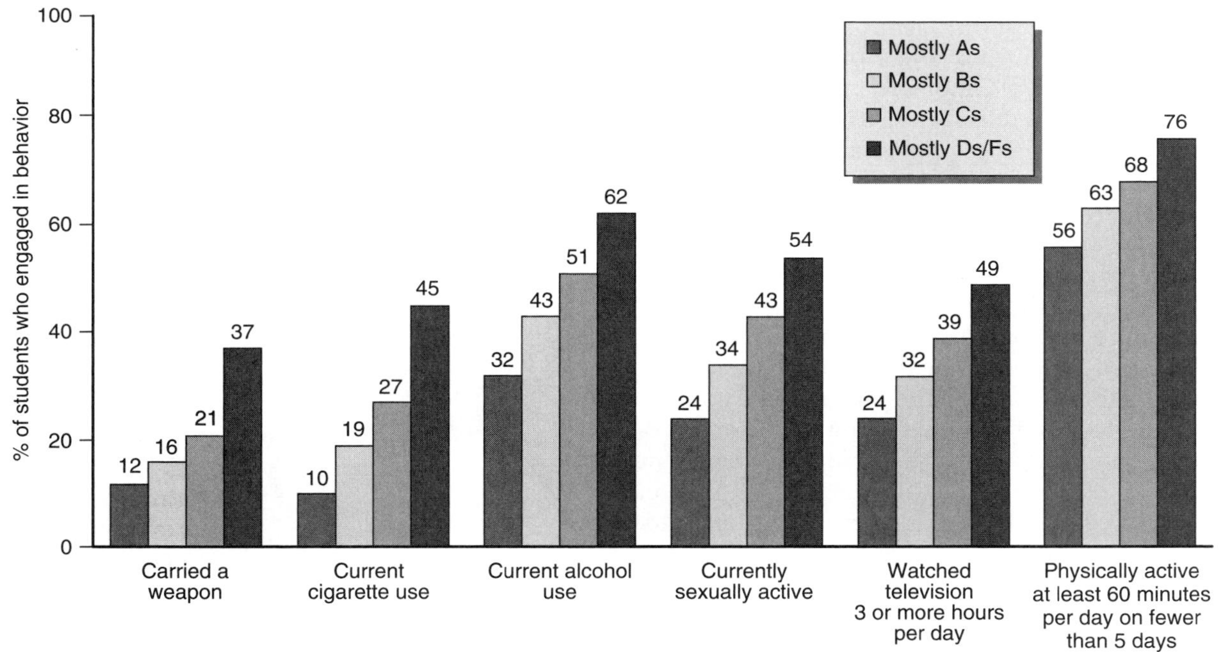

Figure 5.1 Percentage of high school students who participated in health-risk behaviors by types of grades earned.

Adapted from United States Youth Risk Behavior Survey 2009.

- Student success can be improved through strengthened bonds with school, increasing connectedness.
- Students must experience high expectations for academic success, feel supported by staff, and feel safe in their schools.
- Accountability indicators such as academic performance, fighting, truancy, and dropout rates can be influenced by school connectedness.
- Increased school connectedness is related to educational motivation, classroom engagement, and better attendance.
- School connectedness is also related to lower rates of disruptive behavior, substance and tobacco use, emotional distress, and early age of first sexual activity.

The WSCC approach, which involves families, schools, and communities and emphasizes the need for a healthy social and emotional school climate, can help build school connectedness. Regular communication and collaboration between school staff members, school counselors, and school psychologists allow professionals to provide varying levels of assistance and care needed by students. Through the coordination of existing resources and services, school staff can effectively and efficiently meet the needs of students without working outside their areas of experience and while avoiding duplication of services (CDC, 2009).

School health educators also have a role in helping students develop connectedness in schools. The National Health Education Standards (NHES) serve as a framework for curriculum, instruction, and assessment in health education. Reviews of effective health education curricula indicate that students should be given the opportunity to practice and refine key skills reflected in the NHES, such as interpersonal communication skills, refusal skills, and decision-making and conflict resolution skills, in a safe environment while providing constructive feedback for improvement (Joint Committee on National Health Education Standards, 2007). These skills are critical for building effective relationships, creating a safe social and emotional climate, and developing school connectedness (Basch, 2011; Catalano, 2004; CDC, 2009).

Safe classrooms and a positive school climate can also contribute to school connectedness. Basch (2010) recommends an assessment of school climate and school connectedness as part of a school's accountability measures. A poor school climate can dramatically affect connectedness and engagement levels and lead to absenteeism, dropping out, and subsequently poor educational and health outcomes, as illustrated in figure 5.2.

Examples of specific strategies to develop a safe school climate include planned supervision, especially during noninstructional periods (e.g., class changes, before and after school, lunch periods), intentional efforts to greet each student by name, and using physical education classes to develop collaboration skills and promote fair play and conflict resolution (Basch, 2011).

Evaluate Healthy School Community and Academic Connection

The WSCC approach emphasizes the collaboration and communication necessary between students and families, the school, and the community for the development of the whole child. An abundance of research shows the link between physical, mental, emotional, and social health and student growth and academic achievement (Basch, 2010). The Healthy School Communities (HSC) approach is an effort that began with ASCD to promote the integration of health and learning and the benefits of school–community collaboration. The foundation of HSC includes belief in the development of the whole child, best practices in leadership,

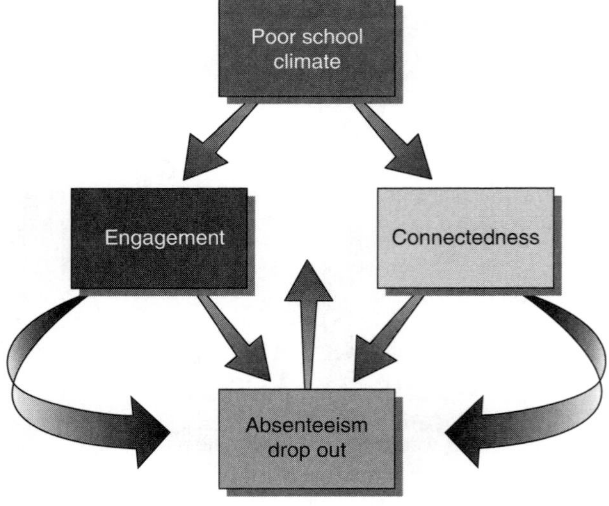

Figure 5.2 A poor school climate causes engagement and connectedness to decrease, which in turn increases absenteeism and dropping out.
Based on Catalano 2004; Klem & Connell 2004; Libbey 2004.

strong collaboration between the school and community, networking with other school communities, use of evidence-supported policies and practices, establishment of a healthy environment, and the use of data to make decisions and identify areas for improvement (ASCD, 2010). By using assessment tools such as the Healthy School Report Card (HSRC), schools can use data to make continuous WSCC improvements to ensure that schools are healthy, safe, engaging, supportive, and challenging places for all students.

Several states are reflecting the WSCC approach in their use of data for school improvement. California is an example of state and district use of continuous assessment for improvement. The California Department of Education requires all public schools to administer the California School Climate, Health, and Learning Survey every two years. These data are used to analyze links between health and wellness behaviors and academic performance. Each school receives a report card listing the results of the survey and strategies for using the results (Carr et al., 2012). The Illinois state report card is required by law to include health and wellness metrics, and the state is working toward developing health and wellness indicators for each school to report. The district report card in Chicago Public Schools indicates whether a school has achieved "Healthy School Certification," based on its progress in the HealthierUS School Challenge (Carr et al., 2012).

Healthy School Communities should be an important consideration of the overall school improvement plan for districts, and the focus of the plan should be those factors identified as the greatest needs (ASCD, 2010). National leaders and health and education experts were convened by the Healthy Schools Campaign and the Trust for America's Health to draft recommendations for improving student health and learning. One of many recommendations to the U.S. Department of Education included the development of state longitudinal health and wellness data and the integration of health and wellness into the federal School Improvement Grant program (Carr et al., 2012). One state is taking the lead in this regard. Legislative mandates in Colorado require health and wellness metrics in school improvement plans. Districts are required to analyze current data, identify needs, and outline how they plan to address those needs each academic year (Carr et al., 2012). These types of shifts in educational planning require strong leadership and professional development for administrators on best practices for promoting student health and wellness and facilitating community engagement (Carr et al., 2012).

Principal leadership in planning was determined by an ASCD Healthy School Communities pilot study as a critical catalyst for creating school change. School administrators should aim to build team leadership and ensure that all stakeholders are heard and valued. In addition to building leadership infrastructure within the school, administrators must actively seek out and access community resources to work in concert with the school to promote and sustain changes that result in healthy schools (ASCD, 2010).

Reduce Aggression and Violence and Address Mental Health Problems

Teachers of all disciplines must make efforts to monitor student behavior in classrooms, hallways, and school grounds to correct inappropriate actions that can be perceived as hurtful or disrespectful by others. Bullying, violence, and aggression in schools threaten students' academic performance, engagement, and sense of connectedness (Woods & Woke, 2004; Baker-Henningham et al., 2009; Forrest et al., 2013). Administrators, faculty, and staff, specifically school counselors, social workers, and school psychologists, must work together to identify, intervene, and prevent violent and aggressive behaviors among students. Schools can adopt and implement policies that establish a climate of high academic standards and zero tolerance for weapons on campus, harassment, bullying behaviors, and undesirable gang activity (Basch, 2011). A comprehensive health education program that helps students build skills in the areas of conflict resolution, negotiation, communication, listening, decision making, self-management, and goal setting is a logical setting for creating a culture of intolerance for violence in the school and community.

In addition to emotional and social well-being and safety, the WSCC approach focuses on mental health promotion. Professional preparation programs for educators and administrators can benefit students by emphasizing the relationship between school climate, student health, and academic achievement. These three factors are intricately linked and key to success in schools. Educators can better serve students when they know how to build relationships with students, can demonstrate a level of cultural competency in their thoughts and actions, and know how to use

School Health *in Action*

Healthier Students Are Better Learners

The October 2011 issue of the *Journal of School Health (JOSH)* is devoted to the linkage between the health of students and learning. The issue features 10 articles authored by Charles E. Basch, PhD, the Richard March Hoe Professor of Health and Education in the Department of Health and Behavior Studies at Teachers College, Columbia University. Although the focus of the articles is on the connection between seven health issues and the health of urban minority youth, the main thrust of this important document, health and learning, is relevant to all children. In the journal preface, Howell Wechsler, former director of the Division of Adolescent and School Health (DASH), CDC, describes the collection of articles by Basch as representing "the most comprehensive, authoritative, and compelling summary of why addressing health-related barriers to learning needs to be a fundamental component of school reform efforts" (p. iii).

The seven health issues, each addressed in a separate article by Basch, include (1) vision, (2) asthma, (3) teen pregnancy, (4) aggression and violence, (5) physical activity, (6) breakfast, and (7) inattention and hyperactivity. These issues were selected because of the extent to which they affect urban minority youth, the evidence of causal effects on educational outcomes, and the feasibility of addressing these issues through school-based programs. Although Basch's focus is on urban minority youth, these issues affect young people from all backgrounds.

Basch summarizes the purpose of the special issues of *JOSH* as a presentation of evidence that can provide a rationale for the importance of school health initiatives. These four points are that (1) urban minority youth are disproportionately affected by both educational and health disparities, (2) healthier students are better learners, (3) school programs and policies can favorably influence educationally relevant health disparities affecting change, and (4) now is an opportune time for change. In the closing article of the journal, Basch presents detailed recommendations that are intended to move this agenda forward.

support services to help students who are facing challenges and crises. Academic and safety concerns support the need for focused mental health resources in schools. Eisenberg, Golberstein, and Hunt (2009) identified depression among college students, independent of other factors, as a significant predictor of lower grade point average (GPA). One study measuring the effect of poor health on academic achievement found that depression could lead to a 0.45 decrease of GPA, reducing performance by at least one standard deviation (Ding et al., 2009). Depression is also associated with an increased probability of dropping out of school. Depression and anxiety are the two most common mental health conditions among adolescents. The co-occurrence of these health problems serves as a significant predictor for lower GPA (Eisenberg et al., 2009; Kessler et al., 2005). Abundant evidence supports the need for earlier identification and intervention for the students' health and future academic performance and education outcomes. Coordinated assistance from guidance counselors, school psychologists, social workers, parents, faculty, and administrators can drastically alter the personal, academic, and economic trajectory of a student suffering from a mental health problem.

Provide Health Services and School-Based Health Centers

The health problems experienced by adolescents can be complex and may require the services of multiple health providers for prevention, intervention, and crisis services. The WSCC approach promotes the coordination of the provision of health services through schools. School-based health centers (SBHCs) are intended to create access to a variety of services, especially for children and adolescents in underserved communities. SBHCs typically provide a combination of medical and preventative care and mental health services to students at school. These services are provided without consideration of a student's financial circumstances. Previous studies have documented the cost effectiveness of SBHCs, which include reducing emergency room visits, improving health outcomes, and increasing school attendance and graduation rates (Allison et al., 2007; Wade & Guo,

2010). When students can seek medical treatment or preventative services without having to leave campus, the positive effect for users and schools can be observed not only through improvements in the health and well-being of students but also in attendance rates and GPA over time (Walker et al., 2010).

Promote Family and Parental Engagement

Family engagement is a critical element of the WSCC approach. Schools cannot effectively address the learning, emotional, social, and developmental needs of students without communication and collaboration with the families of the students they serve. Studies have shown a positive relationship between **parental engagement** in a child's education and academic achievement. Students with engaged parents are more likely to earn higher grades and test scores, attend school regularly, and demonstrate positive social skills and behaviors, regardless of income or background (Henderson et al., 2002). Parental involvement at home appears to demonstrate a protective effect for children. Children are more likely to do better in school and continue their education when families demonstrate interest and involvement in their learning and progress (Henderson et al., 2002). The greater the degree of involvement by parents in all types of learning and at all levels, the greater the academic gains and benefits (Henderson & Berla, 1994; Cotton & Wikelund, 2005). The WSCC approach promotes early family engagement in the education process. Earlier involvement of parents and active involvement by parents (e.g., working with children at home on school assignments and projects, volunteering in the classroom and school building, communicating with teachers and school staff about learning progress) significantly increase the academic gains of students (Cotton & Wikelund, 2005). Programs can effectively connect with families and communities when they welcome parental involvement, listen to and address parent and community concerns, and develop trusting relationships (Henderson et al., 2002). The WSCC approach fosters respecting the needs of the family, which is of great value when connecting with parents. Examples of recognizing the needs of families include providing childcare during meetings and events at school, identifying alternative locations and times for meetings with parents outside the school building, sending educational kits and resources home with students, creating discussion groups with other families, and encouraging family members to send a representative for the family to meetings or trainings when necessary (Starkey & Klein, 2000).

Provide a Healthy Breakfast and Promote Balanced Nutritional Services

Schools and families often need to work together to provide students with one of life's most basic needs—healthy food options. The nutrition environment and services component of the WSCC approach describes a critical intersection of schools, families, and communities working together to address the nutritional needs of students, which can improve their physical, cognitive, social, and emotional well-being. A growing body of research is shedding light on the educational challenges associated with skipping breakfast. Breakfast intake enhances cognitive performance, especially with complex tasks that require extensive processing and visual learning (Rampersaud et al., 2000; Mahoney, Taylor, Kanarek, & Samuel, 2005; Widenhorn-Muller et al., 2008; Hoyland et al., 2009). Breakfast consumption also contributes to lower mental distress, depression, anxiety, and hyperactivity among adolescents (Murphy et al., 1998; Kleinman et al., 2002; Lien, 2007). Some studies suggest that eating breakfast at school results in lower incidents of student tardiness, decreased absences, improved attention and behavior, and increased math grades and test scores (Kleinman et al., 2002; Murphy, 2007; Taras, 2005). Children and adolescents skip breakfast more than they do any other meal (Rampersaud et al., 2000). When students are hungry or have not eaten a nutritious meal, they may experience difficulty concentrating and short-term memory lapse. Schools should try to serve breakfast to all students each day. Creative programs like breakfast bags at the entrance, breakfast carts to serve students in classrooms, and breakfast periods in the school day help students access the nutrients they need to focus, process, and retain new learning each day (GENYOUth Foundation, 2013).

Although breakfast isn't the only nutritional factor that affects cognitive performance and health, it is the one that is most frequently monitored and measured in the research literature because of its importance to educational

School Health *in Action*

Transformative Legislation in the District of Columbia

The District of Columbia passed transformative legislation, the Healthy Schools Act, which took effect in August of 2010, to improve student health, wellness, and academic potential. Schools are provided with financial incentives when at least one component of a reimbursable breakfast or lunch meal is composed entirely of locally grown and unprocessed foods. District-sponsored competitive grants are made available to schools that meet the physical activity requirements and seek to increase the amount of physical activity in which students engage. Local grants are also available to support school gardens.

All schools must meet or exceed the federal nutrition standards of the Child Nutrition Act of 1996 and other applicable federal laws. All meals and snacks served in school and after-school programs must meet standards geared to reducing saturated fat and sodium and eliminating trans fat. Schools must provide free breakfast to all students. Schools in which more than 40 percent of students qualify for free or reduced-priced meals must offer breakfast in the classroom at the elementary level and an alternative model such as grab-and-go carts in high traffic locations at the middle and high school levels to increase breakfast program participation. The legislation requires that schools solicit input from students, faculty, and parents through taste tests, comment boxes, surveys, and a student nutrition advisory council regarding nutritious meals that appeal to students. Food service providers must provide the menu for each meal served, the nutritional value for each menu item, and the location where fruits and vegetables served in schools are grown and processed. All beverages and snack foods sold through vending machines, as fund-raisers, and as after-school meals must meet the United State Department of Agriculture's Healthier U.S. School Challenge Gold Award Level for competitive foods. Foods and beverages that do not meet the nutritional requirements of this legislation cannot be used as incentives, prizes, or awards in schools and may not be advertised or marketed in schools.

By school year 2014–2015, students in kindergarten through grade 5 must receive at least 150 minutes of physical education per week. Students in grades 6 through 8 must participate in an average of at least 225 minutes of physical education per week, and at least 50 percent of physical education class time must be devoted to physical activity.

By the 2014–2015 school year, schools must provide at least 75 minutes of health education instruction per week to students in kindergarten through grade 8. All health and physical education will meet the curricular standards adopted by the board of education. The legislation also mandates that physical activity cannot be used or withheld as a means of punishment for students.

The school environment is also addressed in this legislation. The district is required to develop a master recycling plan, post the results of environmental testing online, use environmentally friendly cleaning supplies, develop a plan to use sustainable products in serving meals to students, and develop an environmental literacy plan that includes relevant teaching and learning standards and professional development for teachers.

Funds are dedicated to implement this legislation and to further improve health, wellness, and nutrition in D.C. public, public charter, and participating private schools.

Examples of individual schools within the district that are implementing the Healthy Schools Act through creative programs and practices can be found at http://dchealthyschools.org/healthy-schools-act-hero-awards. Schools are identified annually for the Healthy Schools Heroes Awards and recognized for their success in putting the Healthy Schools Act into action.

Based on information from the D.C. Healthy Schools Act (n.d.), http://dchealthyschools.org/.

outcomes and its availability at school sites. Fu, Cheng, Tu, and Pan (2007) examined the association between unhealthy eating patterns and unfavorable school performance in children. Poor overall school performance was positively associated with unhealthy eating patterns, which included low consumption of nutrient-dense foods and dairy products and high consumption of non-nutrient sources of food (sweets and fried foods) (Fu et al., 2007). Given that students eat two of the three traditional daily meals at school, school nutrition services can partner with school health specialists to create nutrition education programs that teach students to plan a balanced approach to meal selection that meets dietary recommendations without ignoring their personal taste preferences. Schools can empower students in their meal selections by providing a student voice in the meal planning and food options through the use of comment cards and advisory committee meetings.

Besides considering student interests and cultural influences, school districts should comply with federal standards for school breakfast, lunch, and competitive food sales. Locally grown and raised foods can promote sustainability and lower costs for schools. School and community gardens offer opportunities for parental and community involvement, nutrition education, analyzing the scientific origins and processing of foods, and healthy taste testing for students and families (Carr et al., 2012). One example of including the community in planning to address obesity through the school's nutrition services occurred in Columbus City Schools in Ohio. Leaders in Columbus City Schools brought together school and community school health champions to advance the wellness council process and develop a three-year plan to address high rates of obesity and diabetes among the district's students. The nutrition committee worked with the district's vending company to replace sugar-sweetened beverages with water in vending machines. Significant changes to the school meals menu followed, which removed high-calorie, low-nutrient value vending and à la carte items (GENYOUth Foundation, 2013).

Provide Quality Physical Education and Physical Activity

Schools can provide a healthy and inviting environment for food choices and physical activity. Physical activity in public schools has declined over the last 40 years. Administrators and school officials are keenly aware of the importance of using instructional time wisely to increase students' proficiency in academic standards. Some school administrators fear that dedicating time to nontested disciplines such as physical education may take time away from tested subject areas and subsequently lower standardized test scores used for assessment and accountability purposes. Recent research suggests a positive correlation between the amount of time spent being physically active and academic performance. Students who were more active during school and on weekends received higher standardized test scores in reading, math, and spelling. Even though time was dedicated to physical activity during instructional hours, students still earned higher test scores (Donnelly et al., 2009). Educators should recognize the benefits of physical activity and feel confident that providing opportunities like recess to students on a regular basis can benefit academic behaviors and at the same time facilitate fundamental social skills (National Association for Sport and Physical Education, 2006).

Even short bouts of physical activity can have positive effects. Improved cognition among students has been attributed to physical activity during the school day, and recent research shows that teachers observe additional positive effects on focus and memory (Hillman et al., 2009). Unexpected improvements in attention to task and task performance in preadolescent children were documented following brief bouts of exercise in school (Hillman et al., 2009; Mahar, 2011). Classroom teachers can collaborate with physical education teachers to plan integrated lessons and units, structured recess, and physical activity options before, during, and after school. Donnelly and Lambourne (2011) studied the effect of classroom activities that integrate movement and physical activity with academic lessons. These lessons did not require extensive teacher preparation, were enjoyable for the teacher and student, and resulted in improved academic achievement scores. Figure 5.3 presents a summary of five programs designed to provide classroom physical activity breaks and the effect of each program.

Schools can promote learning and help students develop skills and behaviors that have a lasting effect. The WSCC approach can contribute to increased physical activity and healthy diets for students that are positively associated with children's weight, health outcomes, and fewer academic and behavior problems at school (Shi, 2013, 5). Figure 5.4 highlights improved academic performance as a result of healthy eating and physical activity as recommended by the CDC. More information can be found at cdc.gov and genyouthfoundation.org.

SUMMARY

A mission shared by most schools is to help teachers prepare students so that they can be successful and productive citizens in the world in which they live. Collectively, the evolving body of literature supporting the academic benefits of health promotion can be used to encourage

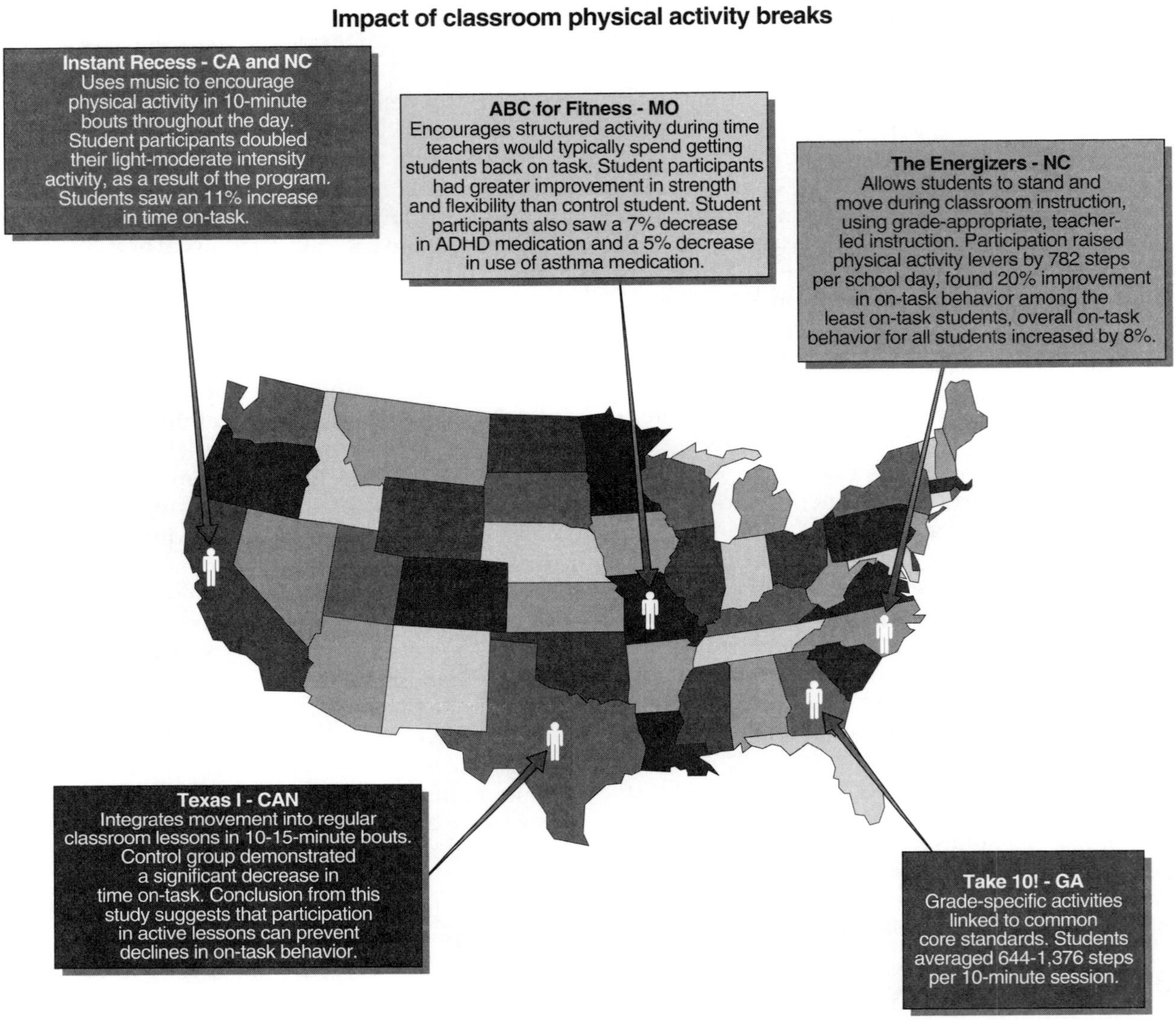

Impact of classroom physical activity breaks

Instant Recess - CA and NC
Uses music to encourage physical activity in 10-minute bouts throughout the day. Student participants doubled their light-moderate intensity activity, as a result of the program. Students saw an 11% increase in time on-task.

ABC for Fitness - MO
Encourages structured activity during time teachers would typically spend getting students back on task. Student participants had greater improvement in strength and flexibility than control student. Student participants also saw a 7% decrease in ADHD medication and a 5% decrease in use of asthma medication.

The Energizers - NC
Allows students to stand and move during classroom instruction, using grade-appropriate, teacher-led instruction. Participation raised physical activity levers by 782 steps per school day, found 20% improvement in on-task behavior among the least on-task students, overall on-task behavior for all students increased by 8%.

Texas I - CAN
Integrates movement into regular classroom lessons in 10-15-minute bouts. Control group demonstrated a significant decrease in time on-task. Conclusion from this study suggests that participation in active lessons can prevent declines in on-task behavior.

Take 10! - GA
Grade-specific activities linked to common core standards. Students averaged 644-1,376 steps per 10-minute session.

Figure 5.3 Effect of classroom physical activity breaks.
Based on Whitt-Glover et al. 2013.

the coordination of school health programs through WSCC. With careful attention to school climate and strategies to create connectedness for students and their families, schools can improve educational outcomes for their students. Administrators and policy makers must focus on health and education outcomes through all grade levels beginning in early childhood. Schools can provide mental, emotional, and physical health education and services; daily opportunities for a balanced and accessible breakfast and food choices; and physical activity through time dedicated to physical education and planned integration of physical activity into the school day. The coordination of these programs and services can benefit students' academic performance, attention to task, cognition, and education and economic outcomes. By coordinating efforts to promote the health and well-being of students, schools and communities are investing in a better future for all.

Glossary

academic achievement—Often considered the outcome of an educational endeavor

Healthy Students Are Better Learners

Healthy eating and engaging in physical activity leads to improved academic performance.

Students who regularly eat breakfast

- earn better grades and higher standardized test scores,
- miss fewer days of school, and
- demonstrate higher levels of concentration and memory.

Students who skip breakfast

- exhibit poor memory and inattentiveness and
- miss more school than students who usually eat breakfast.

Students who are physically active (e.g., during physical education, recess, or classroom-based activities) often

- experience improved academic performances, concentration, and attention;
- have fewer disciplinary problems; and
- are less likely to drop out of school.

Because children and youth spend a majority of the time in school, schools can have a positive impact on the foods they eat and the quality and quantity of physical activity they engage in.

Figure 5.4 The effects of healthy eating and physical activity on students and learning.

(the end of a K–12 education). The extent to which students, teachers, or institutions have achieved their educational goals. Academic achievement is commonly measured by examinations or continuous assessment.

education outcomes—The goals for learning, which can be defined as the knowledge, skills, attitudes, and values that students will need to be successful in work, family, and community. They are what students should know, understand, and be able to do to be an educated person and meet the demands that the future will place on them.

health—The World Health Organization (WHO) defined health as a state of complete physical, mental, and social well-being, not merely the absence of disease or infirmity. The definition of health can also be the physical, mental, and social wellness or a condition of well-being.

health assets—Qualities and characteristics of value or importance to a person's health.

health outcomes—A change in the health status of an individual, group, or population that is attributable to a planned program or intervention, regardless of whether such an intervention was intended to change health status.

Health-risk behavior—An action by an individual that increases the likelihood of diminishment of health status or safety.

parental engagement—Parents and school staff working together to support and improve the learning, development, and health of children and adolescents.

school connectedness—The belief held by students that adults and peers in the school care about their learning as well as about them as individuals.

Application Activities

1. You are responsible for developing a presentation to the local school board meeting on improving academic performance. The board has invited education professionals from various disciplines to address this topic. Your 20-minute presentation should focus on the relationship of students' health to academic success. You should also include in your presentation the role that WSCC can play as a method for promoting academic success. Develop a detailed outline for your presentation.
2. Either through individual discussions or in several small-group discussions, ask other college students to describe a time when their physical, mental, or emotional health affected their academic performance or the academic performance of a friend or family member. As part of the discussion ask them to provide recommendations for how schools can help promote health and academic success. Based on these discussions, write a paper that includes a summary of selected experiences described in the discussion, their recommendations, and your overall reaction to your findings from the discussions.
3. A principal was reassigned to a local middle school, which was recently identified as a low-performing, high-priority school. The principal examined data collected by the school and the district and observed high absentee rates among the student population, poor scores on state achievement tests, and high incidences of reported violent acts in school. A brief focus group with teachers, students, and parents indicated a poor overall climate at the school. The principal had used WSCC strategies with success in previous schools and decided to focus on building a safe and supportive social, emotional, and physical environment within the school and expanding students' opportunities to enhance their personal health during the next academic year. After announcing these priorities, the principal received negative feedback from teachers and parents who were concerned about other pressing issues that need to be addressed. Analyze the Whole Child snapshot for your state using the ASCD website, www.ascd.org/programs/whole-child-snapshots.aspx, and use these data and the challenges of the school (described earlier) to justify the proposal of using a WSCC approach. Include an emphasis on the connection between health and academic success in your justification.

Resources

American Public Health Association. The Center for School, Health, and Education. www.school-basedhealthcare.org

American School Health Association. 2010. *What School Administrators Can Do to Enhance Student Learning by Supporting a Coordinated Approach to Health.* www.ashaweb.org/files/public/miscellaneous/administrators_coordinated_approach_support.pdf

Basch, Charles E. 2011. Healthier Students are Better Learners: High Quality, Strategically Planned, and Effectively Coordinated School Health Programs Must Be a Fundamental Mission of Schools to Help Close the Achievement Gap. *Journal of School Health, 81*(10), 650–662.

California Healthy Kids Resource Center. n.d. *Health and Academic Achievement.* www.californiahealthykids.org/health_and_academic_achievement

Centers for Disease Control and Prevention. 2011. *Health and Academics.* www.cdc.gov/healthyyouth/health_and_academics/index.htm

Centers for Disease Control and Prevention. 2009. *School Connectedness: Strategies for Increasing Protective Factors Among Youth.* Atlanta, GA: U.S. Department of Health and Human Services. www.cdc.gov/healthyyouth/adolescenthealth/pdf/connectedness.pdf

Centers for Disease Control and Prevention. 2010. *The Association Between School Based Physical Activity, Including Physical Education, and Academic Performance.* Atlanta, GA: U.S. Department of Health and Human Services.

Children's Action Alliance. 2012. *Weighing In: Practical Steps Schools Can Take to Improve Student Health and Academic Success.* www.azchildren.org/MyFiles/12Pub/Weighing_In.pdf

Dilley, Julia. 2009. *Research Review: School-Based Health Interventions and Academic Achievement.* Olympia, WA: Washington State Board of Health, Washington State Office of Superintendent of Public Instruction, Washington State Department of Health.

GENYOUth Foundation. 2013. *The Wellness Impact: Enhancing Academic Success Through Health Schools.* www.genyouthfoundation.org/wp-content/uploads/2013/02/The_Wellness_Impact_Report.pdf

Healthy Schools Campaign and Trust for America's Health. 2012. *Health in Mind: Improving Education Through Wellness.* http://healthyschoolscampaign.org/programs/health-in-mind/

References

ASCD. 2010. *Learning, Teaching, and Leading in Healthy School Communities.* The ASCD Whole Child Initiative.

Arendt, Jacob Nielsen. 2005. Does Education Cause Better Health? A Panel Data Analysis Using School Reforms for Identification. *Economics of Education Review, 24*(2), 149–160.

Allison, Mandy A., Crane, Lori A., Beaty, Brenda L., Davidson, Arthur J., Melinkovich, Paul, & Kempe, Allison. 2007. School-Based Health Centers: Improving Access and Quality of Care for Low-Income Adolescents. *Pediatrics, 120*(4), e887–e894.

Baker-Henningham, Helen, Meeks-Gardner, Julie, Chang, Susan, & Walker, Susan. 2009. Experiences of Violence and Deficits in Academic Achievement Among Urban Primary School Children in Jamaica. *Child Abuse & Neglect, 22*, 296–306.

Basch, Charles E. 2010. Healthier Students Are Better Learners: A Missing Link in School Reforms to Close the Achievement Gap. *Equity Matters: Research Reviews*, No. 6.

Basch, Charles E. 2011. Aggression and Violence and the Achievement Gap Among Urban Minority Youth. *Journal of School Health, 18*(10): 619–625.

Basch, Charles E. 2011. Breakfast and the Achievement Gap Among Urban Minority Youth. *Journal of School Health, 18*(10), 635–640.

Basch, Charles E. 2011. Executive Summary: Healthier Students Are Better Learners. *Journal of School Health, 81*(10), 591–592.

Blum, Robert, & Libbey, Heather P. 2004. Executive Summary: Healthier Students are Better Learners. *Journal of School Health, 74*(7), 231–232.

Bond, Lyndal, Butler, Helen, Thomas, Lyndal, Carlin, John, Glover, Sara, Bowes, Geen, & Patton, George. 2007. Social and School Connectedness in Early Secondary School as Predictors of Late Teenage Substance Use, Mental Health, and Academic Outcomes. *Journal of Adolescent Health, 40*, 357e9–357e18.

Carr, Dana, Schaible, Alex, & Thomas, Kadesha. 2012. *Health in Mind: Improving Education Through Wellness.* Chicago: Healthy Schools Campaign and Trust for America's Health.

Case, Anne, Fertig, Angela, & Paxson, Christina. 2005. The Lasting Impact of Childhood Health and Circumstance. *Journal of Health Economics, 24*, 365–389.

Catalono, Richard F., Haggerty, Kevin P., Oesterle, Sabrina, Fleming, Charles B., & Hawkings, David. 2004. The Importance of Bonding to School for Healthy Development: Findings from the Social Development Research Group. *Journal of School Health, 74*(7), 252–261.

Centers for Disease Control and Prevention. 2009. *Health-Risk Behaviors and Academic Achievement. Youth Risk Behavior Survey.* www.cdc.gov/HealthyYouth/health_and_academics/pdf/health_risk_behaviors.pdf

Centers for Disease Control and Prevention. 2012. *MMWR Youth Risk Behavior Surveillance—United States 2011.* www.cdc.gov/mmwr/pdf/ss/ss6104.pdf

Cotton, Kathleen, & Wikelund, Karen Reed. 2005. Parent Involvement in Education. *School Improvement Research Series, 6*, 1–15.

D.C. Healthy Schools Act. n.d. http://dchealthyschools.org

Ding, Weili, Lehrer, Steven F., Rosenquist, J.Niels, & Audrain-McGovern, Janet. 2009. The Impact of Poor Health on Academic Performance: New Evidence Using Genetic Markers. *Journal of Health Economics, 28*, 578–597.

Donnelly, Joseph, Gibson, C.A., Smith, B.K., Washburn, R.A., Sullivan, D.K., Dubose, K., Mayo, M.S., Schmelzle, K.H., Ryan, J.J., Jacobsen, D.J., & Williams, S.L. 2009. Physical Activity Across the Curriculum (PAAC): A Randomized Controlled Trial to Promote Physical Activity and Diminish Overweight and Obesity in Elementary School Children. *Preventative Medicine, 49*(4), 336–341.

Donnelly, Joseph, & Lambourne, Kate. 2011. Classroom-Based Physical Activity, Cognition, and Academic Achievement. *Preventative Medicine, 52*, S36–S42.

Eisenburg, Daniel, Golbertstein, Ezra, & Hunt, Justin B. 2009. Mental Health and Academic Success in College. *B.E. Journal of Economic Analysis & Policy, 9*(1), 1–27.

Forrest, Christopher B., Bevans, Katherine B., Riley, Anne W., Crespo, Richard, & Louis, Thomas A. 2013. Health and School Outcomes During Children's Transition Into Adolescence. *Journal of Adolescent Health, 50*, 186–194.

Fu, Ming-Ling, Cheng, Lieyueh, Tu, Su-Hao, & Pan, Wen-Harn. 2007. Association Between Unhealthful Eating Patterns and Unfavorable Overall School Performance. *Journal of American Dietetic Association*, *107*(11), 1935–1943.

GENYOUth Foundation. 2013. *The Wellness Impact: Enhancing Academic Success Through Healthy School Environments*. www.nationaldairycouncil.org/ChildNutrition/Documents/Wellness%20 Impact%20Report.pdf

Henderson, Anne T., & Berla, Nancy. 1994. *A New Generation of Evidence: The Family Is Critical to Student Achievement* (pp. 1–160). Washington, DC: Center for Law and Education.

Henderson, Anne T., Mapp, Karen, Jordan, Catherine, Orozco, Evangelina, Averett, Amy, Donnelly, Deborah, Buttram, John L., Wood, Lacy, Fowler, Marilyn, & Myers, Margaret. 2002. *A New Wave of Evidence: The Impact of School, Family, and Community Connections on Student Achievement* (pp. 1–244). SEDL Advancing Research Improving Education.

Hillman, Charles H., Pontifex, Mathew B., Raine, Lauren B., Castelli, Darla M., Hall, Eric E., & Kramer, Arthur F. 2009. The Effect of Acute Treadmill Walking on Cognitive Control and Academic Achievement in Preadolescent Children. *Neuroscience*, *3*, 1044–1054.

Hoyland, Alexa, Dye, Louise, & Lawton, Clare L. 2009. A Systematic Review of the Effect of Breakfast on the Cognitive Performance of Children and Adolescents. *Nutritional Research Reviews*, *22*, 220–243.

Joint Committee on National Health Education Standards. 2007. *National Health Education Standards: Achieving Excellent* (2nd ed.). Atlanta, GA: American Cancer Society.

Kessler, Ronald C., Berglund, Patricia, Demler, Olga, Jin, Robert, & Waters, Ellen E. 2005. Lifetime Prevalence of Onset Distributions of DSM-IV Disorders in the National Comorbity Survey Replication. *Archives of General Psychiatry*, *62*(6), 593–627.

Kleinman, Ronald, Green, H., Korzec-Ramirez, D., Patton, K., Pagano, M.E., & Murphy, J.M. 2002. Diet, Breakfast, and Academic Performance in Children. *Annals of Nutrition and Metabolism*, *46*(suppl 1), 24–30.

Klem, Adena M., & Connell, James P. 2004. Relationships Matter: Linking Teacher Support to Student Engagement and Achievement. *Journal of School Health*, *74*(7), 262–273.

Libbey, Heather P. 2004 Measuring Student Relationships to School: Attachment, Bonding, Connectedness, and Engagement. *Journal of School Health*, *74*(7), 274–283.

Lien, Lars. 2007. Is Breakfast Consumption Related to Mental Distress and Academic Performance in Adolescents? *Public Health Nutrition*, *10*(4), 422–428.

Mahar, Matthew T. 2011. Impact of Short Bouts of Physical Activity on Attention-to-Task in Elementary School Children. *Preventative Medicine*, *52*(Suppl 1), S60–S64.

Mahoney, Carolina R., Taylor, Holly A., Kanarek, Robin B., & Samuel, Priscilla. 2005. Effect of Breakfast Composition on Cognitive Processes in Elementary School Children. *Physiology and Behavior*, *85*, 635–645.

Murphy, J. Michael., Pagano, Maria E., Nachmani, Joan, Sperling, Peter, Lane, Shirley, & Kleinman, Ronaled E. 1998. The Relationship of School Breakfast to Psychosocial and Academic Functioning: Cross-Sectional and Longitudinal Observations in an Inner-City School Sample. *Archives of Pediatric & Adolescent Medicine*, *152*(9), 899–907.

Murphy, J. Michael. 2007. Breakfast and Learning: An Updated Review. *Current Nutrition and Food Science*, *3*, 3–36.

National Association for Sport and Physical Education. 2006. *Recess for Elementary School Students* [position paper]. Reston, VA.

Novello, Antonia C., Degraw, Christopher, & Kleinman, Dushanka V. 1992. Healthy Children Ready to Learn: An Essential Collaboration Between Health and Education. *Public Health Reports*, *107*(1), 3–15.

Rampersaud, Gail C., Pereira, Mark A., Girard, Beverly L., Adams, Judi, & Metzl, Jordan D. 2000. Breakfast Habits, Nutritional Status, Body Weight, and Academic Performance in Children and Adolescents. *Journal of the American Dietetic Association*, *105*(5), 743–760.

Shi, Xiangrong, Tubb, Larry, Fingers, Sheryl, Chen, Shande, & Caffrey, James L. 2013. Associations of Physical Activity and Dietary Behaviors With Children's Health and Academic Problems. *Journal of School Health*, *83*(1), 1–7.

Spernak, Stephanie M., Schottenbauer, Michele A., Ramey, Sharon L., & Ramey, Craig T. 2006. Child Health and Academic Achievement Among Former Head Start Children. *Children and Youth Services Review*, *28*, 1251–1261.

Starkey, Prentice, & Klein, Alice. 2000. Fostering Parental Support for Children's Mathematical Development: An Intervention with Head Start Families. *Early Education and Development*, *11*(5), 659–680.

Taras, Howard. 2005. Nutrition and Student Performance at School. *Journal of School Health*, *76*(6), 199–213.

United Health Foundation. 2013. *America's Health Rankings: 2013 Senior Health Disparities*. www.americashealthrankings.org/senior/all/2013.

Wade, Terrance J., & Guo, Jeff Jianfei. 2010. Linking Improvements in Health-Related Quality of Life to Reductions in Medicaid Costs Among Students Who Use School-Based Health Centers. *American Journal of Public Health*, *100*(9), 1611–1616.

Walker, Sarah Cusworth, Kerns, Suzanne E.U., Lyons, Aaron R., Bruns, Eric J., & Cosgove, T.J. 2010. Impact of School-Based Health Center Use on Academic Outcomes. *Journal of Adolescent School Health*, *46*, 251–257.

Wechsler, Howell. 2011.Preface. *Journal of School Health*, *81*(10), iii–v.

Whitt-Glover, Melicia C., Porter, Amber T., Yancey, Toni K., Alexander, Ramine C., & Creecy, Jeskell M. 2013. Do Short Physical Activity Breaks in Classrooms Work? *Active Living Research Brief.* Robert Wood Johnson Foundation.

Widenhorn-Muller, Katharina, Hille, Katrin, Klenk, Jochen, Weiland, Ulrike. 2008. Influence of Having Breakfast on Cognitive Performance and Mood in 13- to 20-Year-Old High School Students: Results of a Crossover Trial. *Pediatrics*, *122*(2), 279–284.

Wingspread Declaration on School Connections. 2004. *Journal of School Health*, *47*(7), 233–234.

Woolf, Steven H., Johnson, Robert E., Phillips, Robert L., & Philipsen, Maike. 2007. Giving Everyone the Health of the Educated: An Examination of Whether Social Change Would Save More Lives Than Medical Advances. *American Journal of Public Health*, *97*(4), 679–683.

Woods, Sarah, & Wolke, Dieter. 2004. Direct and Relational Bullying Among Primary School Children and Academic Achievement. *Journal of School Psychology*, *42*, 135–155.

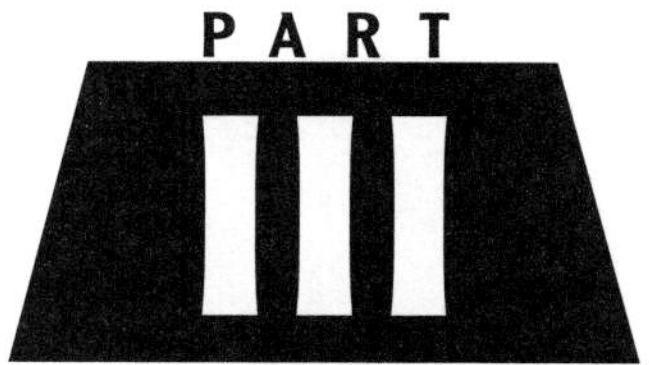

Building Partnerships and Support

6

Role of School Administration

JEREMY LYON

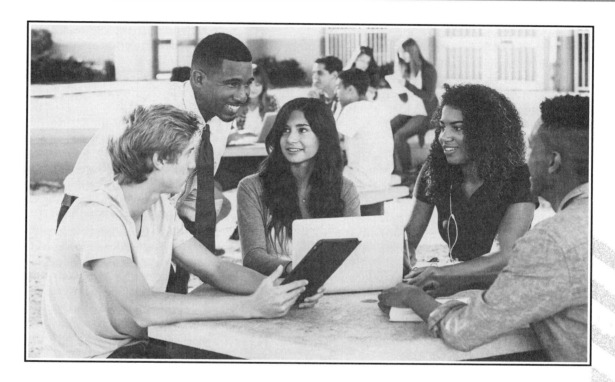

School administrators are empowered, by the nature of their positions, with the opportunity to transform schools and school districts into places where healthy and active children learn that lifestyle habits are important for positive health throughout life (Valois, 2011). The role of the school administrator is perfectly designed to implement Whole School, Whole Community, Whole Child (WSCC) strategies, to cheerlead and encourage healthy lifestyles, to build partnerships for improving student and staff health, and to advocate for practices that exemplify healthy living. An ASCD evaluation of school programs found that when a principal serves as a school health leader, a shift occurs in the school climate to focus more on promoting health. Having an administrator lead, not just support, school health promotion can be a strong catalyst of change for a school or district (Valois, 2011).

School administrators, armed with a job description and leadership role, often have little understanding of the connections between student and staff health and wellness, academic success, productivity, and happiness in life. The Whole Child Initiative launched by ASCD is an attempt to move away from that narrowly defined view to a broader understanding of what children need to be successful. The Whole Child approach supports children by ensuring that they are healthy, safe, engaged, supported, and challenged (ASCD, *The Whole Child*, 2013).

WSCC implementation offers the best pathway toward creating a change in the school culture, and administrators have the greatest authority with schools and districts to activate staff members, students, parents, and community members. Health experts have suggested that our children will live shorter life spans than those that we enjoy (Committee, 2009; Olshansky et al., 2005; Roger et al., 2013). We can make no stronger statement of our collective failure to our children. This chapter identifies specific leadership skills and behaviors of school administrators essential to WSCC implementation as well as actions, both small (single outcomes) and large (systemic changes), that result in improved health and wellness outcomes for students and staff.

NEED FOR SCHOOL HEALTH PROMOTION

On a fall morning a few years ago, before I launched into another busy day as a school superintendent, I read an article in our local newspaper that stopped me short. The headline and subtitle read, "Diabetes cases projected to soar in Texas: Diagnoses to rise by 259 percent to 8 million adults across the state." The first line of the article stated, "About 8 million adult Texans, or 24 percent of the population, will be diagnosed with diabetes by 2040" (Eaton, 2010, para. 1). What struck me was that here I was, about to go spend another day working in the trenches of public education, with other dedicated and talented educators, all working hard to improve student academic achievement. In our district, we were immersed in the work of how to align the curriculum, how to use student data most effectively to improve and modify instruction, and what targeted instructional intervention actions and programs would yield the greatest student achievement results. I was like many other school superintendents, central office administrators, campus principals, assistant principals, and teachers working in our high-stakes accountability environment. We all share a strong desire (and work hard) to help children be more successful.

Yet here was a headline that predicted a societal train wreck of severely unhealthy people that is to happen directly on our watch as torchbearers for the next generation. And that is what stopped me short. We say that we are preparing tomorrow's future today in our schools or a similar slogan indicating that schools embrace their responsibility to children. We say that we love children and are building a future for them. But nurturing and developing the intellectual abilities of children is difficult if they are not healthy. We face the glaring statistic that the life expectancy of America's children is predicted to be less than the life expectancy of their parents (Committee, 2009; Olshansky et al., 2005; Roger et al., 2013). Cultivating a college-ready graduate capable of thinking creatively and critically, ready to self-actualize and contribute to our economy and democracy is difficult when the young person is physiologically or psychologically impaired (Basch, 2010). For students to thrive academically, physical fitness, a nutritious diet, and mental health must play a role (CDC, n.d.b).

For the school administrator skeptical of this kind of thinking, consider the blossoming research linking physical activity, a nutritious diet, and psychologically healthy students to student achievement. The research connecting physically active students with positive academic achievement is coming into focus. In 2010 the U.S. Department of Health and Human Services conducted a **meta-analysis** of 50 studies related to the association between school-based physical activity and academic performance and found that 50.5 percent of the studies yielded positive gains, 48 percent yielded no gains, and 1.5 percent had a negative effect on academic performance (CDC, 2010). The majority of positive associations were made in studies related to increasing physical activity in classrooms (8 out of 9 studies) and participation in extracurricular physical activities (19 out of 19 studies). And if the research on student academic achievement related to exercise is positive, think about the potential positive outcomes related to teacher performance (CDC, 2010).

When an athlete goes into a competition with an injury, sports announcers invariably elaborate on the nature of the injury and predict the degree of impairment that the athlete will exhibit. Imagine that approach in schools: "Well, Chuck, our third-grader, Daniel, is tired and cranky this morning because he has had no physical exercise and he skipped breakfast. We'll see whether Mrs. Rodriguez can somehow get productivity out of Daniel on the vocabulary test, but with Daniel less than 100 percent, he'll have a hard time with anything polysyllabic." If our students are not physically and mentally healthy, all the applied genius and hard work of improving curriculum and instruction will ultimately fall short.

We are failing our mission as educators unless we commit to getting our children healthy, first and foremost. It was this moment of stark realization regarding my failure as an educational leader to create school environments that result in healthy children that changed the way I look at a leader's role in education. An array of research, sociological findings, and observations has huge implications for school systems. The news about the health of America is alarming, whether we are talking about the adult population or children in particular. The decline of the physical health of Americans since the 1980s is staggering. Yet right next to all the reports about our collective lack of physical activity and poor eating habits is a body of research that is equally staggering in positive promise. This research describes the benefits of physical activity and healthy eating on varied aspects of emotional, intellectual, and physical health. In addition, research supports the importance of a school climate that focuses on relationships with students and the reduction of bullying on students' mental health and self-esteem (CDC, 2010).

SCHOOL ADMINISTRATORS AS ADVOCATES FOR WSCC

School administrators do not need to be health promotion experts. Content-area training in health services, health education, physical education, nutrition, and counseling are not necessary to lead planning, implementation, and evaluation efforts. School administrators are viewed as having authority to allocate resources and support key decisions by their staff, students, and parents. Students and adults expect school administrators to be effective communicators and to represent their interests. Trust is developed quickly when an administrator is able to communicate a vision that resonates with internal and external constituents and yields a positive climate within the school or school district. No single model can describe every effective school administrator, but all administrators must be able to convey a vision, best built collaboratively, and apply it in a manner that builds a positive school climate and culture. Within this construct of effective leadership, school administrators have regular opportunities to begin communicating the importance of health and wellness (American School Health Association, 2010). The simple act of infusing health and wellness advocacy into hallway conversations, during speeches and assemblies, within daily announcements, on school marquees, at staff meetings, during parent and PTA meetings, at board meetings and public forums, and at Rotary and Chamber of Commerce events all serve as reinforcement that allows the larger components of WSCC to come into focus (CDC, n.d.a).

When school administrators regularly verbalize and write about the importance of health and wellness, two remarkable things happen simultaneously:

- **Students, staff, and parents begin to view the school administrator as a friendly and positive leader**. When stakeholders see and hear a school administrator verbalizing and expressing an interest in their well-being, it resonates differently than any other function of school administration. This message is personal and helps to present school administrators in a positive light. When a school administrator expresses a commitment to health and wellness and expresses a genuine interest in helping create schools that are healthy places, the paradigm of the school administrator as authoritarian disappears. And the authoritarian paradigm disappears most quickly with students, who are full of wonderfully creative ideas about improving health and wellness in schools if we take the opportunity to listen to them.
- **The school administrator becomes the collecting point where all ideas, big and small, about health begin to reside**. Students, staff, parents, and community partners all begin to view a school administrator who advocates for healthy schools as a sounding board for personal stories, positive ideas, promising practices, new research, and endless community opportunities pertaining to elements of school health promotion. Children and adults, particularly those who have previously separated school from their private values regarding health, see a school administrator who is inviting them to express and implement health values into the educational environment. This viewpoint is powerful because it quickly brings into the forefront a core group of health and wellness champions eager to make a difference.

Having students, staff, and parents who view the school leader as enthusiastic and supportive of health presents a key starting point for WSCC planning. Note that Hodges and Angermeier, in chapter 8, emphasize that visible administrative leadership can be an important factor in school–community collaboration related to WSCC.

Administrative support is also more relevant considering the value and link to academics. The American School Health Association (2010) states that the school administrator needs to take time to communicate and promote the link found in the research between academics and health. Basch (2013), in focusing on the connection between health and academic success, recommended that "leaders communicate clearly and powerfully that school health programs are an essential component of school reform" (p. 655).

EMBRACING THE LEADERSHIP ROLE IN WSCC

School administrators who embrace their leadership role in health and wellness begin to see the opportunities to connect the 10 components of WSCC. This awareness is a threshold event for school administrators. It requires abandonment of a mental model of school administration as managing discreet organizational boxes representing departments by function and adopting an organic and free-flowing mental construction of schools as holistic, unified experiences for students, staff, and parents. Examples of this deep shift in thinking are abundant. For example, serving breakfast in classrooms, implementing physical activity into core instruction, having students engage in physical activity before taking standardized state tests, guiding students to create personal health plans, having snack carts in hallways bring nutritious foods to high school students during class passing times, buying standing desks for staff, and encouraging physical movement during planning periods are examples of taking functions previously isolated by department and blending them together into a systemwide approach.

PROMOTING CHANGE

School administrators who begin to advocate for improved health and wellness within schools and who are able to see the connections of components of WSCC as beneficial to academic performance must confront one more thing—their own personal health and wellness (Directors of Health Promotion and Education, 2007). They do not need to become fitness fanatics and try for a spot on an Olympic team. If that is the outcome, more power to that school administrator, but most of us are just trying to be the best we can be with what we were given. But trying to be our best means that we need to demonstrate positive role-modeling for our students —that improvement is gradual,

School Health *in Action*

Administrative Leadership in CSH

The following two model initiatives showcase efforts made by administrators to address some aspect of the WSCC approach by making physical changes in the school.

Physical education and physical activity: This initiative involved a Texas superintendent who started a daily physical education pilot program at an elementary school by converting an unused classroom into a fitness room. This modification allowed the school to eliminate the logistical barrier of limited gymnasium space and efficiently rotate children through the fitness room throughout the day using existing staff. By demonstrating that it could work, the pilot program inspired other elementary schools to adopt the same strategies.

Counseling, psychological, and social services: This effort involved the creative use of facilities by a principal in upstate New York. The principal changed the physical environment by moving the school social worker and school psychologist into offices in the main office suite. This change sent a message to the staff and community regarding how strongly the administration valued the mental and emotional health of the students. In addition, the change increased the interactions and discussions between administration and the psychologist and social worker, resulting in a stronger sense of shared purpose and support.

and healthy habits don't emerge overnight. School administrators are responsible for creating conditions of trust and respect, for both students and staff. We cannot guilt anyone into better behavior regarding diet and exercise.

Todd Whitthorne of the Cooper Institute explains that the key is to recognize when a person is ready for change and improvement, take some small first steps ("floss just one tooth!" he likes to say), and shape those small steps into habits of personal fitness and wellness. That applies to all of us, beginning with school leadership. For students, apples can't replace cupcakes overnight, and nothing is more sensitive to all of us than comments or observations about our bodies. School administrators must work steadfastly at encouragement and positive reinforcement while having the utmost respect for people's feelings and phobias. When a school administrator successfully nudges a climate of respect and trust forward, students and staff have a chance to thrive. With a spirit of trust and respect, remarkable things are possible. When a school administrator successfully creates an environment of trust and encouragement for improving everyone's health and wellness, personal stories of triumph start to be told. When we begin to share these individual stories of people breaking through past barriers and challenges by accomplishing such feats as completing a structured walk or road race, losing significant weight for the first time in their adult lives, and quitting smoking, we are hearing stories of deep emotional meaning from people we work beside every day. Sharing these stories (with their permission, of course) through faculty meetings, newsletters, and pictures is powerful evidence of trust and camaraderie. When we encourage people to try to be healthier, in a manner that does not reinforce the guilt of our shortcomings, these stories add to the celebration of health and wellness (Directors of Health Promotion and Education, 2007).

SCHOOLS AS CENTERS FOR EMPLOYEE WELLNESS

One of the unintended consequences (among many) of high-stakes testing in America's public schools is the physical and emotional stress that our current system is inflicting on our teachers. Principals often report that teachers come to them in desperation after struggling to keep pace with overwhelming curriculum expectations and unrealistic pressure from parents. The stress of trying to cope with all the job-related demands may cause teachers to compromise their family and social lives. Because teachers often attempt to solve every challenge by simply working harder, we are at a point where many of our most talented teachers, who chose teaching over higher-paying private jobs, are calling it quits because they are compromising their internal standards of excellence. When school administrators are not acutely sensitive to understanding the forces negatively affecting teachers' professional lives, they are asking for low morale, poor staff attendance, and a climate of unhappiness. But schools can become centers of health promotion for teachers and staff members (Directors of Health, 2007).

Teachers who are in poor health or who have family members in poor health will tend to miss work and, like their students, have difficulty with concentration. Health promotion for faculty and staff has shown to increase healthy behaviors, decrease the number of days absent from work, and promote increased ability to concentrate at work. In addition, healthy staff can be good role models for their students (Dilly, 2011). The good news is that between 2000 and 2012, the percentage of school districts that have someone who oversees or coordinates health promotion activities or services for faculty and staff throughout the district increased from 28.2 percent to 40.1 percent. Despite these increases, findings indicate that additional support for faculty and staff health promotion is needed if real advances are to be made (CDC, 2013).

Administrators can provide opportunities for school personnel to engage in those healthy behaviors through a number of avenues. Supporting a healthy worksite might include the following recommendations from the American School Health Association (2010):

- Provide access to school fitness facilities and equipment
- Provide time for physical activity, health education, and other health-related services during staff development days
- Give recognition for participation in individual health risk assessment and health promotion activities
- Consider including a personal health objective as part of professional development plans

IDENTIFYING HEALTH CHAMPIONS

The next step for school administrators is to create the capacity for change by identifying health champions who exist in all schools and districts. Every school and school district has some staff members, parents, and students who get the big picture of CSH but have no outlet for their ideas and actions. Typically, they concentrate their efforts on themselves, their families, or the students they teach, but they see no pathway for having a greater influence, even though they are enthusiastically willing when asked. Everyone applauds their efforts, but those efforts are not systematic or sustainable beyond the individual's tenure. This circumstance can change if we recognize and empower our school, district, and community health and wellness champions.

The first task is to identify those champions. This undertaking can be done simply by calling a voluntary meeting at a school or the district office to invite those interested in health and wellness to have a conversation. By holding these conversational meetings a couple of times over the course of a fall or spring semester, a cadre of champions will soon be identified. Most districts have a formal student health advisory group, sometimes created by legislative mandate. This group of student champions needs to be activated and empowered. Formally activating champions, through an existing or new health council or team, is a start to having focused conversations about conditions and opportunities within a school or district for introducing WSCC efforts.

IDENTIFYING A LEADER

Whenever possible, at the district level, the pathway to successful implementation of WSCC may require a single critical act that costs money. If possible, a paid health coordinator position should be created. Successful implementation of WSCC in a school district requires that someone be hired to champion the effort. The creation of a position so that one person has authority to oversee and manage school health promotion efforts is supported in the American School Health Association document *What School Administrators Can Do to Enhance Student Learning by Supporting a Coordinated Approach to Health* (2010). CDC states that to achieve the goals of school health, identification of either a full-time or part-time school health coordinator is critical to successful implementation of a coordinated approach (CDC, n.d.a).

School Health *in Action*

Students and Teachers Collaborating to Promote Health

School administrators who support faculty and staff wellness can have a positive effect on a number of efforts within the WSCC approach.

At a middle school in Frisco, Texas, a group of health education students decided that as part of a project they would solicit teachers at their school with an offer to develop and implement personal health plans for them. Each staff member involved in the project signed a contract with the students, agreeing to abide by the student-developed fitness program and meal plan. Students then visited the teachers on a regular basis to check on their progress with the contracts.

Each day, the students contacted their clients and asked them whether they had consumed enough water, exercised, and met their calorie limit. They also discussed the need for working out at least three times a week. The program was so popular that some teachers had to be turned away because there weren't enough student coaches. More information about this project is available at www.friscoisd.org/news/2013/04/08/maupin-project.

School administrators need to recognize that they cannot work in isolation and need to consider partnerships and collaborations that team up community agencies with the school district. Medical City Children's Hospital in partnership with the Greater Dallas Restaurant Association ran a program called Kids Teaching Kids. The program fights childhood obesity by providing students with healthy kid-friendly snacks designed by high school culinary arts students. A cookbook is published each year highlighting the best snacks. The culinary arts students showcase the snacks and teach students how to make them throughout the year. See http://kids-teaching-kids.com/.

The complexities of working across traditional boundary lines of authority between central administration, departments, schools, the health and medical community, and the plethora of partners interested in children's health and wellness requires a dedicated position and a person with a special skill set. The superintendent can provide focused and engaged encouragement and tangible support of resources but cannot carry the daily load of implementing WSCC. Without a designated position in place, no one has ultimate ownership for the success or failure of implementation. Without ownership, all efforts are likely to fail over time. According to the CDC's *Profiles 2010: School Health Profiles Characteristics of Health Programs Among Secondary Schools*, the median percentage of secondary schools with a school health coordinator has decreased since 2008. This decrease is of concern because the administration and management of WSCC will require time and expertise (Brener et al., 2011).

When WSCC leadership becomes another duty assigned of personnel within departments such as health education, student services, health services, or curriculum and instruction, decreased buy-in and fragmented implementation is more likely. School superintendents, always mindful of the return on investment of creating new positions in school districts, need to become convinced that this position is as fundamentally necessary as a school principal is. When we empower a qualified professional to work across traditional boundary lines, access up and down the chain of command is provided, including regular access to school decision makers. A full-time coordinator can work to break down the barriers that exist among the 10 areas of WSCC. The coordinator can challenge, collaborate, and conquer internal frameworks and operations that lead to isolated decisions and practices that provide no vision regarding health and wellness outcomes.

A coordinator should have a blend of experience implementing programs within schools coordinated through a central office; some degree of formal education or training in health, kinesiology, nursing, or medicine; and exceptional communication skills. The person also needs to demonstrate and embrace the imperative of improving health and wellness for our children and staff through WSCC efforts. This person needs passion, intelligence, and communication skills to create strong collaborative efforts through positive actions focused on both short-term and long-term results. This person is the key organizer, clearinghouse, moderator, and implementation specialist for WSCC. Figure 6.1 includes a list of CDC suggested responsibilities of a school health coordinator.

FIGURE 6.1

Responsibilities of a School Health Coordinator

Facilitate collaboration among school staff responsible for health and safety of students

Serve as a liaison between the school and those who oversee school health and safety programs at the district level and in other schools

Communicate school health and safety priorities to the principal, staff, parents, community organizations, and students

Help secure funding or other resources to support school guiding health and safety activities

Manage school health funds

Organize and conduct meetings of the school health team

Facilitate the provision of professional development activities for school health and staff

Assist with the assessment of student health needs and evaluation of school health policies and activities

Adapted from Centers for Disease Control 2011.

MOVING FORWARD

Superintendents, principals, and other administrators play a key role in supporting, planning, implementing, and sustaining WSCC. The following recommendations are made to provide direction for administrators to make quality WSCC a reality in their school districts and schools:

- Promote positive relationships that recognize the diversity and value of all stakeholders in the school community
- Incorporate health in the vision, mission statement, and school improvement plan of the school district or school
- Establish a school health team for the school district or school
- Appoint a school health coordinator with specific responsibilities for WSCC
- Monitor best practices in each of the 10 components of WSCC
- Allocate resources for WSCC
- Continually communicate the importance of health promotion to all members of the school community
- Maximize the use of school facilities for health promotion for the school community

SUMMARY

Maintaining and improving the health of students, teachers, and staff working in schools must be aggressively addressed. School administrators are in an ideal position to assume leadership in implementing WSCC programming within schools and school districts. School administrators who are willing to reexamine their responsibility as it relates to student and staff health will discover a pathway that improves the health and academic achievement of their students, results in a happier and healthier staff, and leads to personal improvement as well.

Changing our current practices related to health and wellness in schools is an imperative that strikes at the core of our ethical responsibility to our children. School administrators can make a huge difference by becoming advocates for health within the existing duties of administration, by finding champions, and by implementing collaborative practices that can result in transformative change in schools.

Glossary

ASCD—Founded in 1943, ASCD (formerly the Association for Supervision and Curriculum Development) is the global leader in developing and delivering innovative programs, products, and services that empower educators to support the success of each learner. See www.ascd.org/about-ascd.aspx for more information.

meta-analysis—A method of statistical analysis that is applied to a collection of similar studies in order to make judgments about the overall results of the studies.

Whole Child Initiative—The initiative started in 2007 by ASCD that aims to focus greater attention on a holistic, well-rounded education that caters to each child's social, emotional, mental, physical, and cognitive development.

Application Activities

1. You are a member of a school health committee in a local school district. Your colleagues on the committee have charged you with developing a 15-minute PowerPoint presentation that makes the case for the district to hire a full-time coordinator for WSCC. Develop a draft of the PowerPoint presentation that you will give to present your rationale for the position.
2. Your local school district makes a decision to hire a full-time coordinator for WSCC (see application activity 1). Develop a job description for the position (maximum 100 words) and a list of questions to ask of the candidates invited for an interview.
3. Interview a school or school district administrator. Begin the interview by presenting an overview of WSCC. Develop interview questions that address the administrator's thoughts on WSCC as a school health promotion approach, the administrator's personal perception of the importance and feasibility of hiring a district health coordinator.

Resources

American School Health Association: www.ashaweb.org

Centers for Disease Control and Prevention, *Results From the School Health Policies and Practices Study 2012*. www.cdc.gov/healthyyouth/shpps/2012/pdf/shpps-results_2012.pdf

Centers for Disease Control and Prevention, *How Schools Can Implement Coordinated School Health*. www.cdc.gov/healthyouth/cshp/schools.htm

Medical City Children's Hospital, 2010, *The Partnership That Gets the Whole Thing Cooking. Kids Teaching Kids*. Kids Teaching Kids. http://kids-teaching-kids.com/

National Association for Sport and Physical Education (NASPE), 2009: Standards and Position Statements. www.aahperd.org/naspe/standards/peps.cfm

Staley Students Develop Health and Wellness Plans for Teachers, April 8, 2013, Frisco ISD News, District eNewsletter report on the Maupin Project. www.friscoisd.org/news/2013/04/08/maupin project

References

American School Health Association. 2010. *What School Administrators Can Do to Enhance Student Learning by Supporting a Coordinated Approach to Health*. Kent, OH: American School Health.

ASCD. 2013. *The Whole Child*. www.wholechildeducation.org

Basch, Charles E. 2010. Healthier Students Are Better Learners: A Missing Link in School Reforms to Close the Achievement Gap. *Equity Matters: Research Review*, No. 6..

Basch, Charles E. 2013. Healthier Students Are Better Learners: High-Quality, Strategically Planned, and Effectively Coordinated School Health Programs Must Be a Fundamental Mission of Schools to Help Close the Achievement Gap. *Journal of School Health, 81*(10), 650–662.

Brener, Nancy, Demissie, Zowditu, Foti, Kathryn, McManus, Tim, Shanklin, Shari, Hawkins, Joseph, & Kann, Laura. 2011. *CDC Profiles 2010: School Health Profiles Characteristics of Health Programs Among Secondary Schools*. Atlanta, GA: Centers for Disease Control and Prevention.

Centers for Disease Control and Prevention (CDC). 2010. *The Association Between School Based Physical Activity, Including Physical Education, and Academic Performance*. Atlanta, GA: U.S. Department of Health and Human Services.

Centers for Disease Control and Prevention (CDC). 2011, September 16. School Health Guidelines to Promote Healthy Eating and Physical Activity. *Morbidity and Mortality Weekly Report (MMWR), 60*(5).

Centers for Disease Control and Prevention (CDC). 2013. *Results From the School Health Policies and Practices Study 2012*. www.cdc.gov/healthyyouth/shpps/2012/pdf/shpps-results_2012.pdf

Centers for Disease Control and Prevention (CDC). n.d.a. *How Schools Can Implement Coordinated School Health*. www.cdc.gov/healthyouth/cshp/schools.htm

Centers for Disease Control and Prevention (CDC). n.d.b. *The Case for Coordinated School Health*. www.cdc.gov/healthyyouth/cshp/case.htm

Committee on Childhood Obesity Prevention Actions for Local Governments. 2009. *Local Government Actions to Prevent Childhood Obesity*. Institute of Medicine and the National Research Council Institute.

Dilly, Julia. 2011. *Research Review: School-Based Health Interventions and Academic Achievement*. Washington State Board of Health.

Directors of Health Promotion and Education. 2007. *School Employee Wellness: A Guide for Protecting the Assets of Our Nation's Schools*. www.healthyschoolsms.org/staff_health/documents/EntireGuide.pdf

Eaton, Tim. 2010, November 30. Diabetes Cases Projected to Soar in Texas. *Austin American Statesman*. www.aahperd.org/naspe/standards/peps.cfm

Medical City Children's Hospital. 2010. *The Partnership That Gets the Whole Thing Cooking. Kids Teaching Kids*. http://kids-teaching-kids.com/

National Association for Sport and Physical Education (NASPE). 2009. *Standards and Position Statements, Position Statement: Physical Activity Used as Punishment and/or Behavior Management*.

Valois, Robert E. 2011. *The Healthy School Communities Model Aligning Health and Education in the School Setting*. www.ascd.org/hsc

7

Meeting the Needs of Diverse Students, Families, and Communities

ANGELIA M. PASCHAL

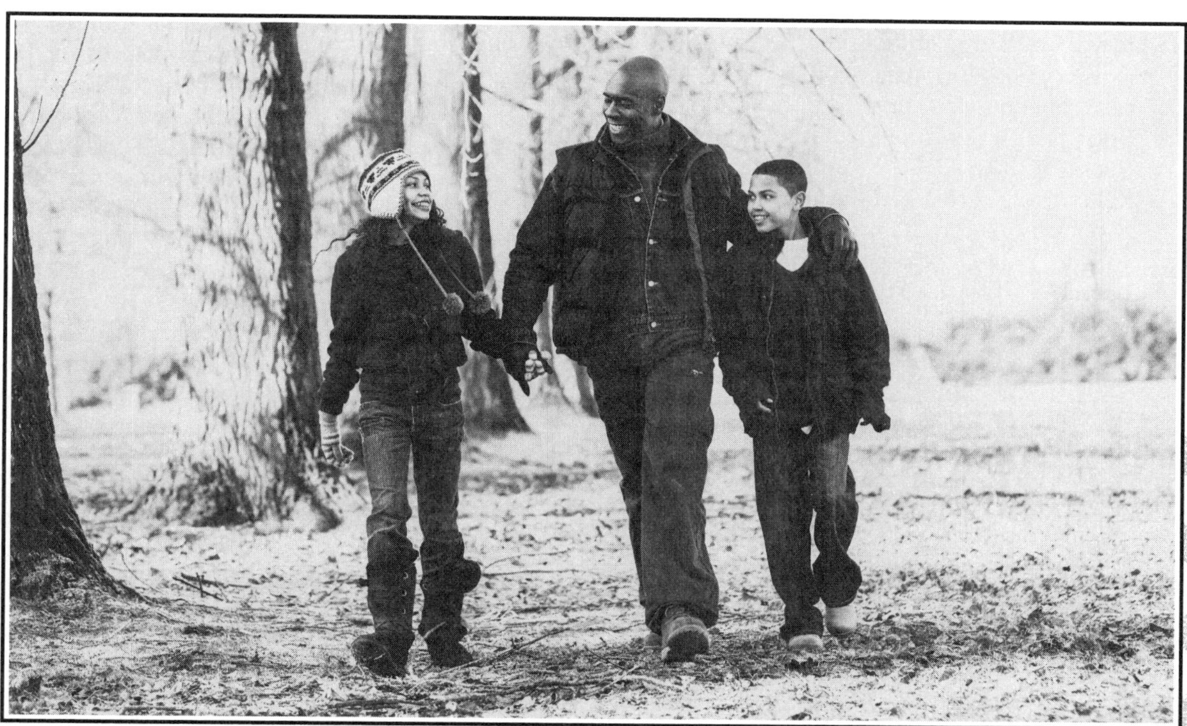

As the United States population continues to change and our society becomes more culturally diverse, school systems need to become more responsive to the needs of their diverse student populations through culturally relevant strategies (Bustamante & Van der Wees 2012; Center for Mental Health in Schools at UCLA, 2011; U.S. Census Bureau, 2010). Many students are faced with multiple and multilayered challenges that traditional methods of student connectedness, family involvement, and community engagement may not adequately address. Addressing these challenges requires significant commitment and resources on behalf of the schools. Yet the majority of students and the broader community can eventually benefit from efforts designed for diverse students.

In this chapter, various issues that diverse students and families experience, as well as the challenges that schools face in addressing those issues, are discussed. Science-based strategies and action steps to increase school connectedness among students are also reviewed. Culturally relevant strategies that can be used to increase family involvement and community engagement among diverse populations are examined. Finally, using the Whole School, Whole Community, Whole Child (WSCC) approach, strategies are presented for addressing the needs of diverse students, families, and communities. Effective school health requires concerted efforts from schools to build genuine, effective partnerships with families and communities to meet the educational and health needs of their students.

DIVERSE STUDENTS AND SCHOOL CONNECTEDNESS

Regardless of curriculum, governance structure, accountability measures, or school policies, if children are not motivated or not able to learn, educational progress will be limited. One of the factors associated with students' ability to learn is health. Various health problems have been associated with factors affecting educational achievement such as sensory perceptions, cognition, school connectedness, absenteeism, and dropping out (Basch, 2011). Poor health outcomes among children have been linked to low socioeconomic status, which highlights the interrelated nature of children's health, their environment, and educational outcomes (Basch, 2011). The complex nature of this interconnection emphasizes the need to address academic, social, emotional, and physical health issues among students. Although such comprehensive efforts will benefit all students, special consideration should be given to diverse student populations whose needs are greater.

The term *diverse students* in this chapter refers to children who are socioeconomically poor; are a racial or ethnic minority; or have physical, emotional, and mental impairments. Diverse students also refer to those with social identities that place them at a social disadvantage, including those who self-identify as lesbian, gay, bisexual, transgender, or queer (LGBTQ). Significant disparities in health, health care, and educational outcomes exist among these diverse children and youths (Basch, 2011; U.S. DHHS, 2010). These interrelated disparities can be illustrated in the case of homeless children, a socioeconomically disadvantaged student population. Often depressed, anxious, and withdrawn, about one in six homeless children experiences emotional disturbances (National Center on Family Homelessness, 2009). This diverse student group is four times more likely to suffer from some physical illnesses (e.g., respiratory infections, ear infections, and stomach problems) compared with other children. Additionally, homeless students are also three times more likely to have behavioral issues related to traumatic stress compared with other students. In addition to experiencing home instability and safety issues, many of these children are exposed to violence (Kilmer, Cook, Crusto, Strater, & Haber, 2012). With approximately 1.5 million homeless children in the United States, many schools must not only meet the educational needs of these students but also address their unique health and social issues (National Center on Family Homelessness, 2009). If inadequately addressed, these issues are likely to hinder academic achievement among homeless students.

Sexual minority youths represent another example of diverse students with special needs. These students are more likely to engage in sexually risky behaviors, such as having sexual intercourse at younger ages, having multiple sex partners, and not using condoms. Sexual minority youths are also more likely to engage in other risky health behaviors including use of tobacco, alcohol, and other drugs. Their social environment also affects their academic experiences. For instance, negative attitudes toward LGBTQ students place them at increased risk for bullying and other forms of violence (Kann, O'Malley, McManus, Kinchen, et al., 2011). Therefore, schools are sometimes unsafe for sexual minority youths, who may have to focus on safety and survival as priorities as opposed to education (Weiler, 2001). Consequently, these risky health behaviors, social disadvantages, and health risks require schools to respond to their unique health and educational needs.

Racial and ethnic minority students also provide examples of diverse students with unique challenges. Disparities in health and health care continue to persist among low-income minority children (Flores and the Committee on Pediatric Research, 2010). Minority children also tend to rate their health-related quality of life relatively low, indicating perceived psychological and physical health issues as early as second grade (Mansour, Kotagal, Rose, Ho, et al. 2003). Therefore, in addition to health disparities and perceived health impairments, many racial and ethnic minority children experience various forms of social and economic disadvantages, such as language barriers, real and perceived discrimination, and poverty. Mansour and colleagues (2003) found that among minority urban students, health-related quality of life was significantly associated with school connectedness and socioeconomic status. These conditions have implications for academic achievement among diverse students and school efforts in addressing them.

The preceding examples demonstrate the challenges that diverse student populations experience and that schools may face in addressing them. The needs of diverse students are substantial and surpass the provision of standard quality education, conventional school services, and traditional family and community engagement in schools. Yet few schools have the resources or time to address the underlying factors and conditions that contribute to the academic issues prevalent in diverse student populations (Anderson-Butcher & Ashton, 2004; Basch, 2011). The WSCC approach can address this gap (Basch, 2011, 2012).

Students are more likely to engage in healthy behaviors and experience academic success if they feel connected to school (CDC, 2009a). **School connectedness** is defined as "the belief by students that adults and peers in the school care about their learning as well as about them as individuals" (CDC, 2009a, p. 3). Some students are less likely to be connected to their schools. Students from families dealing with socioeconomic challenges, for instance, may have certain personal characteristics (e.g., learning disabilities, health problems), contextual and demographic factors (e.g., culture, race and ethnicity, poverty status), and socioenvironmental challenges (e.g., overcrowding at home, parents with limited educational ability to provide support, limited community resources) that impede their ability to feel connected (Mendez, 2010). Thus, school connectedness among diverse students might require better or different strategies.

Four factors associated with increased school connectedness among students are described in *School Connectedness: Strategies for Increasing Protective Factors Among Youth* (CDC, 2009a): adult support, belonging to a positive peer group, commitment to education, and a positive school environment. These factors are further addressed in six recommended strategies:

- Create decision-making processes that facilitate student, family, and community engagement; academic achievement; and staff empowerment.
- Provide education opportunities to enable families to be actively involved in their children's academic and school life.
- Provide students with the academic, emotional, and social skills necessary to be actively engaged in school.
- Use effective classroom management and teaching methods to foster a positive learning environment.
- Provide professional development and support for teachers and other school staff to enable them to meet the diverse cognitive, emotional, and social needs of children and adolescents.
- Create trusting and caring relationships that promote open communication among administrators, teachers, staff, students, families, and communities.

These six strategies include specific actions that schools can take, and several include culturally relevant approaches. Although the strategies are meant to increase school connectedness among all students, they can be effective in meeting the needs of diverse students, families, and communities. The culturally relevant action steps are presented in figure 7.1. Culturally relevant themes include shared decision making; collaboration and partnerships; open and frequent communication; and education and awareness about student and family needs, concerns, and preferences.

DIVERSE FAMILY ENGAGEMENT

Central to meeting the needs of diverse students is family involvement. The benefits of family involvement to student academic success and school readiness are well documented (CDC, 2009a; Mendez 2010). **Family engagement**, also called family involvement, partnership, and collaboration, refers to "a wide range of activities through which parents, grandparents, older siblings, tribal members, and other members of students' extended family contribute to and support student learning" (Brewster & Railsback, 2003, p. 9). The importance of these activities is illustrated through the WSCC approach that includes a separate component, family engagement. In the CSH model, family involvement was included in a component with community involvement. School expectations for family involvement are generally classified in the following areas over and above the family's central role of parenting: communication with schools, volunteerism, support of the student's learning needs at home, participation in school governance and decision making, and playing a role in school–community collaborations (Epstein et al., 2009).

Diverse families are more likely to experience barriers to becoming involved with their children's schools. For example, many diverse families may not be able to communicate adequately with teachers and other school personnel because of language barriers or communication styles. In addition, they may not have sufficient time to volunteer, or they may not possess the skills and knowledge to support learning at home or to participate in other expected roles (Brewster & Railsback, 2003). Thus, schools need to focus on the sociocultural factors that can affect diverse

FIGURE 7.1

Culturally Relevant Strategies for Fostering School Connectedness

1. **Create decision-making processes that facilitate student, family, and community engagement, academic achievement, and staff empowerment.**
    - Engage teams of students, faculty, staff, parents, and community members to plan school policies and activities.
    - Empower students to communicate openly with school staff and parents, such as through parent–teacher–student conferences and teacher evaluations.
    - Engage community partners to provide health and social health services at school that students and their families need, such as dental services, vaccinations, and child care.
    - Brainstorm and get involved in taking steps to improve the school climate and students' sense of connectedness to school. Involve diverse groups of school staff, students, and families in these efforts.
2. **Provide education opportunities to enable families to be actively involved in their children's academic and school life.**
    - Offer workshops and trainings for parents to increase their ability to be actively involved in their children's school life and to help their children develop academic and life skills.
    - Create opportunities to involve and accommodate parents with varied schedules, resources, and skills to help them participate in meaningful school and classroom activities as well as share their culture and expectations.
    - Translate materials into languages spoken in students' homes and provide interpreters at events when needed.
    - Encourage students to talk openly with school staff and parents. Involve students in parent–teacher conferences, teacher evaluation, curriculum selection committees, and school health teams.
    - Seek opportunities for parents and students to share their culture with others in school.
3. **Provide students with the academic, emotional, and social skills necessary to be actively engaged in school.**
    - Translate materials into languages spoken in students' homes.
    - Request interpreters as needed to ensure clear communication and to avoid misunderstandings arising from language barriers.
    - Provide opportunities for students to improve their interpersonal, stress management, and decision-making skills.
    - Allow and encourage students to identify, label, express, and assess their feelings.
4. **Use effective classroom management and teaching methods to foster a positive learning environment.**
    - Provide opportunities, such as service learning, creative projects, and extracurricular activities, that promote meaningful student involvement, learning, and recognition.
    - Clearly communicate expectations for learning and behavior that are developmentally appropriate and applied equitably. Describe the goals of the lesson and relate them to the students' lives and the real world.
    - Be flexible with instructional strategies to allow for teachable moments and personalization of lessons.
    - Use student-centered pedagogy and appropriate classroom management and discipline strategies that meet students' diverse needs and learning styles.

- Engage students in appropriate leadership positions and decision-making processes in the classroom and school.
- Encourage open, respectful communication about differing viewpoints.

5. **Provide professional development and support for teachers and other school staff to enable them to meet the diverse cognitive, emotional, and social needs of children and adolescents.**
   - Educate school staff on strategies for communicating with parents and involving them in the children's school life.
   - Further develop staff expertise in adolescent development and share lessons learned with other school staff to increase understanding about the needs of students.
   - Attend workshops and trainings on communicating effectively with and involving parents in school activities and share ideas for involving parents with school staff members.
6. **Create trusting and caring relationships that promote open communication among administrators, teachers, staff, students, families, and communities.**
   - Allow students and parents to use the school facility outside school hours for recreation or health promotion programs.
   - Apply and fairly enforce reasonable and consistent disciplinary policies that are jointly agreed on by students and staff.
   - Hold schoolwide, experience-broadening activities that enable students to learn about different cultures, people with disabilities, and other topics.
   - Support student clubs and activities that promote a positive school climate, such as gay–straight alliances and multicultural clubs.
   - Involve students in parent–teacher conferences, curriculum selection committees, and school health teams.
   - Challenge all school staff to greet each student by name.
   - Encourage teachers, counselors, health service professionals, coaches, and other schools staff to build stronger relationships with students who are experiencing academic or personal issues or social problems, such as bullying or harassment.

Adapted from Centers for Disease Control and Prevention 2009.

family involvement. These cultural and family considerations include but are not limited to socioeconomic status, language, literacy levels, communication styles, nontraditional family structures, work schedules, and educational skills or abilities. These factors might require schools to reconsider their approaches to family involvement to facilitate the partnership needed to support their students. WSCC can be instrumental to meeting the needs of diverse students, families, and communities and generating effective partnerships with schools.

Research indicates that three practices have guided the efforts of schools that have successfully demonstrated diverse family engagement: a focus on trust and collaborative relationships; concerted attempts to recognize, respect, and address the needs of diverse families, including their socioeconomic and cultural differences; and a philosophy that embraces shared power and responsibility with families (CDC, 2009a; Brewster & Railsback, 2003; Henderson and Mapp, 2002). In other words, instead of resorting to assumptions that many diverse families do not want to be engaged, these schools have instead embraced core values (trust, respect, shared power, and responsibility) that resulted in effective partnerships with diverse families.

To illustrate the effect of certain family characteristics on parents' ability or willingness to be involved in schools, socioeconomic status will be discussed. Socioeconomically poor families are less likely to be engaged compared with those who are not poor (Austin, Nakamoto, & Bailey, 2010). Diverse families, especially racial and ethnic minority families, are disproportionately poor. Many families that are socioeconomically poor do not have flexible jobs, are employed in jobs that are physically demanding, or work in positions that require work during hours or shifts when their children are not in school (afternoons, evenings, and nights). Moreover, stress and depression have been linked to racial and ethnic minority parents living in poverty (McLoyd, 1998). Collectively, these factors have implications for family attendance at school events, ability to pay for their children's activities, volunteering at school, and being involved in other school-related activities and meetings. These parents may not only have limited time but also insufficient energy or literacy skills needed to assist their children with homework and other educational needs. Therefore, schools may need to consider creative volunteer opportunities, varying times for school events, low-cost school activities or financial assistance for students, and alternative methods to provide academic support to students without overburdening diverse parents who would otherwise help or be involved but can't. The WSCC approach can be used to address these needs.

Literacy and language issues among diverse families provide additional examples of how various issues affect families' ability or willingness to be involved in schools. **Literacy** is defined as "using printed and written information to function in society, to achieve one's goals, and to develop one's knowledge and potential" (Kutner, Greenberg, & Baer, 2006). A significant proportion of American adults have literacy challenges, which makes it difficult for them to understand and use information provided by their children's schools. For example, approximately 43 percent of adults find it difficult to perform prose tasks (ability to search, comprehend, and use information from continuous texts). About 34 percent find it difficult to perform document tasks (ability to search, comprehend, and use information from noncontinuous texts in various formats). More than half (55 percent) find it difficult to perform quantitative tasks (identify and perform computations, either alone or sequentially, using numbers embedded in printed materials). Many people with limited literacy skills are racial and ethnic minorities (e.g., black and Hispanic), people who did not graduate from high school, adults who did not speak English before going to school as a child, and people who are unemployed (Kutner, Greenberg, & Baer, 2006). Thus, family engagement is likely to be affected by parents' literacy levels. Yet several strategies can be implemented to address parental literacy issues. For example, schools could strive to develop and use materials

School Health *in Action*

Addressing Health Disparities Benefits All

Focused on health disparities among its racial and ethnic students, Gasden County, Florida, used culturally relevant strategies to implement districtwide Coordinated School Health (CSH). Specifically, community participatory approaches were used by the CSH planning and advisory committee, the Gasden County Wellness Approach to Community Health (G-WATCH), to develop and implement several CSH activities. For example, G-WATCH used public service announcements (PSAs) produced by students. As such, the messages conveyed in the PSAs were more likely to be meaningful and effective among students. Health education activities that involved parents were promoted, as were health education curricula relevant to students. Moreover, collaborations were established among community partners (health service providers, city government, county recreation department) to enhance health services provided to students, increase family involvement in school activities, and promote healthy behaviors among families and community members.

The effect of G-WATCH's efforts was evident after two years of its implementation. Among the overall CSH outcomes were a districtwide policy regarding physical fitness and not withholding physical activity as punishment, a districtwide policy of daily 15-minute recess for students in grades pre K through 5, prohibited sales of carbonated beverages during meal periods, and meal schedules that complied with Florida's guideline of a 20-minute seated eating time.

Although the focus of G-WATCH was on health disparities and academic challenges among diverse student groups, the CSH efforts and outcomes were a benefit to all students. Thus, this effort demonstrates how WSCC could be used to meet the needs of diverse students (including families and community members) and achieve outcomes that benefit the majority of students (CDC, 2007).

written at low literacy levels. In addition, use of pictures or other illustrations when appropriate is also recommended. Audiovisuals and other formats used in meetings should also be considered. Finally, schools could collaborate with local organizations (e.g., adult basic education programs) to offer literacy, health literacy, Graduate Record Examination (GRE) courses, and other needed support services to families.

Similar to socioeconomic status and literacy level, language barriers may decrease the likelihood of parents' ability or willingness to be involved in their children's schools (Austin, Nakamoto, & Bailey, 2010). In schools that have a disproportionate numbers of immigrant children or children of immigrants, English may not be the primary language spoken at home. Although schools collect information on primary language spoken in the home, being cognizant of these findings when designing and implementing school activities is important. For instance, parents would need to know that volunteers at school events could aid them in their communication (Brewster & Railsback, 2003). In addition, providing bilingual forms and information as often as possible is suggested.

As indicated earlier, *School Connectedness: Strategies for Increasing Protective Factors Among Youth* (CDC, 2009a) describes six science-based strategies to increase school connectedness, including family involvement and community engagement. Several action items are indicated for each strategy. Many of these action steps are culturally relevant and could be instrumental to meeting the needs of diverse students and families (e.g., create opportunities to involve and accommodate parents with varied schedules, resources, and skills to help them participate in meaningful school and classroom activities as well as share their culture and expectations). Refer to figure 7.1.

DIVERSE COMMUNITY INVOLVEMENT

Communities and the organizations within them can be valuable assets to schools and to the children and families they serve. Research has demonstrated the benefits of community engagement and its effect on student achievement and health outcomes (Basch, 2011; Krishnaswami, Martinson, Wakimoto, & Anglemeyer, 2012). Communities offer a wealth of resources that can contribute to curriculum and other educational needs of diverse students and families. Therefore, community engagement is important. Community participatory approaches can be used to help promote community engagement.

Picturing community engagement as a continuum, community participatory approaches would be near the higher end of the gradient (see figure 7.2). **Community participatory approaches** involve community members or their representatives in some or all phases of a project or activity (e.g., development, implementation, or evaluation of a project). On the extreme end of the community engagement continuum is **community-based participatory research (CBPR)** in which the community or its representatives is an equal partner and is involved in each phase of the research project, from its conceptualization to the dissemination of

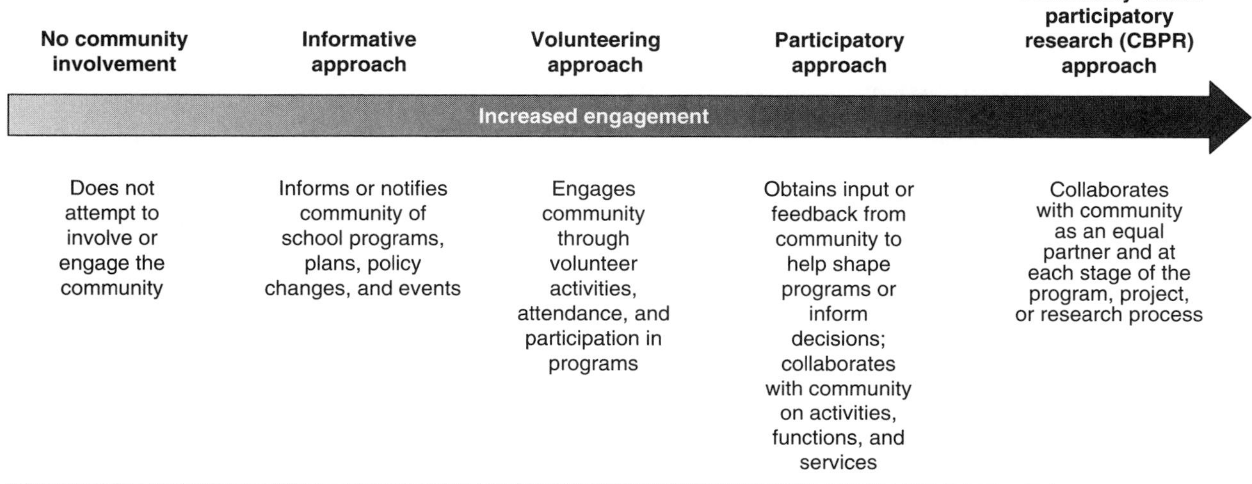

Figure 7.2 Community engagement continuum.
Data from Epstein et al. 2009; Minkler and Wallerstein 2008.

information. The extent to which the community is involved in the individual phases of the study or project can vary from project to project or community to community. Regardless, the CBPR relationship is characterized by genuine collaboration in which the power relationship is equalized, colearning occurs, capacity building among community members is encouraged, project results are used to benefit both partners, and a long-term partnership commitment is established (Minkler & Wallerstein, 2008; Wallerstein & Duran, 2010).

Using community participatory approaches has many benefits. Krishnaswami and colleagues (2012) found better outcomes among programs and interventions that used community participatory approaches. Community participatory approaches have been especially effective in working with racially and ethnic diverse groups (Krishnaswami et al., 2012). Using CBPR in particular, in which the community is involved in each stage of a research or project, has resulted in increased participation of minority communities, more meaningful and relevant projects, and successful project outcomes (Krishnaswami et al., 2012). As a culturally competence strategy, CBPR and other general community participatory approaches can be effective in promoting community engagement.

Community engagement strategies can be either formal or informal and can include partnering with the community to sponsor school and community events, instituting a community advisory board, focusing curricula on issues that the community has deemed important, or inviting community members to provide presentations to students and families. In addition, employing school personnel who reflect the diversity of the community is regarded as an important cultural competency strategy (Wallerstein & Duran, 2010). This community diversity should also be reflected in the school or school district health committee or council. Building a base of community school volunteers to reflect community diversity is another important strategy. Examples of community organizations that could be involved in the school and the WSCC approach include local nonprofit social service agencies to help provide counseling services; planned parenthood and local departments of health to assist with sexual health curriculum; collaboration with Big Sisters, Big Brothers for mentoring programs for school youths; and college or university partnerships to incorporate expertise in practice, research, and service (Anderson-Butcher & Ashton, 2004).

CULTURAL COMPETENCE STRATEGIES

Understanding the broader sociocultural context within which students live and operate is necessary to achieve adequate involvement and support from their families and communities. Although the aim of nearly all educators is to provide the best education and support they can to students, many may lack the knowledge and skills needed to work with diverse students, families, and community members (Brewster & Railsback, 2003). Cultural competence is important to addressing their needs. **Cultural competence** is defined as "a set of values, behaviors, attitudes, practices, and policies within an organization or program or among staff that enables people to work effectively with diverse groups" (Vaughn, 2008, p. 46).

Many educators would be considered **culturally sensitive**, which means that they are aware of and respect cultural differences. But cultural competency goes beyond cultural sensitivity to include behaviors or actions that result in effective interactions with or service provision to diverse populations. Although cultural sensitivity may be a starting point, subsequent steps should be taken in schools to learn more about diverse students, families, and communities (to include understanding the diversity between and within groups and without stereotyping) and to develop skills to ensure effective interactions and work with diverse groups (i.e., cultural competency). Schools should consider cultural competency training for school personnel that includes general information about the diverse students and families, their strengths and challenges, community assets and needs, and effective strategies to use in interacting and working with them.

Cultural competence implies that the issues, assets, needs, supporting factors, and barriers of diverse students, families, and communities have already been identified. In the context of education, some of these issues and barriers pertain to language, literacy levels, incomes and family resources, communication styles, age, job factors (e.g., schedules, part-time or full-time status), and so on (Vaughn, 2008). Other issues or unique needs may exist. Schools can conduct assessments to identify issues, assets, barriers, needs, preferences, and recommendations for various factors that can help them become more effective in providing services to diverse students and families. Such assessments could be conducted formally

School Health *in Action*

Culturally Relevant Ways to Address Youth Tobacco Use

Wisconsin's Coordinated School Health efforts included initiatives to address tobacco use, physical activity, and healthy eating among its students (CDC, 2009b). An important aspect of the School Tobacco Prevention Program was a concerted effort to address tobacco control issues among youth populations that were disproportionately affected by tobacco use. Culturally relevant curricula and programs specific to gender and racial and ethnic groups were used. For example, the American Lung Association's school-based, 10-session tobacco cessation program, Not on Tobacco (N-O-T), was implemented in many school districts (American Lung Association in Wisconsin, 2013; Wisconsin Department of Public Instruction, 2005). Besides smoking cessation, the N-O-T program promotes healthy lifestyle behaviors and builds life skills among students. The curriculum is gender sensitive and is tailored for some racial and ethnic student populations.

Another culturally relevant strategy used in Wisconsin's CSH effort was student involvement in the development and implementation of tobacco prevention and cessation programs and activities (Wisconsin Department of Public Instruction, 2005). In some districts, high schools students were trained as peer helpers, and many trained other students on the dangers of secondhand smoke. Peer education programs were common in Wisconsin. In some school districts, students served on tobacco coalitions. Moreover, in some schools students led and implemented all efforts pertaining to tobacco cessation campaigns and advocacy. This community participatory approach, using extensive student input and involvement, was a theme among several school districts across the state. Similarly, several districts collaborated with families and community organizations (e.g., racial- and ethnic-oriented health coalitions, health care organizations, county government) to address tobacco prevention and control among families and the broader community (Wisconsin Department of Public Instruction, 2005).

Wisconsin's overall efforts to reduce smoking among students generated positive results. For instance, six to eight weeks after completing the N-O-T program, students showed a 36 percent quit rate. In addition, overall smoking rates among students have decreased significantly since the implementation of the statewide CSH tobacco prevention program, from 38 percent in 1999 to 20 percent in 2007 (CDC, 2009b). The Wisconsin School Tobacco Prevention Program is an example of how culturally relevant strategies using appropriate outreach and involvement among students, families, and communities can lead to positive and meaningful outcomes.

or informally by employing culturally competent strategies. Informally, for example, parents could simply be asked about their preferences regarding certain issues when talking with them during enrollment, parent–teacher meetings, or during an after-school activity. In some cases, non-English speaking parents may use family spokespersons for communication if no interpretation is available. Formal assessments could include a survey, putting additional questions on an existing form, or conducting a focus group with parents and community members.

Conducting assessments are more likely to result in relevant and meaningful activities, programs, procedures, and polices (Brewster & Railsback, 2003). Determining preferred types of volunteer activities, modes of communication, and the appropriate family member to contact about school issues are examples of questions that could be explored in assessments and used to help promote family involvement and community engagement. Including family and community members in developing assessments or conducting them can also increase engagement (Krishnaswami et al., 2012). Being culturally competent in working with diverse students, families, and communities requires identifying and understanding their issues, assets, needs, barriers, preferences, and recommendations.

Cultural competence also involves showing respect for the cultural practices, beliefs, and values of diverse students, families, and communities. Yet many schools fail to recognize the social assets of diverse cultural groups. Nontraditional attitudes, beliefs, and practices are often regarded negatively and are perceived as barriers to providing quality education as opposed to being viewed as strengths (Fuller & Coll, 2010). For example,

Latino families who are less acculturated are generally cohesive as family units. In turn, such cohesion has been associated with providing strong support to their children. Serving as a protective factor, such strong family bonds promote academic achievement, especially among those who are first-generation Latino (Fuller & Coll, 2010). On the other hand, some diverse families have parenting styles or education beliefs that are not conducive to traditional forms of family involvement at schools (Mendez, 2010). For instance, many parents may believe that schools have the primary, if not the sole, responsibility of educating their children, as opposed to viewing education as a shared responsibility. Although such attitudes may impede family involvement, identifying and respecting such beliefs marks the genesis of a trusting, respectful relationship (Brewster & Railsback, 2003). Next, going beyond cultural sensitivity and respect to learning more about the cultural values, behaviors, and beliefs among diverse families and communities is important. Subsequently, evaluating alternative methods and culturally sensitive approaches to increase family involvement should be considered in this example.

WHOLE SCHOOL, WHOLE COMMUNITY, WHOLE CHILD APPROACH

The Whole School, Whole Community, Whole Child (WSCC) approach can help improve the education, health, and well-being of diverse students and families (ASCD, 2014). Comprehensive in its approach, WSCC includes 10 components: health education; physical education and physical activity; health services; nutrition environment and services; counseling, psychological, and social services; employee wellness; family engagement; community involvement; physical environment; and social and emotional climate. The varying needs of diverse student populations can be addressed through WSCC. Two examples of the use of CSH to address the needs of diverse populations are given: the districtwide CSH in Gasden County, Florida (CDC, 2007), and the Wisconsin Coordinated School Health Program (CDC, 2009b). Sidebars in this chapter describe both models in detail.

As another example of CSH, a school-based project in Michigan was developed to address the needs of diverse students by providing cultural competency training for staff (CDC, 2013a). In this example, the Michigan Department of Education (MDE) convened a work group to address the safety issues of LGBTQ students. In collaboration with the Calhoun Intermediate School District (ISD), the MDE developed a resource guide, "A Silent Crisis: Creating Safe Schools for Sexual Minority Youth," that was used by teachers, counselors, administrators, parents, and other professionals. In addition, the MDE conducted 44 workshops using the source, and more than 100 high schools in Michigan established gay–straight alliances. Other outcomes from this project included in-service programs with staff, revised policies and curricula, and service referrals (CDC, 2013a). Again, this example shows how school efforts that focus on the needs of diverse students can be effective and have far-reaching effects. The implications for CSH programming using culturally relevant strategies are evident.

A school project in North Carolina further illustrates how culturally competent education and training can be used to affect the health of diverse student populations. Funded in part through CDC's Division of Adolescent and School Health, the North Carolina Department of Public Instruction Healthy School Program partnered with the North Carolina Division of Public Health Youth Suicide Prevention program to create a five-hour training program, "How to Be an Ally" (CDC, 2013b). The target audience for the training was counselors, social workers, teachers, and administrators. Survey results indicated that school personnel that participated in the training became more aware of the mental and emotional needs and health issues of LGBTQ students. They were also more appreciative of the need for allies in schools and were committed to demonstrating support as allies for these vulnerable students (CDC, 2013b). This example demonstrates how cultural competency training and partnerships could be effective in improving attitudes and support for diverse student groups. Using cultural relevant strategies, including cultural competency training, is important in designing WSCC programs that would be effective in meeting the needs of diverse students, families, and communities.

Considering the multitude of issues that affect many diverse groups, a multilevel approach is needed. For example, many homeless students may have to deal with both academic issues and exposure to violence and substance abuse (Kilmer, Cook, Crusto, et al., 2012). Therefore, their needs may require not only academic attention but also psychological, medical, and social services. In its fullest form, WSCC can be designed to provide such comprehensive support. Cultural considerations and appropriate strategies for serving diverse students, families, and communities should be considered for each component of WSCC.

Often used as a framework for prevention, the **social ecological model** is a useful framework to identify, understand, and address the range of cultural considerations for each component of WSCC. The social ecological model takes into account the complex connections and interplay between factors at the individual, relationship, institutional, community, and societal levels (McLeroy, Bibeau, Steckler, & Glanz, 1988). Examples of factors at each level of the model include individual-level factors (e.g., child's personal characteristics and demographics); relationship-level factors (e.g., characteristics of the family, relationship with teachers, peers); institutional-level factors (e.g., characteristics of a school or health care organization including its procedures, practices, policies); community-level factors (e.g., relationships between the school and the neighborhood); and societal-level factors (e.g., social and cultural norms, health, economic, educational, and social laws and policies). In figure 7.3 the social ecological model is used as a framework to indicate specific cultural considerations for each of the 10 components of the WSCC approach.

FIGURE 7.3
Cultural Considerations for WSCC Components

Health Education

INDIVIDUAL LEVEL

- Education among health education teachers about particular health beliefs, practices, and attitudes of diverse students, families, and community
- Cultural competency training provided to health education teachers

INTERPERSONAL LEVEL

- Communication with students and families about health issues, needs, barriers, preferences, and strategies
- Participation among students in the development and implementation of health education activities (e.g., student peer trainers as part of a tobacco cessation program)

ORGANIZATIONAL LEVEL

- Implementation of new forms of health education practices that appeal to current generation of students and young parents (e.g., using text massages as form of communication with parents or students)
- Brochures, pamphlets, videos, written materials, documents, and so on that depict diverse groups or individuals in health education materials
- Materials written at low literacy levels
- Bilingual health education materials

COMMUNITY LEVEL

- Partnership with community organizations to promote health education (e.g., partnering with local university black sorority/fraternity groups to conduct a smoking cessation campaign at a high school)

(continued)

Figure 7.3 *(continued)*

POLICY LEVEL

- Assessment of policies and practices that affect students, families, and communities as they pertain to physical education and physical activity
- Family and community involvement in the assessment, development, implementation, or monitoring of school physical education and physical activity policies

Physical Education and Physical Activity

INDIVIDUAL LEVEL

- Education and awareness among physical education teachers about health beliefs, practices, and attitudes of diverse students, families, and community and physical activities
- Cultural competency training provided to physical education teachers

INTERPERSONAL LEVEL

- Communication with students and parents about physical education and physical activity
- Participation among students in the development and implementation of physical education and physical activity programs and projects

ORGANIZATIONAL LEVEL

- Incorporation of nontraditional, interesting, stimulating forms of physical education and physical activity (e.g., yoga, music)
- Physical education- and physical activity-related brochures, pamphlets, videos, and written materials and documents that depict diverse groups or individuals

COMMUNITY LEVEL

- Partnership with community organizations that serve diverse populations (e.g., YMCA, students from local Historically Black College or University's Physical Education program, a tribal organization's Pow Wow)

POLICY LEVEL

- Assessment of policies and practices that affect students, families, and communities as they pertain to physical education and physical activity
- Family and community involvement in the assessment, development, implementation, and monitoring of school physical education and physical activity policies

Nutrition Environment and Services

INDIVIDUAL LEVEL

- Education among nutrition administration and staff and cafeteria staff about nutrition and dietary beliefs, practices, and attitudes of students, families, and community
- Supplementary nutrition and cooking classes and training for cafeteria staff as needed to facilitate the inclusion of culturally diverse foods and cuisines in school menu

INTERPERSONAL LEVEL

- Communication with students and families about nutrition issues, needs, concerns, barriers, preferences for food options, and strategies

ORGANIZATIONAL LEVEL

- Integration of various cultural foods into school menu (e.g., healthily cooked chicken such as oven-fried chicken; various cuisines offered once a month)

COMMUNITY LEVEL

- Partnership with or involvement of diverse community groups, organizations, or services (e.g., a Lebanese family-owned restaurant catering food at a school event; church league providing baked items for sale at a school carnival)

POLICY LEVEL

- Assessment of school nutrition policies and practices designed to meet the needs of diverse student groups
- Family and community involvement in the assessment, development, implementation, or monitoring of school nutrition policies

Health Services

INDIVIDUAL LEVEL

- Education among health services staff about health beliefs, practices, and attitudes of diverse students, families, and communities
- Cultural competency training among health services staff

INTERPERSONAL LEVEL

- Communication with students and families about health issues, needs, barriers, preferences, and current services
- Faculty, staff, and volunteers who meet linguistic needs of students and parents, especially at school events

ORGANIZATIONAL LEVEL

- Organizational self-assessment of cultural and linguistic competence (e.g., assessment of linguistic services, bilingual clinic forms, depiction of diverse groups on clinic brochures and pamphlets, culturally trained staff)
- Participation among students in the development and implementation of health services (e.g., student representatives on the school's health and health services committee)

COMMUNITY LEVEL

- Partnership with community organizations to enhance or supplement services to meet needs of diverse students (e.g., collaboration with clinic that serves primarily Latinos to provide cultural competency to school staff
- Involvement and input from community (e.g., diverse community advisory group or board for health services)

(continued)

Figure 7.3 *(continued)*

POLICY LEVEL

- Assessment of health services policies and practices that affect students, families, and communities
- Family and community involvement in the assessment, development, implementation, or monitoring of school health services policies

Counseling, Psychological, and Social Services

INDIVIDUAL LEVEL

- Education among counseling, psychological, and social services school personnel about psychosocial beliefs, practices, and attitudes of diverse students, families, and community
- Cultural competency training among counseling, psychological, and social services school personnel

INTERPERSONAL LEVEL

- Communication with students and families about counseling, psychological, and social service issues (e.g., school psychologist's meeting with middle school parents to discuss how to identify and address depression in children)

ORGANIZATIONAL LEVEL

- Use of nontraditional sources of assistance (e.g., consulting with traditional health healers)
- Inventory of diverse community services that could help meet the cultural, socioeconomic, and social environmental needs of students and their families
- Participation among students in the development and implementation of certain counseling, psychological, or social service programs and activities (e.g., a student peer-led support group for children with learning disabilities)

COMMUNITY LEVEL

- Partnership with community organizations (e.g., having a domestic violence prevention organization that targets young low-income families to talk to students about domestic and intimate partner violence)

POLICY LEVEL

- Assessment of current policies and practices designed to meet the needs of diverse student groups regarding counseling, psychological, and social services
- Family and community involvement in the assessment, development, implementation, or monitoring of school policies that promote culturally relevant counseling, psychological, and social services

Social and Emotional Climate

INDIVIDUAL LEVEL

- Education among appropriate school personnel about social and emotional issues that affect diverse student, family, and community members

- Cultural competency training provided to appropriate school personnel to assist in communicating with and understanding the social and emotional needs of diverse students

INTERPERSONAL LEVEL

- Participation among students in the development and implementation of activities that promote healthy social and emotional school environments (e.g., a student advocacy project)
- Meetings that include students, families, or community members to address social and emotional health concerns that affect special student populations (e.g., fifth-grade parent group led by counselor to discuss bullying among immigrant children)

ORGANIZATIONAL LEVEL

- Regular input obtained from students and families about the school's social and learning environment (e.g., annual questionnaire)
- Organizational self-assessment of cultural and linguistic competence (e.g., assessment of interpreter services; depiction of diverse groups on school brochures, pamphlets, and videos)

COMMUNITY LEVEL

- Partnership with community organizations to promote a healthy social and emotional school environment (e.g., collaboration with LGBTQ organization to talk with students about bullying)

POLICY LEVEL

- Assessment of policies and practices that affect the social and emotional environment of students (e.g., examining policies that promote nonviolent interaction on the playground, in class, and among students while taking student culture into account)
- Family and community involvement in the assessment, development, implementation, or monitoring of school policies that promote healthy social and emotional environments

Physical Environment

INDIVIDUAL LEVEL

- Education and awareness among appropriate school personnel about physical environmental health issues common to diverse students (e.g., health risks associated with poor indoor air quality in schools located in poor, rural communities)
- Cultural competency training provided to school personnel to assist in communicating about physical environmental issues and concerns to diverse students, families, and communities

INTERPERSONAL LEVEL

- Involvement of families in projects that address physical environmental health issues (e.g., a parent–teacher organization project to promote safer routes and

(continued)

Figure 7.3 *(continued)*

personal safety among students who walk to schools in neighborhoods with high crime rates)

- Participation among students in the development and implementation of a healthy physical environment (e.g., a student-driven awareness campaign about maintaining clean and properly functioning gym equipment)

ORGANIZATIONAL LEVEL

- Regular input obtained from students and families about the school's physical environment
- Visual depictions and representations of diverse student groups and populations in promoting a healthy environment (e.g., diverse students in a flyer about litter prevention)

COMMUNITY LEVEL

- Partnership with community organizations to promote a healthy physical school environment (e.g., collaboration with transportation agency or law enforcement to provide safe passages between homes and schools for children)

POLICY LEVEL

- Regular assessment of physical environmental policies and practices regarding biological, physical, and chemical threats that put diverse students at risk
- Community involvement in establishing policies and practices needed to promote healthy physical environments

Employee Wellness

INDIVIDUAL LEVEL

- Education and awareness among faculty and staff of health and wellness activities that could positively influence students and families (e.g., providing examples of how to model healthy and culturally inclusive health behaviors to students)

INTERPERSONAL LEVEL

- Involvement of students and families with faculty and staff wellness activities (e.g., annual 5K walk)

ORGANIZATIONAL LEVEL

- Regular input obtained from students and families about strategies that can facilitate their involvement with joint health and wellness activities

COMMUNITY LEVEL

- Partnerships with community organizations to sponsor or help organize wellness activities that include families and community members

POLICY LEVEL

- Assessment of school policies and practices that encourage collaborative health and wellness activities between faculty and staff and others (students, families, communities)

Family Engagement

INDIVIDUAL LEVEL

- Education and awareness among school personnel about issues and needs that are important to students and families
- Periodic cultural competency training provided to school personnel about effective strategies to use in communicating with diverse families and communities

INTERPERSONAL LEVEL

- Family participation in programs and activities (e.g., parents serving on a planning committee for a family fun day at school)
- Parent helpers and school volunteers that represent race and ethnicity of student populations

ORGANIZATIONAL LEVEL

- Regular input obtained from families about needs and strategies to address them
- Diverse family participation in parent–teacher organizations
- School personnel or volunteers to meet linguistic needs of students and parents, especially at school events
- Literacy-appropriate information distributed to parents
- Appropriate, feasible days and times for school activities and events (e.g., evening hour activities, occasional Saturday events)
- Inventory of family-related resources to make available to families (e.g., domestic violence shelters, sources for homeless families, soup kitchens, social service and government agencies)

COMMUNITY LEVEL

- Partnerships with family-oriented agencies in community (e.g., counselor's collaboration with local therapy clinic in hosting evening session on stress management)

POLICY LEVEL

- Assessment of policies and practices regarding family engagement
- Family involvement in the assessment, development, implementation, and monitoring of school policies that promote family engagement.

Community Involvement

INDIVIDUAL LEVEL

- Education and awareness among school personnel about issues and needs that are important to the community
- Periodic cultural competency training provided to school personnel about effective communication and collaboration with diverse communities

(continued)

Figure 7.3 *(continued)*

INTERPERSONAL LEVEL

- Participation of community members in the development and implementation of school programs and activities (e.g., students serving on a planning committee for a family fun day at school)
- Community volunteers that represent race and ethnicity of student populations

ORGANIZATIONAL LEVEL

- Accessible space or facilities (e.g., allowing monthly meeting of a civic group in school's cafeteria)
- Regular input obtained from community (e.g., school or district's community advisory committee)

COMMUNITY LEVEL

- Connection of school activities to community cultural events (e.g., cultural arts festivals, Dr. Martin Luther King celebrations, Cinco de Mayo)
- Collaboration with community organizations to provide important resources or opportunities (e.g., literacy, health literacy, Graduate Record Examination (GRE) classes, and so on)

POLICY LEVEL

- Assessment of current policies and practices regarding community engagement
- Community involvement in the assessment, development, implementation, and monitoring of school policies

Based on McLeroy et al. 1998.

SUMMARY

As the United States becomes more culturally diverse (U.S. Census Bureau, 2010), school systems need to become responsive to the needs of diverse students. In addition, as disparities in health among children continue to rise (e.g., obesity, autism), other models of involvement might be required. Currently, many diverse students are faced with complex, multilevel, interrelated challenges that hinder the effectiveness of traditional methods. Effective strategies to address these issues call for genuine collaborations, cultural sensitivity, and culturally appropriate strategies. Sufficient student connectedness, family engagement, and community involvement among diverse populations require mutual respect, trust, and shared power and decision making (Brewster & Railsback, 2003). Although schools must devote significant effort and time to these efforts, the majority of students and the broader community could benefit. Using culturally competent approaches within WSCC to promote school connectedness among diverse students, strengthen family involvement, and increase community engagement will be an important step.

Glossary

community-based participatory research (CBPR)—The community or its representatives are equal partners and are involved in each phase of the research project, from conceptualization to dissemination of information.

community participatory approaches—Community members or their representatives are involved in some or all phases of a project or activity (e.g., development, implementation, or evaluation of a project).

cultural competence—A set of values, behaviors, attitudes, practices, and policies within an organization or program or among staff that enables people to work effectively with diverse groups.

culturally sensitive—Being aware of and respecting cultural differences.

family engagement—A wide range of activities through which parents, grandparents, older siblings, tribal members, and other members of students' extended family contribute to and support student learning.

literacy—Using printed and written information to function in society, to achieve goals, and to develop knowledge and potential.

school connectedness—Belief held by students that adults and peers in the school care about their learning as well as about them as individuals.

social ecological model—An approach for health education and health promotion that takes into account the connections and interplay between factors at the individual, relationship, institutional, community, and societal levels.

Application Activities

1. Write an article for a newspaper that describes a hypothetical school that uses the culturally relevant strategies presented in figure 7.1. Write the article as if you visited the school and observed the use of specific strategies in various components of the WSCC approach.
2. Using the information from figure 7.2, interview a school administrator to determine a school or school district's application of the social ecological model to the WSCC approach to school health promotion. Develop a written report with your observations about the application at each level for each component and, if appropriate, provide recommendations for improvement for each component. This activity could be a group activity in which several students conduct the interview and each student writes a selected component of the report.
3. Search the Internet for a website that you believe can be a valuable tool for school faculty and staff in the development and enhancement of cultural competency. Provide a brief summary of the content on the site and the way in which that information can be useful to schools.

Resources

Centers for Disease Control and Prevention. 2009. *School Connectedness: Strategies for Increasing Protective Factors among Youth.* Atlanta, GA: U.S. Department of Health and Human Services. www.cdc.gov/healthyyouth/adolescenthealth/pdf/connectedness.pdf

Hutchins, Darcy J., Greenfeld, Marsha D., Epstein, Joyce L., Sanders, Mavis G., & Galindo, Claudia L. 2012. *Multicultural Partnerships: Involve All Families.* New York: Routledge.

Klotz, Mary Beth. 2006, March. Culturally Competent Schools: Guidelines for Secondary School Principals. *Student Counseling, PL*, 11–14.

References

ASCD. 2014. *Whole School, Whole Community, Whole Child: A Collaborative Approach to Learning and Health.* Alexandria, Virginia: ASCD. www.ascd.org/ASCD/pdf/siteASCD/publications/wholechild/wscc-a-collaborative-approach.pdf

American Lung Association in Wisconsin. 2013. *Not on Tobacco (N-O-T).* www.lung.org/associations/states/wisconsin/events-programs/not-on-tobacco-n-o-t/

Anderson-Butcher, Dawn, & Ashton, Deb. 2004. Innovative Models of Collaboration to Serve Children, Youths, Families, and Communities. *Children and Schools*, *26*, 39–53.

Austin, Greg, Nakamoto, Jonathan, & Bailey, Jerry. *Racial/Ethnic Differences in School Performance, Engagement, Safety, and Supports. CHKS Factsheet #9.* Los Alamitos, CA: WestEd. http://chks.wested.org/using_results/publications

Basch, Charles E. 2011. Healthier Students Are Better Learners: A Missing Link in School Reforms to Close the Achievement Gap. *Journal of School Health*, *81*, 593–598.

Basch, Charles E. 2011. Healthier Students Are Better Learners: High-Quality, Strategically Planned, and Effectively Coordinated School Health Programs Must be a Fundamental Mission of Schools to Help Close the Achievement Gap. *Journal of School Health*, *81*, 650–662.

Brewster, Cori, Railsback, Jennifer, and Office of Planning and Service Coordination. 2003. *Building Trust With Schools and Diverse Families: A Foundation for Lasting Partnerships.* Portland, OR: Northwest Regional Educational Laboratory.

Bustamante, Arturo Vargas, & Van der Wees, Philip J. 2012. Integrating Immigrants Into the U.S. Health System. *Virtual Mentor*, *14*, 318–323.

Center for Mental Health in Schools at UCLA. 2011. *Immigrant Children and Youth: Enabling Their Success at School*. http://smhp.psych.ucla.edu/pdfdocs/immigrant.pdf

Centers for Disease Control and Prevention, Division of Adolescent and School Health. 2007. *Interventions and Strategies to Improve Health and Increase Academic Performance Among Groups Experiencing Health Disparities: Gasden County, FL*. www.cdc.gov/healthyyouth/stories/pdf/2007/success_cshp.pdf

Centers for Disease Control and Prevention. 2009a. *School Connectedness: Strategies for Increasing Protective Factors Among Youth,* Atlanta, GA: U.S. Department of Health and Human Services.

Centers for Disease Control and Prevention, Division of Adolescent and School Health. 2009b. Wisconsin: Building Healthier Schools to Foster Healthier Students. In *School Health Programs: Success Stories From the Field 2009.* www.cdc.gov/nccdphp/publications/aag/pdf/dash_success.pdf

Centers for Disease Control and Prevention, Division of Adolescent and School Health. 2013a. Michigan: Establishing Safe and Supportive School Environments. In *2012 Success Stories: State and Local Organization Examples* (pp. 8–9). www.cdc.gov/healthyyouth/stories/pdf/ss_booklet_0713.pdf

Centers for Disease Control and Prevention and Division of Adolescent and School Health. 2013b. Allies Matter: Creating Safe School Environments for North Carolina's LGBT Youth. In *2012 Success Stories: State and Local Organization Examples* (pp. 11–12). www.cdc.gov/healthyyouth/stories/pdf/ss_booklet_0713.pdf

Epstein, Joyce L., Sanders, Mavis G., Sheldon, Steven B., Simon, Beth S., Salinas, Karen Clark, Jansoon, Natalie Rodriguez, Van Voorhis, Francis L., Martin, Celia S., Thomas, Brenda J., Greenfeld, Marsha D., Hutchinson, Darcy J., & Williams, Keyatta J. 2009. *School, Family, and Community Partnerships: Your Handbook for Action*. Thousand Oaks, CA: Corwin Press.

Flores, Glenn, and the Committee on Pediatric Research. 2010. Racial and Ethnic Disparities in the Health and Health Care of Children. *Pediatrics*, *125*, e979.

Fuller, Bruce, & Coll, Cynthia Garcia. 2010. Learning from Latinos: Contexts, Families, and Child Development in Motion. *Developmental Psychology*, *46*, 359–365.

Henderson, Anne T., & Mapp, Karen L. 2002. *A New Wave of Evidence: The Impact of School, Family, and Community Connections on Student Achievement*. Austin, TX: Southwest Educational Development Laboratory, National Center for Family, and Community Connections With Schools.

Kann, Laura, O'Malley, Emily, McManus, Tim, Kinchen, Steve, Chyen, David, Harris, William A., & Wechsler, Howell. 2011. Sexual Identity, Sex of Sexual Contacts, and Health-Risk Behaviors Among Students in Grades 9–12—Youth Risk Behavior Surveillance, Selected Sites, United States, 2001–2009. *Morbidity and Mortality Weekly Report*, 60, 1–133.

Kilmer, Ryan P., Cook, James R., Crusto, Cindy, Strater, Katherine P., & Haber, Mason G. 2012. Understanding the Ecology and Development of Children and Families Experiencing Homelessness: Implications for Practice, Supportive Services, and Policy. *American Journal of Orthopsychiatry*, *82*, 389-401.

Krishnaswami, Janani, Martinson, Marty, Wakimoto, Patricia, & Anglemeyer, Andrew. 2012. Community-Engaged Interventions on Diet, Activity, and Weight Outcomes in U.S. Schools. *American Journal of Preventive Medicine*, *43*, 81–91.

Kutner, Mark, Greenberg, Elizabeth, & Baer, Justin. 2006. *1992 National Adult Literacy Survey and 2003 National Assessment of Adult Literacy* (NCES 2006-470). Washington, DC: National Center for Education Statistics, Institute of Education Sciences, U.S. Department of Education.

Mansour, Mona E., Kotagal, Uma, Rose, Barbara, Ho, Mona, Brewer, David, Roy-Chaudhury, Ashwini, Homung, Richard W., Wade, Terrance J., & DeWitt, Thomas J. 2003. Health-Related Quality of Life in Urban Elementary School Children. *Pediatrics*, *111*, 1372–81.

McLeroy, Kenneth R., Bibeau, Daniel, Steckler, Allan, & Glanz, Karen. 1988. An Ecological Perspective on Health Promotion Programs. *Health Education Quarterly*, *15*, 351–377.

McLoyd, Vonnie C. 1998. Changing Demographics in the American Population: Implications for Research on Minority Children and Adolescents. In Vonnie C. McLoyd & Laurence D. Steinberg (eds.), *Studying Minority Adolescents: Conceptual, Methodological, and Theoretical Issues* (pp. 3–28). Mahwah, NJ: Erlbaum.

Mendez, Julia L. 2010. How Can Parents Get Involved in Preschool? Barriers and Engagement in Education by Ethnic Minority Parents of Children Attending Health Start Programs. *Cultural Diversity and Ethnic Minority Psychology*, *16*, 26–36.

Minkler, Meredith, & Wallerstein, Nina. 2008. *Community-Based Participatory Research for Health: From Process to Outcomes*. San Francisco: Wiley.

National Center on Family Homelessness. 2009. *Annual Report of the National Center on Family Homelessness*. Newton, MA: Author. www.familyhomelessness.org/media/88.pdf

U.S. Census Bureau. 2010. *American Fact Finder 2010*. http://factfinder.census.gov

U.S. Department of Health and Human Services, Office of Disease Prevention and Health Promotion. 2010. *Healthy People 2020*. Washington, DC: Author. http://healthypeople.gov/2020

Vaughn, Emogene Johnson. 2008. Cultural Competence and Health Education. In Miguel A. Perez & Raffey R. Luquis (Eds.), *Cultural Competence in Health Education and Health Promotion* (pp. 43–65). San Francisco: Jossey-Bass.

Wallerstein, Nina, & Duran, Bonnie. 2010. Community-Based Participatory Research Contributions to Intervention Research: The Intersection of Science and Practice to Improve Health Equity. *American Journal of Public Health, S1*, S40–S46.

Weiler, Erica. 2001. Safe and Affirmative Schools of Sexual Minority Youth. *Pathways to Tolerance*, 1–3.

Wisconsin Department of Public Instruction. 2005. *Wisconsin Success Stores: Tobacco Free Youth*. Madison, WI: Author.

8

Community Involvement

BONNI C. HODGES • LISA ANGERMEIER

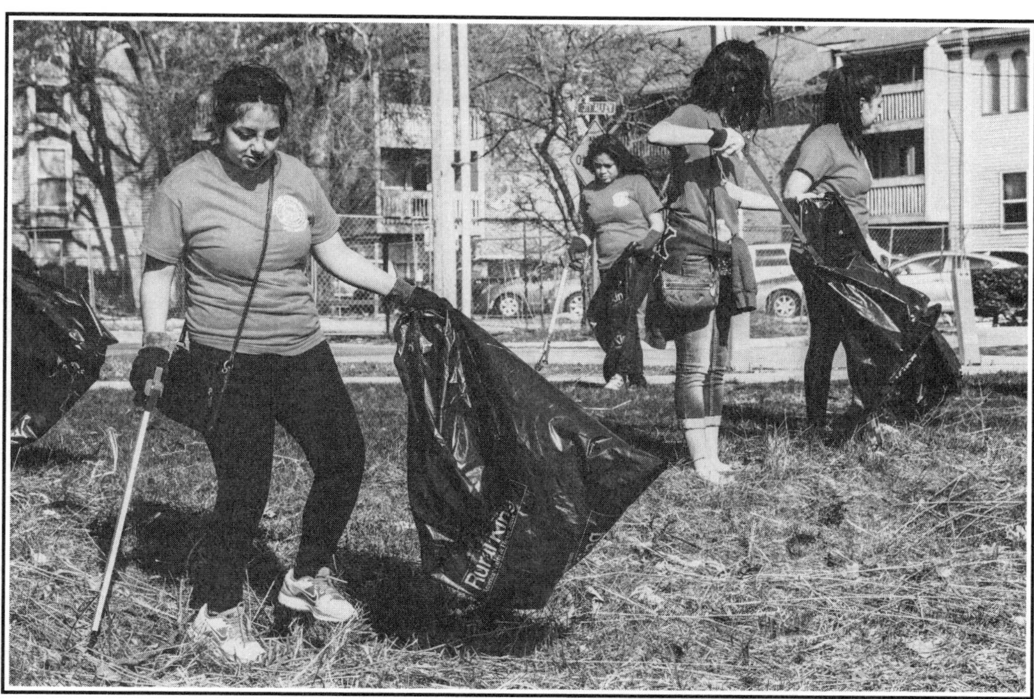

Community involvement is essential to the Whole School, Whole Community, Whole Child (WSCC) approach. With the increasing recognition of the value of a broad ecological approach to youth development concerning both health and academic success, community involvement becomes more prominent as an important strategy (CDC, 2012, 2009; Bronfenbrenner, 1979). Engaging community members and community agencies allows schools and communities to address their health and academic challenges more effectively (Adelman & Taylor, 2011). Historically, many implicit and explicit barriers have worked against integrated planning between schools and community agencies and institutions for youth health and well-being (Hodges et al., 2011).

Strong collaborations among schools, community agencies, and community members are the foundation of ASCD's Whole Child approach and Healthy School Communities initiative (Valois et al., 2011; ASCD, n.d.a, n.d.b). ASCD's Whole Child approach, "ensuring that each child, in each school, in each community, is healthy, safe, engaged, supported and challenged," includes community collaboration as one of its primary indicators (ASCD, n.d.c, p. 1). The Healthy School Communities effort seeks to create environments that support the Whole Child concept through school–community collaborations, strong school leadership, a systems approach to supporting physical and emotional well-being of those in school buildings, the creation of a healthy environment, and data-driven decisions (ASCD, n.d.b). Adelman and Taylor point to the need for a paradigm shift from "marginalized and fragmented set of student services" (2011, p. 9) to a multifaceted system of coordinated and interconnected supports to provide students ways to get around the myriad and complex barriers that interfere with learning.

One of ASCD's nine levers of school change, community stakeholder engagement and collaboration, is seen as a necessary component to creating and using a systems approach to school improvements (ASCD, n.d.b). These community stakeholders need to be engaged in meaningful dialog and problem solving through all phases of planning, implementation, and evaluation.

This chapter addresses advantages to school–community collaborations, stages of collaboration, and barriers to school–community collaboration and provides direction and examples for building strong collaborations.

NEED FOR SCHOOL–COMMUNITY COLLABORATIONS

School–community collaborations can increase and improve the efficiency and effectiveness of programs and services for all collaborators and creates structure supporting the Whole Child concept (ASCD, n.d.a, n.d.b). Quality collaborations involve representation across all areas of the **socioecological framework** (see figure 8.1) (Bronfenbrenner, 1979), which creates connectedness and increases the credibility, buy-in, follow-through, and **institutionalization** of the resulting collaborative programs and services (Hodges et al., 2012). The socioecological framework nests the child in the center of layers of broadening environments that have direct and indirect effects on the child's development. The layer that immediately surrounds the child, the microsystem, directly affects the child's development. This layer consists of such elements as the child's family, peers, and school. The interactions of elements within this layer create the next outward layer, the mesosystem. The mesosystem also has a direct effect on the child. Surrounding these two layers is the exosystem and the macrosystem. One can think of these systems as containing the many systems that shape how we experience our lives but with which the child has no direct interaction. But the actions of the systems in this layer have an indirect effect on the child. Looking at the area of nutrition and diet, the socioecological framework suggests to us that what

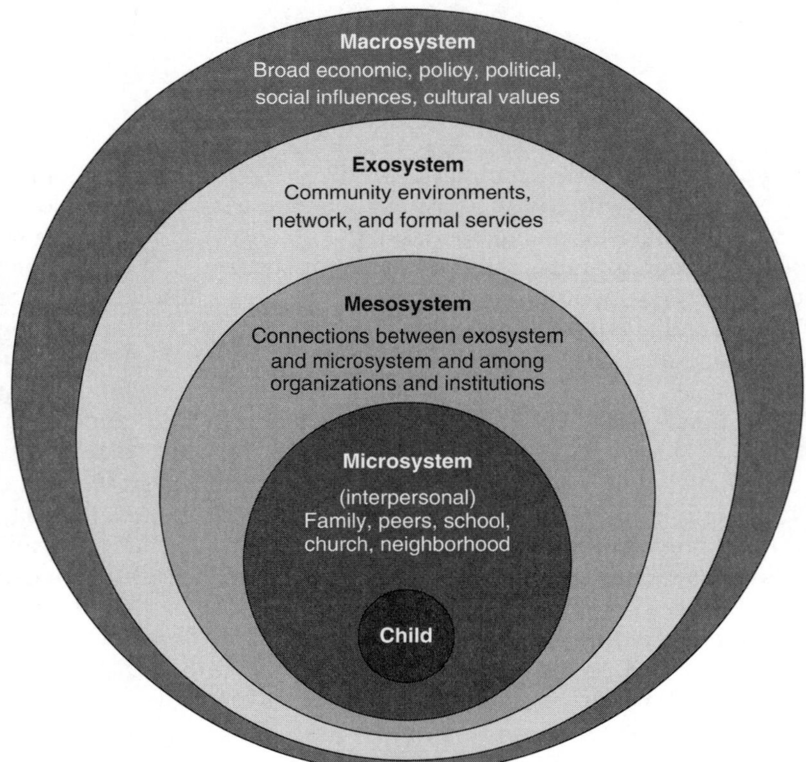

Figure 8.1 Bronfenbrenner's socioecological framework.

Adapted, by permission, from U. Bronfenbrenner, 1979. Available: http://faculty.weber.edu/Hday/human.development/ecological.htm

an elementary-school-aged child eats is directly affected by what the parents and the school serve the child at meal and snack times (microsystem), that what is appropriate for school snack time can be affected by the collaboration of parents and the school to determine a healthy snack policy (mesosystem), and that what is served for school lunches can be affected by school lunch services (exosystem) and cultural norms (macrosystem). The WSCC surrounds the "whole child" with the school health components, which in turn are surrounded by the community. This notion clearly shows the influence of Bronfenbrenner's ideas. The positive effects of these systems on the health and academic development of children are greater when the systems are in alignment and working together.

Beyond these outcomes, increased efficiency arises through sharing services, staff, expertise, funding, space and facilities, and programming among community members and with community organizations. This sharing assists schools and community organizations in their ability to use resources available to them for the support of health and academic growth and overall development of youth (Ferguson et al., 2010).

Well-planned and well-executed school–community collaborations have the potential to develop program goals and objectives collaboratively and increase the effectiveness of efforts to improve health and academic performance. The inclusion of a broad representation of stakeholders allows collaborators to take into account a multitude of factors and perspectives when developing goals and objectives and planning programs and services. Moreover, when designed appropriately, school–community collaborations create and sustain community-wide structures and systems that reflect the Whole Child approach. These collaborations support positive health and academic growth and development wherever a person might be in a community and throughout the person's lifetime by purposefully connecting the home, the school, and the wider community (Ferguson et al., 2010; Henderson et al., 2007; Weiss et al., 2009).

STAGES OF COLLABORATION

To realize the full benefits of the WSCC approach, a variety of collaborators need to work together. Benham-Deal and Hodges (2009) have identified the following practices to consider in creating successful collaborations:

- Those who embody the 10 components of the WSCC within an individual school or school district community need to collaborate on the development and coordination of policies, practices, and processes; those who lead health promotion efforts need to collaborate with classroom teachers and other staff in delivering policies, programs, and services.
- Faculty and staff need to collaborate with administrators and school board members.
- Those in schools need to collaborate with parents and guardians.
- Those in schools need to collaborate with people and institutions in the community.

To define collaboration further, Gardner (1998) provides a useful way to think about various levels of collaboration (figure 8.2).

The first stage of Gardner's collaboration is information exchange and relationship building. During this stage collaborators learn about each other as people and organizations, learn to communicate using terms that are understandable by all partners and free of jargon, and explore opportunities for collaboration (Gardner, 1998). This stage begins when one or more leaders of a potential collaborator initiate a meeting or create a structure for relationship building among one or more collaborators. For example, the school health coordinator convenes a meeting of the

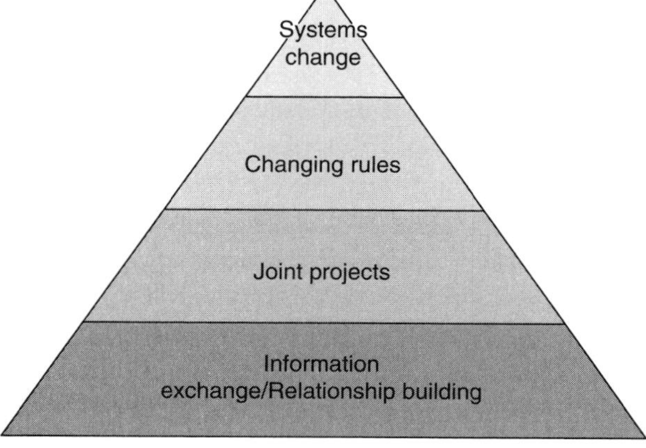

Figure 8.2 Gardner's four stages of collaboration.

Gardner, 1998, "Beyond collaboration to results: Hard choices in the future of services to children and families," (Arizona Prevention Resource Center and the Center for Collaboration for Children), 6–9.

district health council consisting of representatives of all 10 WSCC components, administrative leadership, and other key stakeholders from the community to explore how they may assist one another.

When collaborators identify specific actions that can be taken together, the collaboration moves to the joint projects level. Key to this stage is the dedication of resources from each collaborator for a shared purpose or project (Gardner, 1998). The focus at this stage is on the partners' implementation of a project designed to achieve one or more goals and objectives of the collaboration. Resources may include money, facilities, staff, and access to populations. Consider these examples:

- A health care organization and a school may collaborate on a school-based health clinic in which the school provides the facility (space in the school) and the health care organization provides the staff and the service.
- A school may provide access to students, families, and facilities to a community organization for after-school literacy and wellness programs.
- A school district may share access to its families with a public health department for a program to get families enrolled in health insurance plans.

Collaborative projects can be beneficial and supportive of WSCC yet still suffer from a lack of **sustainability**, an inability to expand, or difficulty in achieving larger goals and objectives. Numerous barriers and challenges to school–community collaborations and sustainability of joint projects have been identified (Hodges & Videto, 2012), but longstanding collaborations and joint projects do provide a foundation for moving up Gardner's pyramid by building on and expanding these existing relationships. **SEDL** (Ferguson et al., 2010) points out the need for a "shift from a patchwork of random acts of involvement to a systematic approach" (p. 18).

The next two levels of collaboration work to create a situation in which partners can more fully integrate into each other's environments by allowing for joint projects that then arise from mutual perspectives rather than complementary perspectives. At the changing rules level, collaborators engage in broad policy changes that are intended to eliminate barriers to collaboration and collaborative projects and to support mutually determined and mutually beneficial goals and objectives. This level often includes cross-training of staff or joint funding of staff (Gardner, 1998). For example, a school strengthens its wellness policy so that it supports the local health department's nutrition goals. This action alone not only changes the rules to support community health goals, but it also opens the way for the local health department to work with school personnel on such joint projects as faculty and staff nutrition education and school lunch program initiatives.

Systems change is created over time with top-down support that signals and reinforces a cultural shift (Gardner, 1998). For systems change to occur, the leaders of the collaborative partners need to embrace the cultural shift, articulate the shift and its vision to all staff, actively seek knowledge of barriers to achieving goals, and seek and receive strategies for overcoming them. Collaborative goals and objectives are identified, measured, reported, and discussed across all collaborators, indicating the institutionalization of the goals and objectives across levels of organizational staff.

SEDL (Ferguson et al., 2010) notes the difference between random involvement and systematic involvement. Random involvement is an individual or small committee, often handpicked, that develops a policy that is shared in consideration for adoption. In contrast, systematic involvement is an individual or committee that uses an inclusive process to build a policy, shares drafts widely, and refines those drafts based on sincerely sought feedback from a wide variety of stakeholders. Systematic involvement requires that stakeholders work together to determine what needs to be done and that all stakeholders benefit rather than one of the stakeholders (the school) asking the others (the community agencies) to do something specific for them.

Thus, school health systems create overarching prevention and youth development goals and address them through integrated efforts both within and across school and community entities. The WSCC approach provides structure for school health systems change within schools and school districts. In addition, it provides the foundation for school–community collaboration around the Whole Child concept (ASCD, n.d.a) through its community involvement component.

BARRIERS TO COLLABORATION

A review of the literature on school–community collaboration suggests that much of the collaboration is occurring at the lowest two of Gardner's stages (Sulkowski, 2011; Grier & Bradley-King, 2011) and often does not evolve beyond the information-sharing stage (Hodges et al., 2011, 2012). It is useful to identify and important to understand common barriers and challenges to effective school–community collaboration. A number of barriers have been identified from the work of those trying to improve school–community collaborations (see figure 8.3).

Broad barriers and challenges exist around the **siloing** that often occurs within schools and school districts, as well as between schools and community agencies and institutions. This separation tends to takes place in an environment where people focus narrowly on their piece or what they think their piece is, thus missing opportunities to enhance their abilities to realize common goals and objectives that have a positive effect on outcomes for which they are directly responsible (Hodges et al., 2011, 2012). The siloing within school districts creates several disincentives for school–community collaborations (Hodges et al. 2011, 2012; Weist et al., 2012). Community agencies have reported that obtaining the multiple approval levels (e.g., building-level individuals or committees, district level, board of education) often required to do work in the schools can be a lengthy process that can have a deleterious effect on timely program and policy development and implementation and serves as a disincentive to working in collaboration with schools (Hodges et al., 2011, 2012). Some perceive that schools and school districts choose to remain in their silos and connect with community organizations only when those organizations can do something for the school or district.

The first step in moving out of the silo should be for schools to have a stronger, more active presence in existing coalitions or other groups in which schools have current representation. Community groups have reported that schools have a seat on most community coalitions that involve youth development and health but are often not active with those groups (Hodges et al., 2011, 2012). Schools can seek collaborations with relevant and appropriate groups and stakeholders to engage in two-way relationship building. Schools seeking collaborations need to be inclusive and involve a wide range of stakeholders in planning potential collaborations. After establishing these collaborations, the partners should work toward moving beyond the joint projects stage.

Lack of clear administrative leadership for school health is a barrier both to school–community collaborations and to establishing a fully functioning WSCC approach within a district (Hodges et al., 2011, 2012). This lack of administrative leadership may take the form of a clear separation between the WSCC components, such as with health-related services and classroom health education, or the absence of a full and functioning school health team. Without clear administrative leadership, potential collaborators do not know with whom they need to connect. Moreover, without school health leadership, promising collaborative initiatives are not seen as a priority for implementation and can get lost in

FIGURE 8.3

Barriers to School–Community Collaboration

School district in a silo
Unclear or undefined leadership for school health; school health efforts individual driven, not district driven
Not recognizing shared vision, values, and goals
Lack of effective communication
Perceived and real budgetary constraints
Protecting turf
Past negative experiences
Failure to recognize health systems and links to academic success
Implementation issues

a maze of approvals and requests for resources. Lack of clear administrative leadership creates school health initiatives that are individual driven rather than district driven. Individual-driven initiatives result in school health that is neither collaborative nor systematic, decreasing the effect and greatly hampering the ability to sustain successful initiatives.

As part of their role and responsibilities in active leadership of WSCC, school administrators and school boards are vital to fostering welcoming structures for school–community collaborations. School boards and school administrators can provide leadership for collaboration in school health by creating policies and structures that enable WSCC to be fully implemented (Adelman & Taylor, 2011; CSBA, 2009). Communicating the roles and responsibilities and identifying those in charge of and involved with the WSCC approach, both within and outside the school structure, provides entry points for those seeking to collaborate. School administrators are key players in identifying and connecting with potential collaboration partners.

Lack of recognition of shared vision, values, and goals among schools and community agencies and organizations presents another barrier to collaboration (Hodges et al., 2011, 2012; Weist et al., 2012; Mastro et al., 2006; CSBA, 2009). This lack of recognition may be the result of various types of terminology that causes an appearance of a difference in vision, values, and goals. Without this common vision, a climate can be created that prevents schools from recognizing how numerous institutions are charged with and trying to improve the health of youth and children. Schools that expand the concept of school to include the community are more likely to look for and to see where community groups share vision, values, and goals. Active participation in community coalitions by school representatives can help schools see commonalities. Schools and community agencies and groups should work to help each other understand the meanings of discipline and group-specific jargon and work toward the development of a common terminology for their work so that all stakeholders can understand.

Lack of effective communication among school staff, community members, and community organization staff makes it difficult to establish and sustain collaborations and initiatives (Hodges et al., 2011, 2012; Grier and Bradley-King, 2011; Weist et al., 2012). This barrier may take the form of lack of communication within and outside the organization or school about vision, values, and goals, making it difficult to see where they may be shared; not involving a wide enough representation of stakeholders early in any visioning or planning process; or communicating through ineffective channels for the target of the message. Transparent and wide communication among all stakeholders within and outside the schools, including community organizations, requires communication to be delivered through multiple channels and in ways and at levels that will be received by those for whom it is intended. Schools and organizations should work to determine and update the best channels of communication with intended audiences and with each other. Follow-up systems should be created to confirm that messages have been received and understood by the intended audience.

Budgetary constraints, both real and perceived, may prevent the establishment of school–community collaboration (Hodges et al., 2011, 2012; Grier & Bradley-King, 2011; Weist et al., 2012; Rickard et al., 2011, Tracy & Castro-Guillen 2008). Rather than seeing collaboration as a means to use resources efficiently and as an avenue to gain funding for school and community health goals, many stakeholders think that schools and community agencies do not have funds for nonacademic initiatives in the schools. Funding, in fact, may not be available, but school health–community collaborations can make a powerful argument for funding allocation through planned school health advocacy. Real budgetary constraints may exist but should not provide barriers to relationship building, and collaborative joint projects may create efficiencies that can relieve some budgetary constraints for all involved. The examination of shared vision, values, and goals that is part of relationship building will clarify perceptions and assist in identifying where joint projects may bring budgetary efficiencies.

Schools and community agencies are sometimes reluctant to engage with others because they believe that they must protect their turf (Hodges et al., 2011, 2012; Weist et al., 2012). In times of economic challenge and budget constraints, many in schools and community agencies think that collaboration may indicate that their job or program is not necessary, can be taken over or outsourced by someone, or something else. Those working in schools may also think of the schools as a safe space for children and that collaboration with others outside the school compromises that safe space (Hodges et al., 2011, 2012). With a focus on the broader common goal of healthy youth and communities, collaboration and shared resources can make programs stronger and broader in scope while providing support for institutionalization.

For some, one or more negative past experiences in trying to collaborate creates reluctance to do so again (Hodges et al., 2011, 2012; CBSA 2009). Potential collaborators should review historical records for evidence of past collaborative efforts and their outcomes and engage in open communication about experiences in collaboration, both good and bad. The best approach is to acknowledge the past but focus on the present and future with open communication, systematic planning, and shared decision making.

Community members may not see a place for themselves in working with the schools because they are not parents or family members of school-aged youth. Even though they may not have children in the schools, helping community members see the value of their role in developing and supporting the whole child is important in establishing collaborative relationships.

The failure of those working in schools and community agencies to recognize health systems and links to academic success makes it difficult to see the need to collaborate (Hodges et al., 2011). Many within and outside schools perceive that knowledge-focused health education class is what constitutes school health, therefore thinking that school health has nothing to do with their roles or with broader academic success (Hodges et al., 2011, 2012). The development of school–community collaboration can be assisted by advocating for and implementing strong health promotion policies, practices, and processes. Raising awareness of the links between the health status of children and families and academic success within both school district systems and the community can also assist in the creation of school–community collaborations by helping academic and health stakeholders see shared outcomes.

Real and perceived implementation issues can prevent collaborations from forming and prevent existing ones from moving beyond the information-sharing stage (Hodges et al., 2011, 2012; Tracy & Castro-Guillen, 2008). Putting policy and initiatives into action is hard work that requires good planning, teamwork, and coordination with others outside the collaborative partners. Many stakeholders have been involved in collaborations that saw unrealized goals and initiatives that may have been developed but never enacted. These potential collaborators may see new collaborative initiatives as a waste of time. In these cases, new leadership and newly constituted collaborations may entice partners. Once operational, the collaboration needs to work together to prioritize goals and objectives, focus on small achievable steps, and celebrate and publicize achievements.

Recently, a school district that one of the authors works with decided to reinvigorate its district wellness council. Two new leaders, an administrator and a teacher, worked together to identify and invite a number of community partners to

School Health *in Action*

Engaging Community Partners to Address Student Health Issues

Batesville Community School Corporation (BCSC) in Indiana is a rural corporation with about 2,100 students, of whom about 26 percent are eligible for free or reduced lunch. It had a community partner, a local physician, on its school health leadership team who also happened to be a parent of a BCSC student. BCSC has a person dedicated to oversee CSH in the corporation.

BCSC began to notice high rates of binge drinking and obesity in its students. This mind-set became a priority for the school health council.

Although the school health council had some community partners, the need to expand beyond just those represented on the advisory board was noted. The council publicized the work that they were doing (in print, on the radio, and around town) to create a buzz and generate interest from more people in becoming part of the effort to address binge drinking and obesity. The resulting collaboration included both community partners and corporate sponsors, and it generated donations of time, space, and funding. These new partners ultimately helped the sustainability of CSH and its efforts.

collaborate on school health initiatives through the structure of the council. The council reviewed assets and needs assessment data and developed a set of prioritized goals and objectives related to school health. The first priority became updating the district's wellness policy. Many community collaborators indicated that a clear, well-publicized policy would assist them in cooperative planning of initiatives in support of the policy, including after-school programs, recreation programs, youth sport programs, and so on.

CHARACTERISTICS OF EFFECTIVE SCHOOL–COMMUNITY COLLABORATIONS

SEDL has outlined characteristics of effective school–family–community collaborations (Ferguson et al., 2010, pp. 15–18). By adapting these characteristics to WSCC, the potential exists to create effective CSH school–community collaborations that result in the following:

- **Shared responsibility for the health of youth and children among school staff, families, and the larger community**. Institutions, organizations, and individuals acknowledge and support that they all, individually and collectively, have a responsibility and a role in fostering healthy youth and children. These stakeholders demonstrate this shared responsibility by engaging in shared planning and decision making (CSBA, 2009). The vision of the school is expanded to include the community (O'Keefe, 2011), and schools and community entities reach out to each other. The Communities That Care (CTC) (2013) coalition system exists for use by communities that realize that prevention of underage drinking, tobacco use, violence, delinquency, school dropout, and substance abuse is a community-wide responsibility. CTC community groups and schools work together through a coalition structure to determine their community's priority prevention needs in these areas and the best way to employ their collective resources.
- **Seamless and continuous support for developing good health and health-enhancing behaviors from birth to career in the schools, at home, and in the community**. Opportunities to practice health and academic skills intended to develop self-efficacy and reinforce knowledge are created and embedded throughout the community. The ability to practice health-related skills in a variety of real-world situations is an important factor in becoming confident and comfortable in using the skills (Bandura, 1986). School–community collaborations are an important tool for creating formal and informal opportunities to practice these skills across socioecological levels (Bronfenbrenner, 1979).
- **Pathways that honor and attend to the dynamic and multiple factors that contribute to health**. Complex interrelated challenges require comprehensive solutions, and these solutions need to be integrated into school improvement plans (Adelman & Taylor, 2006). School–community collaborations provide those working in schools the opportunity to work with noneducators to create new pathways to support health and healthy behaviors. For example, a school health team can work with local grocery stores to create learning centers within the stores for youth and their parents to apply skills and knowledge, or the team can work with the local restaurant association to improve children's menus and have placemats with health-related learning activities for children to play with while waiting for food. By engaging a wide variety of community partners in the determination and creation of these pathways, the entire community may see improved health (Jehl, 2007), thus reinforcing the goals of WSCC.
- **Supportive culture for health both in the classroom and throughout the community**. Collaborations do a better job of creating community-wide social norms for health behavior than single entities do because community collaborators reinforce a universal message with their nonstudent employees, clients, customers, and so on.
- **Opportunities and processes to foster advocacy for student health and healthy**

communities. Collaborations foster opportunities for all stakeholders to advocate for health and can be powerful tools for creating healthy communities. Family members, community members, youth, and educators can all be advocates for health and the WSCC approach with the schools and the community.

- **Quality health status and health behaviors for every child**. The WSCC approach can help create structural supports and systems within and outside school buildings through collaborations. The work of the Anne E. Casey Foundation (Jehl, 2007) underscores the importance of partnerships in aligning curricula across grades, identifying and aligning additional services to support students and their families, and strengthening communication among school and parent systems that support quality health status and health behaviors. Collaborators both within and outside the school should understand that school health is not just what happens in the health education classroom.

How a collaboration functions has an important influence on its effectiveness. The following

School Health *in Action*

Community Partnership Ideas

Besides monetary support from private foundations, the CSH-led school–community collaboration with the Batesville Community School Corporation was able to develop the following partnerships:

- A local gym donated space for healthy activities after high school football games.
- A local movie theater donated movie and concessions coupons for healthier social opportunities as an alternative to underage drinking.
- The YMCA opened its doors for healthy activities after sporting events.
- Faith-based organizations donated time and space for students to play active video games (Dance Dance Revolution and Guitar Hero).
- A local hospital and farmer's market provided money and support for healthier food options, such as a garden behind the school and local fresh foods (fruits, vegetables, and beef) on a seasonal basis.
- The community supported the Girls on the Run program.
- A community and school group of walkers and runners participated in the Indianapolis Mini-Marathon and the Cincinnati Flying Pig Run.
- The CHOICES program used a three-pronged approach that included a parent pledge, educational programs for teens and parents, and healthy alternative activities for teens. The goal of the program is to ensure that every student and parent is offered multiple opportunities to learn more about the effects of drug and alcohol use. The program is open to all families in the Batesville area, even if their children do not attend the public schools.
- After a Batesville High School student died from a heroin overdose, the superintendent cofounded the Drug Free Coalition of Batesville, a group dedicated to addressing drug issues in the Batesville community. He now serves on the executive board.
- BCSC adopted a new vending machine policy to promote healthier food and drink choices and four years later revised the policy and negotiated a new vendor contract.
- BCSC partnered with the local hospital to implement the CATCH program, which promoted physical activity and healthy food choices for children in grades K through 5.
- BCSC changed how it did fund-raising at the schools. They changed their tradition of having students raise money by selling candy to doing a walk-a-thon fund-raiser. For each lap that a student walked, he or she got to vote on a teacher to kiss a pig. They raised nearly $18,000 and used money to fund reading tutors.

actions represent highly functioning collaborations:

- Seek a broad representation of partners and solicit input and feedback from a broad array of stakeholders
- Engage in open, multidirectional communication using a variety of communication channels and techniques
- Develop vision, goals, and outcomes mutually agreed on by all collaborators
- Recognize organizational limitations and understand that partners will not necessarily bring equal contributions
- Determine clear roles and responsibilities for partners
- Select creative leaders that are in a position of authority to act
- Develop new and multifaceted roles for professionals who work in schools and communities, as well as family and community members willing to assume leadership roles
- Weave together a critical mass of resources and strategies to address goals
- Engage in **capacity building** activities as necessary

Who to pursue for creating collaboration is also an important consideration. Following are some community agencies that may participate in school–community collaborations:

- Youth bureaus
- Health care practitioners, practices, and facilities
- Public safety
- Catholic charities
- Other faith-based organizations
- Mental health prevention and treatment organizations
- Restaurant associations
- Chambers of commerce
- Health-related voluntary organizations (e.g., American Heart Association)
- Health-related government organizations (e.g., health department)
- Service organizations (e.g., Rotary International)
- Area colleges and universities
- Local businesses
- Youth sport organizations and facilities
- Parks and recreation departments
- Neighborhood associations

SUMMARY

School–community collaborations are an integral element in implementing, institutionalizing, and sustaining the WSCC approach. Embodying ASCD's Whole Child approach (ASCD, n.d.a), school–community collaborations embody the broad ecological approach necessary to fostering the health and academic success of today's youth. Schools and community organizations need to move beyond "a patchwork of random acts" to working systematically in identifying, measuring, reporting, and discussing mutually determined and mutually beneficial goals and objectives related to health and academic success (Weist, et al 2012).

A number of barriers and challenges exist to moving toward more systematic and purposeful school–community collaborations. Schools and community groups should examine which barriers and challenges exist for them and work toward decreasing them. In addition, school–community collaborators should strive to foster the characteristics of effective collaborations.

Glossary

capacity building—Capacity building is an ongoing process through which individuals, groups, organizations, and societies enhance their ability to identify and meet challenges. Capacity building is a long-term, continuing process in which all stakeholders of an organization or community participate. Capacity development and organizational development are terms often used to mean capacity building.

institutionalization—To become embedded in the organization so that the program or policy continues after the initial effort.

integrated planning—A structured planning network that involves joint planning and ensures participation of all stakeholders and affected departments or units in a collaborative effort, such as planning that takes place between schools, community agencies, and institutions for youth health and well-being.

multifaceted system of coordinated and interconnected supports—A coordinated effort in which systems work together to provide resources and services to help students overcome barriers that interfere with learning.

SEDL—Formally known as the Southwest Educational Development Laboratory, SEDL is a nonprofit education research, development, and dissemination organizations based in Austin, Texas. The name was changed to SEDL in 2007.

siloing—To contain information or content in one knowledge area or discipline (as in a silo) that is therefore isolated from other groups, such as when teachers at one school do not share information with teachers at another or when math teachers do not share information with English teachers.

socioecological framework (Bronfenbrenner, 1979)—CDC (2014) describes the frameworks as a four-level socioecological model. This model considers the complex interplay between individual, relationship, community, and societal factors. See Bronfenbrenner's use of the socioecological framework in his work.

stakeholders—Individuals or groups that have interest or concern in an organization or system and will be most affected by a program or intervention.

sustainability—The ability of a school to maintain an initiative or program long term beyond implementation or the initial phase that was funded or supported by an outside agency.

systems approach—The application of systems thinking to a problem or a process to understand the complex functioning of a system such as a school district or a community.

Application Activities

1. Interview representatives from several health-related community agencies about the development of collaborations with other agencies. Part of the interview can involve questions that allow you to determine the agency staff's perceptions of the actions for and characteristics of positive collaboration that were presented in this chapter. In addition, discuss their experiences with collaborative activities with both schools and other organizations. Based on the interview, develop a report that includes a summary of the interviews and your reaction to their perceptions and experiences.
2. Your school is part of a collaborative project with several community agencies. The purpose of the project is to increase parent engagement in helping elementary and middle school children learn about the value of physical activity. The community agencies include the local Boys and Girls Club, several faith-based organizations, and the local library. Identify and describe three collaborative methods that involve the community partners and can be used to promote engagement in activity and education.
3. Identify and review two TED talks on developing partnerships or collaborations (the talks can be located at www.ted.com/topics/collaboration). After you have reviewed the talks, write an outline of a talk that you would give on the topic of building collaborations for the development of healthy and successful youth.

Resources

Centers for Disease Control and Prevention. 2012. *Parent Engagement: Strategies for Involving Parents in School Health*. Atlanta, GA: U.S. Department of Health and Human Services. www.cdc.gov/healthyyouth/AdolescentHealth/pdf/parent_engagement_strategies.pdf

Ferguson, Chris, Jordan, Catherine, & Baldwin, Marion. 2010. *Working Systematically in Action: Engaging Family and Community*. Austin, TX: SEDL. www.sedl.org/ws/ws-fam-comm.pdf

Ferguson, Chris. 2005. *Beyond the Building: A Facilitation Guide for School, Family and Community Connections*. National Center for Family and Community Connections With Schools. Southwest Educational Development Laboratory. Austin, TX: SEDL. www.sedl.org/connections/toolkits/beyond-the-building.pdf

References

Adelman, Howard, & Taylor, Linda. 2011. Expanding School Improvement Policy to Better Address Barriers to Learning. *Policy Futures in Education, 9,* 431–436.

Adelman, Howard S., & Taylor, Linda. 2006. School and Community Collaboration to Promote a Safe Learning Environment. *State Education Standard: Journal of the National Association of State Boards of Education, 7,* 38–43.

ASCD. n.d.a. *About the Whole Child Approach.* www.wholechildeducation.org/about

ASCD. n.d.b. *Healthy School Communities.* www.ascd.org/ASCD/pdf/siteASCD/products/healthy schools/ltl_may2010.pdf

ASCD. n.d.c. *Whole Child Tenets and Indicators.* www.wholechildeducation.org/assets/content/mx-resources/wholechildindicators-all.pdf

Bandura, Albert C. 1986. *Social Foundations of Thought and Action: A Social Cognitive Theory.* Englewood Cliffs, NJ: Prentice-Hall.

Benham-Deal, Tami, & Hodges, Bonni C. 2009. *The Role of 21st Century Schools in Promoting Health Literacy.* Proceedings from the Symposium on Health Literacy in the 21st Century: Setting an Education Agenda. Commissioned by NEAHIN, Washington, DC, and the United Health Foundation, Minnetonka, MN. www.neahin.org/healthlit
eracy/index.html

Bronfenbrenner, Urie. 1979. *The Ecology of Human Development: Experiments by Nature and Design.* Cambridge, MA: Harvard.

California School Boards Association (CSBA). 2009. *Building Healthy Communities: A School Leader's Guide to Collaboration and Community Engagement.* West Sacramento, CA: California School Boards Association. www.saferoutespartnership
.org/sites/default/files/pdf/Lib_of_Res/SCHBD_4.pdf

Centers for Disease Control and Prevention (CDC). 2009. *School Connectedness: Strategies for Increasing Protective Factors Among Youth.* Atlanta, GA: U.S. Department of Health and Human Services. www.cdc.gov/healthyyouth/adolescenthealth/pdf/connectedness.pdf

Centers for Disease Control and Prevention (CDC). 2014. *The Social-Ecological Model: A Framework for Prevention.* Atlanta, GA: Injury Prevention & Control: Division of Violence Prevention. www.cdc.gov/ViolencePrevention/overview/social
-ecologicalmodel.html

Centers for Disease Control and Prevention (CDC). 2012. *Parent Engagement: Strategies for Involving Parents in School Health.* Atlanta, GA: U.S. Department of Health and Human Services. www.cdc.gov/healthyyouth/AdolescentHealth/pdf/parent_engagement_strategies.pdf

Communities That Care (CTC). www.sdrg.org/ctcresource/About_CTC_NEW.htm

Ferguson, Chris, Jordan, Catherine, & Baldwin, Marion. 2010. *Working Systematically in Action: Engaging Family and Community.* Austin, TX: SEDL. www.sedl.org/ws/ws-fam-comm.pdf

Gardner, Sid. 1998. *Beyond Collaboration to Results: Hard Choices in the Future of Services to Children and Families* (pp. 6–9). Arizona Prevention Resource Center and the Center for Collaboration for Children.

Grier, Betsy C., & Bradley-King, Kathy L. 2011. Collaborative Consultation to Support Children With Pediatric Health Issues: A Review of the Biopsychoeducational Model. *Journal of Educational and Psychological Consultation, 21,* 88–105.

Henderson, Anne, Mapp, Karen, Johnson, Vivian. R., & Davies, Don. 2007. *Beyond the Bake Sale: The Essential Guide to Family-School Partnerships.* New York: New Press.

Hodges, Bonni, Videto, Donna, & Greeley, Aimee. 2011, October. *Working to Create Limitless Possibilities in Limited Environments.* Paper presented at the 85th American School Health Association Conference, Louisville, KY.

Hodges, Bonni, & Videto, Donna. 2012, November 12. *Connecting Silos: Uniting Institutions for Healthy Schools and Communities.* Webinar. American Association for Health Education.

Jehl, Jeanne. 2007. *Connecting, Schools, Families, and Communities: Stories and Results From the Annie E. Casey Foundation's Education Investments.* Baltimore, MD: Anne E. Casey Foundation. www.aecf.org/upload/PublicationFiles/ED3622H5045.pdf

O'Keefe, Brendan. 2011, October 19. *Five Steps to Better School/Community Collaboration.* Edutopia Teacher Leadership (blog). www.edutopia.org/blog/school_community_collaboration__brendan_o'keefe

Mastro, Elizabeth, Jalloh, Mary, & Watson, Felicia. 2006. Come on Back: Enhancing Youth Development Through School/Community Collaboration. *Journal of Public Health Management and Practice, 12*(6) (suppl), S60–S64.

Rickard, Megan L., Price, James H., Telljohann, Susan K., Dake, Joseph A., & Fink, Brian N. 2011. School Superintendents' Perceptions on

Schools Assisting Students in Obtaining Public Health Insurance. *Journal of School Health, 81*(12), 756–763.

Sulkowski, Michael L. 2011. Response to Intervention and Interdisciplinary Collaboration: Joining Hands to Support Children's Healthy Development. *Journal of Applied School Psychology, 27*(2), 118–123.

Tracy, Elizabeth M., & Castro-Guillen, Evelyn. 2008. *Roles of School and Community Providers in the Delivery of School Based Mental Health Services*. Oxford, OH: Miami University of Ohio Effective Practice Intervention Council, The Center for School-Based Mental Health Programs at Ohio University. www.units.muohio.edu/csbmhp/consultsvcs/EPIC_Tracy_Concept_Paper_4-16%20FINAL.pdf

Valois, Robert F., Slade, Sean, & Ashford, Ellie. 2011. *The Healthy Schools Communities Model: Aligning Health and Education in the School Setting*. ASCD: Washington, DC.

Weiss, Heather, Little, Priscilla, Bouffard, Suzanne M., Deschenes, Sarah N., & Malone, Helen J. 2009. Strengthen What Happens Outside School to Improve What Happens Inside. *Phi Delta Kappan, 90*(8), 592–596. www.hfrp.org/content/download/3362/97494/file/StrengthenWhatHappensOutsideSchool.pdf

Weist, Mark P., Mellin, Elizabeth A., Chambers, Kerri L., Lever, Nancy A., Haber, Deborah, & Blaber, Christine. 2012. Challenges to Collaboration in School Mental Health and Strategies for Overcoming Them. *Journal of School Health, 82*(2), 97–105.

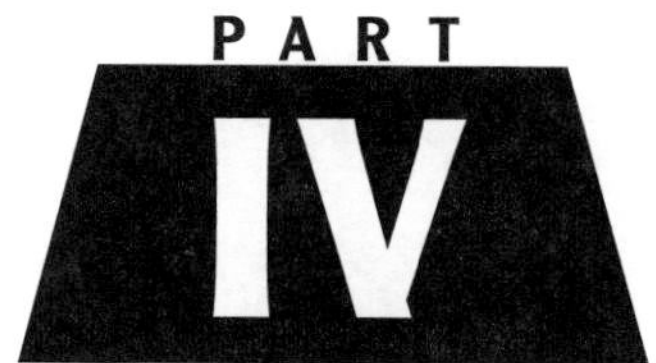

Planning, Implementation, and Evaluation

9

Planning for WSCC

BONNI C. HODGES • DONNA M. VIDETO

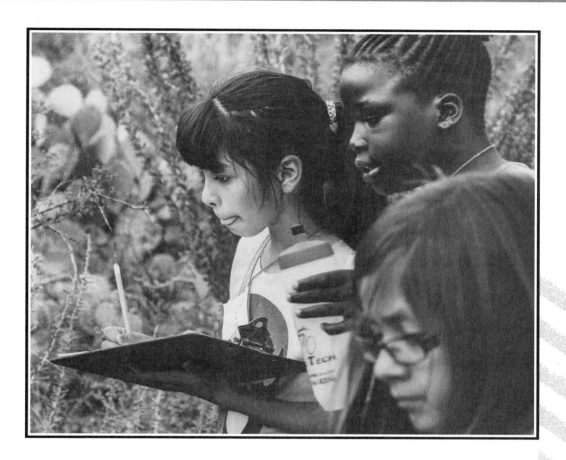

This chapter describes how to create a comprehensive school district health and wellness profile for use as a foundation for planning Coordinated School Health (CSH) programming, now the Whole School, Whole Community, Whole Child approach (WSCC). The chapter also identifies avenues for linking school health and academic performance. Implementation of Race to the Top (United States Department of Education, n.d.), the Common Core Standards (National Governors Association and State Education Chiefs, n.d.), and other education reforms provide a tremendous opportunity for school health, through the framework of the WSCC approach, to be embedded across and within the various systems in today's educational environments. The approach described in this chapter was originally developed to provide the necessary data to use in CSH planning but can be used for WSCC planning as well.

A recommended set of actions are presented to help planners identify data sources, obtain and collect data, and analyze and interpret data holistically and realistically. The chapter demonstrates how to organize the needed data through the employment of the PRECEDE (Green & Kreuter, 2005) framework so that planning for WSCC can incorporate a broad socioecological framework (Bronfenbrenner, 1979)

NEED FOR SYSTEMATIC PLANNING

A critical first step for school districts in identifying avenues for linking school health and academic performance is to create a comprehensive profile of the school district's health and wellness systems. Multiple strategies for collecting baseline data are needed to begin defining the existing health systems as a way to determine what the schools and the district already have in place before recommendations and implementation of action steps (Fetro, Givens, & Carroll, 2009). A variety of existing tools that provide relatively user-friendly frameworks for looking at particular components of school health are described and discussed in some detail in the appendix. It has been the authors' experience as practitioners, consultants, researchers, and professors in school health that popular tools such as the **Youth Risk Behavior Survey** (Centers for Disease Control and Prevention, 2014), the Wellness School Assessment Tool (WellSAT) (Yale Rudd Center, 2013), the School Health Index (SHI) (Centers for Disease Control and Prevention, 2014), and the Healthy School Report Card (HSRC) (ASCD, 2012), although valuable, are used in isolation. A district or a school may use one or two of these tools to assist in school health planning, but rarely do they use these tools together to contribute to a holistic look at school health promotion. In addition, these tools and their data are often not shared or used beyond those most directly involved with school health. Thus, they are rarely considered and applied when setting broader school building and district-level goals (Hodges, Videto, & Greeley, 2011; Hodges & Videto, 2011).

A comprehensive school district health and wellness profile includes community, health, and academic data compiled from a variety of tools and sources. The profile identifies school health and community assets and needs that are suggested by these varieties of data. It can assist in illustrating connections between health and academic performance, reveal district and community assets that can be built upon to improve health and academic performance, and provide a platform for the establishment of more efficient and effective school health systems and collaborations.

The job of constructing an extensive health systems and wellness profile of a school district and the communities it serves may seem overwhelming to school district personnel. This task should not be the responsibility of one person. School districts should use their school health council or other similar group to plan and direct the construction of the profile. In addition, collaborations between school districts and higher education institutions can provide the guidance and assistance needed to undertake the assessment and then develop the profile as well as explore models for institutionalization following the profile construction (Butler, Fryer, Reed, & Thomas, 2011; Videto & Hodges, 2009; Schwartz & Laughlin, 2008).

CREATING A COMPREHENSIVE PROFILE

Comprehensive school district health and wellness profiles need to identify and include many factors that contribute to the health and academic success of students. The PRECEDE portion of the **PRECEDE–PROCEED framework** (Green & Kreuter, 2005) and **Bronfenbrenner's ecological systems theory** (Bronfenbrenner, 1979) provide useful guidance in identifying the most important factors in determining school health-related assets and needs for school districts. Bronfenbrenner's concept of concentrically embedded systems suggests that to get a better understanding of district level school health and wellness, it is necessary to look beyond the confines of the school district system to learn about the structure and functioning of local and state health departments, local governments, and the state education department (Bronfenbrenner, 1979).

PRECEDE provides guidance in the identification of specific data points needed for inclusion in the profiles. Figure 9.1 shows examples of such data points (adapted from Green & Kreuter, 2005). From PRECEDE there are four phases of data gathering useful for collecting information to develop a comprehensive school health and wellness profile.

Because school districts are both part of communities and can be considered communities unto themselves, it is useful to gather social indicator information for the communities that a district serves as well as school-specific district indicators to identify social assets and needs that represent or are affected by health-related situations in the school and the community. Under **social assessment** (phase 1) in figure 9.1 a list of community and school-specific data is presented that can reveal broad assets and needs within a community and a school district. Both current data and trend data from the last several years are important. Trend

FIGURE 9.1

PRECEDE Framework Sample Data Points

Social Assessment Data Points (Phase 1)

COMMUNITY

- demographic data and trend data
- socio-economic data and trend data
- employment rates and trend data
- crime rates and trend data
- housing characteristics
- land area and geographic characteristics
- local government structure
- community resources: health, educational, other
- community engagement: e.g. voting rates, civic organization membership, community events attendance

SCHOOL DISTRICT

- district student demographic information and trend data
- district and school building needs designation
- free/reduced lunch enrollment and trend data
- academic performance and trend data
- students with disabilities classification rates and trend data
- students with special needs rates and trend data
- graduation and college enrollment rates and trend data

Epidemiological, Behavioral, Environmental Assessment Data Points (Phase 2)

- Morbidity and mortality data
- Behavioral Risk Factor Surveillance System and Youth Risk Behavior Surveillance System data
- Environmental contributors to morbidity and mortality priorities

Educational and Ecological Assessment Data Point (Phase 3)

PREDISPOSING:

- knowledge of school health
- attitudes toward school health
- perceptions of role of schools in health of youth
- perceptions of the role of schools in health of community
- strength of belief of tie between health and academic performance

REINFORCING

- Attitudes of school administrators and staff, community organizations, and community members toward school health
- Attitudes of school administrators, staff and parents regarding the role of being healthy in student academic success
- Support of school administrators, staff, parents, and community members of school health initiatives

(continued)

Figure 9.1 *(continued)*

ENABLING

- Resources designated for school health
- Opportunities for students to practice healthy behaviors during the school day
- Intra-school and extra-school communica tion systems and efficacy
- School health coordination skills
- Enforcement of existing school health-related policies and procedures

Administrative and Policy Diagnosis Data Points (Phase 4)

- School district structure
- School health structure and leadership
- Coordinated School Health Implementation and Function
- Integration level of school health with academic mission and planning
- School Health Resources: faculty/staff, funding, collaborations, educational resources

Based on Green and Kreuter 2005

data allow a look at whether a situation is getting better, worse, or staying the same and are important in determining priorities.

Epidemiological, behavioral, and environmental assessment (phase 2) indicates the need to gather specific health-related data. Information about the types and spread of illness and other health problems in school district communities, as well as causes of death and death rates for specific health problems, provides a sense of health priorities and the health environment from which students come. School nurse data on conditions, screening results, and the like will provide a more specific picture of the health status of youth in the schools. Data that provide information on the incidence and prevalence of mental and emotional health diagnoses of students receiving special education services would also be included here. Likely environmental and behavioral contributors to these health conditions should also be determined. Documenting the level of functioning of the WSCC approach and the behaviors, including decision making of administrators and others in positions to create an environment supportive and conducive to WSCC aligns with PRECEDE.

Keeping in mind that the purpose of the assessment is to plan health promotion policies and programming that will have a positive effect on the health status and academic performance of students in the **educational and ecological assessment** (phase 3), it is suggested that the assessment of the state of school health involves looking at data from the previous assessment—epidemiological, behavioral, and environmental assessment (phase 2)—to help explain the current level of CSH or WSCC implementation. The educational and ecological assessment examines knowledge, attitudes toward, and perceptions of school health by school faculty, staff, school administrators, students, parents, and community members to help explain the existing level of CSH or WSCC. Among the questions to be pursued are the following: Is there accurate understanding of what school health is and can be? What is the existing level of support for school health? What resources are currently available for school health? What skills do those directly and indirectly associated with school health have or need that can be built on or developed?

The **administrative and policy assessment and intervention alignment** (phase 4) provides direction for looking at current structures within the district, policies, leadership, existing collaborations, and resources. In addition, an examination of the degree to which school health has been integrated into the academic mission and planning of the school district is pursued.

ACTIONS FOR COLLECTING PROFILE DATA

The asset and needs assessment data points identified in the PRECEDE framework can be collected through a series of four actions for collecting the data:

- Developing community understanding
- Conducting a wellness policy review
- Reviewing the Coordinated School Health implementation

- Conducting a school health function assessment

The data points are used throughout all the action steps, although they do not correspond directly from phase 1 to action step 1 and so on.

The four actions identified here to collect the needs and asset data are suggested as ways to organize and conduct the assessment and complete the data collection for the school district health and wellness profile, thus setting the stage for informed policy and program planning. Data-gathering strategies need to provide breadth and depth, yet both also need to be acceptable to and achievable in schools. A review of the professional literature, consultation with state education department stakeholders, and discussions with public school administrators and staff are useful avenues for informing the data-gathering procedure decisions. Table 9.1 provides an overview of a general process that has been used by the authors in several public school districts to collect the necessary information.

Action 1: Developing Community Understanding

Developing an understanding of the school district, the youth, and the surrounding communities is needed to understand the context in which the school district functions. Community assets can be leveraged by school health programs through collaborations to assist in addressing the needs of the school and the nearby communities. This action begins by generating a list of necessary information about the school district and the communities it serves. Figure 9.1 and table 9.1 serve as general guidelines, but data specific to the communities and district need to be identified within the broad categories listed. After the data list is finalized, potential sources for the information on the list are brainstormed. State education department, school district, and local government and health-related agency stakeholders should be consulted to refine, validate, and finalize potential sources of information. Community understanding

Table 9.1 Actions for Developing a School District Health and Wellness Profile

Actions	Data Gathering Activities
Developing a Community Understanding	Public Domain Document Review, Existing Data Reports Review • Demographic information • Vital statistics • Crime rates • Local government structure • Community issues and initiatives • Epidemiological data • Health & Human Services Resources • School structure and function • Academic performance data • Windshield Tour
Conducting a Wellness Policy Review	WellSAT Assessment
Reviewing CSH Implementation	Assessment with School Health Index
Conducting a School Health Function Assessment	Existing Report Review Key Informant Interviews • School District Personnel • Parents • Community Members Focus Group Discussions • School District Personnel • Parents • Community Members

can be built largely through existing documents and information in the public domain pertaining to the previous 5 to 10 years. Connecting with stakeholders will usually reveal sources of information and documents not generally known but that will be useful, such as internal reports from community agencies not readily available online. After the data list and sources have been finalized, the data can be obtained. Community demographic and public health data are easily obtained through federal, state, and local government websites such as those for the Department of Labor, city or county legislatures, and state and local health departments. Websites or paper materials of the local chamber of commerce, local and regional newspapers, local health and human service agencies, local health care providers, and local telephone books are also good sources.

Given the nature of school district structure and functioning, some school-district-related data are publically available and easy to find and obtain, but not all. For example, **academic performance data** (such as student assessment results) can often be obtained either through the district website or state education department school report cards. School district websites should be accessed and reviewed for other pertinent information. When available, district or school newsletters and board of education minutes for the past three to five years should be reviewed for trends, issues, and initiatives. Providing a list of information needed from a school district to several key administrators and staff will often produce the required data.

School districts should be asked to provide information and documents related to school district and school health structure and functioning. Specifically, requests should be made to districts for the most current district wellness policy; any policies related to alcohol, tobacco, and other drugs; policies on parent involvement; school health services policies and any additional local health-related policies; a diagram of the reporting hierarchy and governance structure of the district; recent YRBSS data or reports; available district data on student health; and the most recent SHI or HSRC data and report if one has been done.

Systematic **windshield tours** of school districts and the communities associated with them provide a way to get a sense of the physical environment and to confirm some of the existing data. Windshield tours are conducted by driving throughout the community and recording notable observations about the environment (Hodges, Videto, & Greeley, 2011). Before conducting a windshield tour, a windshield tour documentation sheet should be developed to direct observers to note specific items along with general impressions and observations. Observations related to the condition and use of areas around school buildings, neighborhoods in the communities, downtown or village areas, parks and other recreational areas, and health care facilities and services should be noted. Figure 9.2 is a windshield tour template developed for a community assessment conducted as part of a larger school health systems assessment project.

Photographs to illustrate observational details are recommended as part of the windshield tour. PhotoVoice, which involves the use of digital participatory storytelling, is also a consideration to be used in some combination with the windshield tour. For more information on PhotoVoice, visit www.photovoice.org/about. Following the research and the windshield tour, the community understanding data at this point provides an overview of general community characteristics; health, health-related behaviors, and environment status of the community with a focus on youth; and school district characteristics and performance data (see table 9.2).

Action 2: Conducting a Wellness Policy Review

The Child Nutrition and WIC Reauthorization Act, mandated by Congress in 2004 (Child Nutrition and WIC, 2013), required school districts that participate in federal school meal programs to create and implement school wellness policies by 2006. The policies needed to address nutrition education, nutrition standards for foods sold, and physical activity. All policies needed to include measures for evaluating the effectiveness of the policy (Yale Rudd Center, 2013). One tool for conducting this evaluation is the WellSAT. Developed by the Rudd Center at Yale University, the WellSAT assessment can provide districts with guidance and resources for making improvements to existing wellness policies (see the appendix for more information on the WellSAT) (Yale Rudd Center, 2013).

Wellness policies are available either through school district websites or district office administrators. Although one person can conduct the review using the WellSAT, the policy should ideally undergo two independent assessments. The WellSAT scores are then compared, and a con-

FIGURE 9.2

Windshield Tour Template

General impressions of the community:

Repeat each section as needed. **School:** ____________ Area surrounding schools (sidewalks, litter, traffic) Fast-food and alcohol outlets (proximity to school)	**School:** ____________ Area surrounding schools (sidewalks, litter, traffic) Fast-food and alcohol outlets (proximity to school)
Downtown/Other Business District Where do students and youth spend their time? Vacant buildings (density and location) Overall atmosphere (sidewalks, litter, traffic)	**Downtown/Other Business District** Where do students and youth spend their time? Vacant buildings (density and location) Overall atmosphere (sidewalks, litter, traffic)
Neighborhood: ____________ Overall condition Yard size, spacing of homes	**Neighborhood:** ____________ Overall condition Yard size, spacing of homes
Park: ____________ Overall condition Size, location, accessibility **Other recreational facilities:** ____________ Overall condition Location, accessibility	**Park:** ____________ Overall condition Size, location, accessibility **Other recreational facilities:** ____________ Overall condition Location, accessibility
Healthcare facility or hospital: ____________ Overall condition Size, location, accessibility	**Healthcare facility or hospital:** ____________ Overall condition Size, location, accessibility

Table 9.2 Action 1: Developing a Community Understanding

Community Understanding Action	Samples of Types of Data Collected
Community Characteristics	• Population Demographics & Trends Socio-economic Indicators & Trends • Geographic Landmarks • Outdoor recreation and leisure facilities • Housing, Crime, Restaurants, • Civic & Service Organizations • Voting Rates
Youth Health Status	• Epidemiological Data • Youth Risk Factors, YRBSS Data • Free & Reduced Lunch Data
School District Characteristics & Performance Data	• Graduation Rates • College Enrollment & Degrees Earned • School Absenteeism & School Drop-out Rates • State School Report Card Data

School Health *in Action*

Using Windshield Tours for Data Collection

In a CSH project in central and upstate New York involving five school districts, the chapter authors conducted a series of assessments that included windshield tours. A systematic windshield tour was conducted at each school district by pairs of trained project personnel. The tour involved driving through the communities served by each school district and noting health-related environmental assets and challenges. Particular attention was paid to the areas within a radius of about 1 mile (1.6 km) of each district school building. Notes were entered onto a windshield tour template, and digital photographs were taken to capture notable community features, both positive and negative. Examples of what was noted include number of, access to, and condition of recreational spaces and facilities (ice rinks, pools, playgrounds, walking paths, children's museums, arcades, miniature golf); access to, number of, and type of health care facilities; types of restaurants and fast-food outlets; churches and other religious facilities; type and relative location of grocery stores, convenience stores, liquor stores, and gas stations; general physical condition of neighborhoods (including needed repairs, number of homes for sale); primary language of neighborhood signs; availability and condition of sidewalks; exterior condition of housing and other buildings; and vitality of local businesses.

In at least one community a lack of sidewalks or sidewalks in poor condition surrounding the schools were found, thus indicating few opportunities for walking programs or other community-wide physical activities. In another community the only grocery store had priced the limited fresh produce higher than the price at full-service grocery stores, making it more difficult to get access to healthier foods.

sensus is reached on ratings for each of the five sections. The WellSAT sections include nutrition education and wellness promotion, standards for USDA child nutrition programs and school meals, nutrition standards for competitive and other foods and beverages, physical education and physical activity, and evaluation (Yale Rudd Center, 2013).

Action 3: Reviewing the Coordinated School Health Implementation

A specific systematic assessment of the current or potential level of implementation and functioning is a critical component of planning for CSH. Either the CDC's School Health Index (SHI) or the ASCD's Healthy School Report Card (HSRC) is recommended at this time. The SHI is an assessment and planning tool that districts or schools can use to improve health and safety policies and programs by using eight self-assessment modules that reflect the eight components of the CSH framework. The SHI also takes the district and school through a process that involves planning for making improvements to the existing CSH (Centers for Disease Control and Prevention, 2013). The other suggested option currently available for assessing CSH implementation levels is the HSRC, an online tool from ASCD. The HSRC is a mechanism to assess CSH as well as the whole school improvement process. The primary use of the HSRC is to assess as well as to impact the school's practices, identify and prioritize changes that can be made, and incorporate those changes into a school's improvement plan (Lohrmann, 2013).

New or revised assessment tools may eventually be offered that better reflect the new WSCC approach and would then be more appropriate for use in such a comprehensive review. The assessment tools discussed in this chapter provide a thorough and systematic look at CSH and can be adapted for use with WSCC until updated tools are developed. The SHI, for example, is aligned with the 8 components of CSH rather than the 10 components of WSCC. Yet within the SHI module School Health, Safety, and Policies, assessment items regarding the WSCC components of physical environment and social and emotional climate are included to some extent. Yet schools or districts might also look at the School Counseling, Psychological, and Social Services module for additional information on the WSCC social and emotional climate component. Also within the SHI are assessment items for the two WSCC components of family engagement and community involvement combined in the SHI module Family and Community Involvement. The HSRC is designed to assess the health of the school and the community with 11 components rather than the CSH's 8. The focus on the community in addition to the school or school district is more closely reflective of the WSCC model, and less adaption may be necessary. HSRC also currently addresses the whole child, which is at the core of the WSCC model. Regardless of which tool a school or district selects, a recent completed assessment can be used in conjunction with the other profile data as part of the planning process.

Districts and school buildings that have either never undertaken an assessment using SHI or HSRC or have not completed one in the last three years should conduct an assessment. Again, with the implementation of the WSCC collaborative approach to health and learning, new or revised assessment tools aligned specifically to the WSCC approach may be more appropriate for use in a school district and community assessment when made available.

Action 4: Conducting a School Health Function Assessment

The first three actions described provide a broad picture and can be used for basic program and policy planning, but action 4 provides a depth of information not available through the other three. Taking the time to talk with people about school health can unearth previously unidentified assets and needs, reveal potential barriers to expanding or institutionalizing school health within the school structure and community, and provide context for priority setting. **Key informant interviews** and **focus group discussions** involving people from the school district and the communities it serves are suggested. A list of suggested questions for use with key informant interviews and focus group discussions in school health planning assessment are provided in figures 9.3 and 9.4.

Key Informant Interviews

Key informant interviews are a common practice when collecting baseline data or conducting a needs assessment (Hodges & Videto, 2011). A key informant is a person in the community or school district who has direct knowledge of that group or has access to information about that group (WHO, 2000). A school district can be asked to provide a list of names of people who represent the key school, parent, and community contacts for interviews. Some recommended participants for interviews include the following.

- School district superintendent
- School nurses (one from the elementary school, one from the middle school, and one from the high school)
- At least one elementary school principal
- At least middle school principal
- At least one high school principal
- Faculty leader(s)
- Head of school nutrition (food) services
- PTA or PTO officers (one from the elementary level and one from the secondary level)

FIGURE 9.3

Key Informant Interview Questions

All (except student questions; see Student-Specific Questions)

Q1: When I say the term "school health," what do you think I am referring to?

Q2: On a scale of 1 (horrible) to 5 (outstanding), where would you place the general health of students in your district? Faculty and staff? Greater community? Why?

Q3: What policies does the district have that support a broad range of health and wellness programs and services?

Q4: Does the district or your school building use a shared decision-making process? If yes, is shared decision-making done with school health issues? Describe how that might be done.

Q5: Does the district actively plan and build partnerships with the community (groups)? If so, would you consider it systematic planning? Why or why not? If so, are there any partnerships that are associated with school health? What are they?

Q6: Can you point to and share examples of how the current school health system contributes to positive health outcomes for students? Faculty and staff? Parents? Greater community?

Q7: Can you point to and share examples of something that you believe might have a negative effect on student learning that occurs within the current school district or building?

Q8: With regard to school health in this district or building, what works particularly well? What is in particular need of improvement?

Q9: How important do you think having good health is for students to be successful in school?

Q10: Does the district or specific buildings have health or wellness councils? If so, who (titles and types) sits on them? Who facilitates them?

Q11: Does the district or specific buildings have leadership teams that meet on a regular basis to address health, mental health, and safety issues? How does this leadership group differ from any health or wellness council? What types of issues do they address?

Q12: Do health or wellness school teams write annual or five-year program plans that contain goals and objectives? If so, describe how goals and objectives are selected.

Parent-Specific Questions

PQ12: Describe how your child's school contributes to his or her health.

PQ13: How important do you think having good health is for students to be successful in school?

PQ14: How are parents involved in creating a healthy school building or district?

PQ15: What makes it easy to get involved in creating a healthy school building or district?

PQ16: What makes it difficult to get involved in creating a healthy school building or district?

PQ17: What do you see as the role of school districts or buildings in creating healthy youth and adolescents?

PQ18: What do you see as the role of school districts or buildings in creating healthy communities?

Community-Leader-Specific Questions

CLQ12: How are community members who are not parents of students involved in creating a healthy school building or district?

CLQ13: What stands in the way of community members who are not parents of students from getting involved in creating a healthy school building or district?

CLQ14: What do you see as the role of school districts or buildings in creating healthy youth and adolescents?

CLQ15: What do you see as the role of school districts or buildings in creating healthy communities?

Student-Specific Questions

SQ1: When I say the term "school health," what do you think I am referring to?

SQ2: On a scale of 1 (horrible) to 5 (outstanding), where would you place the general health of other students in your district? Faculty and staff? Greater community? Why?

SQ3: Can you point to and share examples of how the current school health system contributes to positive health outcomes for students? Faculty and staff? Parents? Greater community?

SQ4: Can you point to and share examples of something that you believe might have a negative effect on student learning that occurs within the current school district or building?

SQ5: With regard to school health in this district or building, what works particularly well? What is in particular need of improvement?

SQ6: What do you see as the role of school districts or buildings in creating healthy youth and adolescents?

SQ7: What do you see as the role of school districts or buildings in creating healthy communities?

SQ8: How important do you think having good health is to being a successful student?

SQ9: Does the district or specific buildings have health or wellness councils? If so, who (titles and types) sits on them? Who facilitates them?

SQ10: How are students involved in creating a healthy school building or district?

SQ11: What makes it easy to get involved in creating a healthy school building or district?

SQ12: What makes it difficult to get involved in creating a healthy school building or district?

- Informal leaders (parents suggested by other parents)
- Athletic director and coaches (one representing female sports and one male sports)
- Arts director or advisor (e.g., music department head, theater director, secondary art teacher)
- Mayor or head local government official
- At least one nonprofit organization representative (e.g., executive director)
- Business community representative
- Head of the chamber of commerce
- At least one local health care representatives (e.g., physician, dentist, nurse practitioner)
- Local public health director

FIGURE 9.4

Focus Group Questions

1. When I say the term "school health," what do you think I am referring to?
2. Keeping in mind that health has physical and psychological aspects, on a scale of 1 (horrible) to 5 (outstanding), where would you place the general health of youth and adolescents in your city or town? Why?
3. We want to get a sense of how you think the schools in this district contribute to the health of youth in this community.
   - What are some examples of how the schools positively contribute to the health of youth in this community?
   - What are some examples of how the schools may interfere with or hinder the health of youth in this community?
4. Do you have any suggestions on how the schools might better address the health needs of children in this community?
5. Do you think that healthy children or youth are more likely to be successful students? Why do you think the way that you do?
6. [Show and briefly explain CSH model]. When you think about school health as including all these pieces, which pieces do you see as working particularly well in this school or this district? Why?
   - Can you provide one or two specific examples?
   - What is in particular need of improvement? Why?
   - Can you provide one or two specific examples?
7. How are community members who are not parents involved in creating a healthy school building or district?
8. What might community members who are not parents do to be more involved in creating a healthy school building or district?
9. On a scale of 1 (low responsibility) to 10 (high responsibility), how much responsibility should the public schools have in creating healthy youth and adolescents? Why did you pick that number? Can you identify one or two specific examples of how public schools should be creating healthy youth and adolescents?
10. On a scale of 1 (low responsibility) to 10 (high responsibility), how much responsibility should the public schools have in creating healthy communities? Why did you pick that number?
11. Can you identify one or two specific examples of how public schools should be creating healthy youth and adolescents?

- Students (identified by teachers and administrators, leaders in student government, athletes, members of student clubs, suggested by other students)

These people are then contacted for interviews that typically last from 30 to 60 minutes depending on the number of questions. Interviews may be conducted face to face or by telephone. Face-to-face interviews should be conducted by two interviewers, one to pose the questions and the other to take notes and audiotape the conversation. Audiotapes of the interviews are recommended so that during data analysis, exact responses are available through the recordings or transcripts of the recording.

Focus Groups

Frequently used in health education, a focus group is a qualitative approach to learning about the intended audience (Goldman & Schmalz, 2001; Torabi & Ding, 1998). Hodges and Videto (2011) recommend running several focus groups representing subgroups of the population as part of the needs assessment process. School district and community agency personnel can be requested to provide contacts for setting up focus group discussions with groups representing members of the community; parents and guardians; and school faculty, staff, and administrators using a **snowball sampling technique** (Hodges & Videto, 2011). Focus group questions are developed to elicit participants' understanding and perceptions of the strengths and challenges of school health.

Focus groups of parents and school faculty, staff, and administration should be conducted at both the elementary and secondary levels. Focus groups of students at the elementary and secondary levels can also be helpful. Those who provide key informant interviews should not be eligible to participate in the focus group discussions. Focus group facilitators should have training in how to conduct a focus group. They should understand when and how to use follow-up questions, the need to ask primary questions in a uniform way, and the importance of confidentiality. Two facilitators should be employed for each focus group—one to pose questions and facilitate discussion and the other to make notes on nonverbal cues, perceived attitudes, and mannerisms and to audiotape the focus group discussion for future transcription. Each focus group should be planned to take 60 to 90 minutes.

Analyzing the Key Informant and Focus Group Data

Before reading transcripts of key informant and focus group interviews, a set of key words based

School Health *in Action*

Using Comprehensive School Health and Wellness Profiles

Looking at a variety of health status, school health, and academic data together allows school district decision makers and stakeholders to move the concept of the connections between health and academic performance from something abstract to something with real implications for their school districts. Comprehensive school health and wellness profiles can bring into view a number of existing situations for support or alteration that are often hidden when health and academic data are segregated (within school districts and between school districts and community health-related agencies). For example, focus group and key informant interview data with school personnel in two school districts in New York suggested a negative impact from mental health issues in the student and student family populations on students' ability to make academic progress. Parent interview data suggested a negative impact of student mental health issues on the classroom and school environment with regard to their children's ability to learn.

Community health status data supported mental health as an issue in youth and adult populations, identified inadequate access to diagnosis and treatment of mental health issues, particularly in youth, and suggested likely sociocultural contributors to mental health issues. The school districts had processes to consider the influence of mental health on the academic performance of individual students with IEPs, yet there appeared to be no mechanism to address possible mental health issues in the student population. For example, there were neither districtwide goals related to improving the mental health of the student population nor any mention in school improvement plans of mental health. The current silo structure in these communities and within the structure of the school districts appeared to have created the following situation:

- Community health agencies and organizations and schools worked largely in isolation on what is a communal problem at a time when resources are scarce.
- Classroom teachers felt unprepared and unsure of their role in managing students who exhibited socioemotional mental health issues and assisting those students with their struggles, even though the effect of their struggles on academic performance was apparent.
- Community mental health agencies, for the most part, were reluctant to approach school districts to explore collaborative interventions because of past negative experiences working with school districts and a feeling of being unwelcome.

After the school health assets and needs presentations, those in attendance discussed how it was clear that the mental health status of the student population was having a deleterious effect on academic performance and that to do something about it, the district would have to look for help from outside agencies and organizations.

on school health and education literature should be generated. A suggested list of key words follows.

Academic success	Health teacher
Alcohol	Healthy
Community partners	Mental
Counseling	Nurse
Dentist	Nutrition
Dental	Physical examinations
Doctor	Physical activity
Drugs	Physical education
Eating	Recess
Emotional	Safe
Engaged	School lunches
Food	Screening
Guidance	Social
Gym	Supported
Health	Test scores
Health class	Vending machines
Health education	Wellness
Health services	

Transcripts of all individual and group interviews are reviewed independently by two or three people for common themes indicated by the key words and phrases. During the first reading, other potential key words suggested by the transcripts are noted and shared. A second reading focusing on the additional key words is then completed. Consensus among the readers as to the collective answers to individual questions across interviewees and focus groups, as well as common themes that emerge from the responses are then determined and recorded as the results of the interviews.

The community profile, SHI or HSRC data and recommendations, academic performance data, WellSAT results, and results of the key informant and the focus group interviews are reviewed collectively by the assessment group to develop a list of school health assets and needs for the district. If desired, assessment group members can first develop individual assets and needs lists and then engage in a modified **nominal group process** (Hodges & Videto, 2011) to create a final list of the district's assets and needs with regard to school health.

Assets would be items such as a community physical environment conducive to physical activity and recreation; abundant health resources in the community; varied cultural opportunities; diverse, active parent groups; willingness of community agencies to partner with schools; existence of present or past success with school community partnerships; physical education that meets or exceeds recommended minutes; and existing resources and processes within the school structure for supporting students experiencing health issues.

Needs would be items such as low socioeconomic status; limited access to health care in the community; lack of effective communication across schools and between central administration and schools; lack of institutional belief in connection between health and well-being and academic performance; lack of evidence of using health data in decision making (policy, programs, strategic planning); no CSH or WSCC structure or only partial implementation of CSH or WSCC.

School health assets and needs identified through the process should be disseminated to districts through presentations to administrative and instructional personnel selected by the district and accompanied by a written report.

Each district presentation should prompt a discussion about the realities of what the data suggest compared with the perceptions of school personnel, any disconnect between school health and academic initiatives, and the effect that CSH or WSCC could have on academic performance. These discussions should be followed up with priority setting and action planning initiatives. The data are used to drive the development of goals and objectives for school health councils and teams, to shape programming and policy development, to make decisions related to the selection of curricula, to support internal and external funding requests, and to shape the mission and school improvement plans of schools and districts. For example, schools and districts with whom the authors have been involved have used school health and wellness profiles to advocate for the inclusion of school health goals and objectives in school improvement plans, to seek external funding for school health initiatives and school–community health partnership initiatives, to support redirecting additional resources to school health services, and to begin the infusion of health literacy skills across disciplines in support of achievement of Common Core Standards.

IMPLICATIONS FOR WSCC

The process involving the four actions outlined earlier provides a means for school districts to identify a set of assets and needs related to WSCC. The process is useful for exploring and tracking school health functioning and for making data-driven decisions about school health and academic performance before deciding on what policies or programs are needed. Moreover, based on feedback from school district personnel who attended district assets and needs presentations given by the authors in various school districts, the comprehensive school district health and wellness profile can raise awareness of the importance of functioning school health systems to academic performance and the interaction of the health and wellness status of students, staff, parents, and the surrounding community. Given the continuing budgetary challenges that school districts are wrestling with, data-based processes that provide an ecological scan can be used as an objective framework for having the difficult discussions of how best to move forward toward meeting academic performance mandates amidst declining funding.

One of the discussions that has been repeatedly prompted by the authors' use of this process is the disconnect between the perceptions of the schools, community organizations, and agencies about their actual and potential roles in assisting with school health and wellness. For the most part, schools saw themselves as being in partnership with many community institutions, whereas community organizations perceived school districts as unwelcoming and viewed any "partnerships" as one-sided in favor of school districts (Hodges & Videto, 2011). Exploration of shared resources in health-related areas between school districts and community organizations may result in more efficiency and effectiveness in improving the health and wellness of youth and adults in school district communities.

SUMMARY

Data-driven school health planning provides a strong foundation for updating or implementing WSCC, and using the four phases of PRECEDE to determine needs and assets is valuable in that process. Moreover, a broad ecological scan of school and community data can illuminate the importance of school health to the health of the community and to academic performance. As schools shift resources toward Race to the Top (United States Department of Education, n.d.) and the implementation of the Common Core Standards (National Governors Association and State Education Chiefs, n.d.), an opportunity is available to demonstrate a place at the table for school health. In addition, as resources are shifted and budgets reduced, the need for true collaborations seems even more critical. Use of the four actions to create a profile—by developing community understanding, conducting a wellness policy review, reviewing the Coordinated School Health implementation, and conducting a school health function assessment—can provide a formula for profiling student health and wellness. School districts can use the resulting profile and suggestions as a way to illustrate the connections between health and academic performance, reveal district and community assets that can be built on to improve health and academic performance, and provide a platform for the establishment of more efficient and effective school health systems and collaborations.

Glossary

academic performance data—Data related to the performance of schools or youth that indicate how well they are doing in regard to a set of academic standards (for example, student assessment results or state-issued report cards).

Bronfenbrenner's ecological systems theory—Also called the human ecology theory, identifies environmental systems with which a person interacts. Bronfenbrenner believed that a person's development was affected by everything in his or her surrounding environment. He divided the person's environment into five levels: the microsystem, the mesosystem, the exosystem, the macrosystem, and the chronosystem.

focus group discussions—A qualitative approach to learning about a group of people, often used in health education and health promotion to collect information for program planning. Participants in the group are usually alike on one or more characteristic, although the composition of the group depends on the purpose of the discussion.

key informant interviews—A key informant is a person in the community or school district who has direct knowledge of a group or has access to information about a group. In a key informant interview, the identified person is interviewed to provide information to the person collecting the data for the purposes of developing or assessing a program or policy.

nominal group process—Nominal group process or nominal group technique (NGT) is described by CDC as a structured variation of a small-group discussion to reach consensus. NGT gathers information by asking participants to respond to questions posed by a moderator and then to prioritize the ideas or suggestions of the group members.

PRECEDE–PROCEED framework—A planning model developed by Green and Kreuter that offers a framework for identifying intervention strategies for achieving objectives. The model provides a comprehensive structure for assessing health and quality-of-life needs and for designing, implementing, and evaluating health promotion and other public health programs to meet those needs. PRECEDE (predisposing, reinforcing, and enabling constructs in educational diagnosis and evaluation) outlines a diagnostic planning process to assist in the development of targeted public health programs. PROCEED (policy, regulatory, and organizational constructs in educational and environmental development) guides the implementation and evaluation of the programs designed using the PRECEDE part of the model.

school district health and wellness profile—A comprehensive school audit that provides an overview of a school district's health and wellness standing. The profile may include community, health, and academic data compiled from a variety of tools and sources. It identifies school health and community assets and needs that are suggested by these kinds of data.

snowball sampling technique—A method of sampling in which existing study subjects recruit future subjects from among their friends and acquaintances. The recruits grow in snowball fashion, hence the name of the technique.

windshield tours—A process of collecting data through direct observation (driving a car) of a community or area where a program or intervention is being developed or assessed.

Youth Risk Behavior Survey—The YRBS, or Youth Risk Behavior Surveillance System (YRBSS), monitors priority health-risk behaviors and the prevalence of obesity and asthma among youth and young adults. The YRBSS includes a national school-based survey that is conducted by CDC. State, territorial, tribal, and district surveys exist that are conducted by state, territorial, and local education and health agencies and tribal governments.

Application Activities

1. Follow the recommendations given in the chapter for collecting data for developing community understanding and develop a community profile paper for a local school district. Use only public domain and public access sources to obtain the data needed to develop that profile. See the information presented in table 9.2 to assist you in determining what you need to include in your paper.
2. As part of a small-group activity, have students conduct a windshield tour of the local community or city. Identify and map schools, parks, recreational and health facilities, restaurants, and grocery-shopping facilities for a review (see figure 9.2). A review consists of driving by the various facilities, taking photos (of one or two representative locations), and providing a written description of the facilities in regard to how the citizens of the community would be able to access the facility (walk, sidewalk quality, or driving and parking conditions).
3. Identify an issue of concern for your campus that all students or a group of students would be interested in discussing (e.g., Do students feel safe walking to and from town at night? How well is the tobacco-free campus policy being implemented?). Then develop a series of questions that you could ask students on campus in a focus group to determine what students know or believe regarding that issue. If possible, you and a class partner can hold a focus group discussion and record both verbal and nonverbal responses from the participants.

Resources

CDC's Youth Risk Behavior Survey (YRBS) home page. www.cdc.gov/HealthyYouth/yrbs/index.htm

Common Core State Standards Tool Kit. www.nea.org/home/ccss-toolkit.htm

Hodges, Bonni C., & Donna M. Videto. 2011. *Assessment and Planning in Health Programs* (2nd ed.). Sudbury, MA: Jones and Bartlett Learning.

NEA Today: http://neatoday.org/2010/06/02/must-reads-race-to-the-top/

Theory at a Glance: A Guide for Health Promotion Practice (2nd ed.). 2005. National Cancer Institute. www.cancer.gov/cancertopics/cancerlibrary/theory.pdf

WellSAT. Home page of the WellSAT, the Wellness Assessment Tool. http://wellsat.org/

References

ASCD. 2012. *Healthy School Report Card.* www.healthyschoolcommunities.org/HSRC/pages/reportcard/index.aspx

Bronfenbrenner, Urie. 1979. *The Ecology of Human Development: Experiments by Nature and Design.* Cambridge, MA: Harvard.

Butler, James, Fryer, Craig S., Reed, Ernestine A., & Thomas, Stephen B. 2011. Utilizing the School Health Index to Build Collaboration Between a University and an Urban School District. *Journal of School Health*, *81*(12), 774–782.

Centers for Disease Control and Prevention. 2014. *School Health Index.* www.cdc.gov/HealthyYouth /SHI/

Centers for Disease Control and Prevention. 2014. *Youth Risk Behavior Surveillance System.* www.cdc.gov/yrbs/

Child Nutrition and WIC Reauthorization Act of 2004. 2013. www.fns.usda.gov/tn/healthy/108-265.pdf

Fetro, Joyce V., Givens, Connie, & Carroll, Kellie. 2009. Coordinated School Health: Getting It All Together. *Educational Leadership*, *67*(4), 32–37.

Goldman, Karen D., & Schmalz, Kathleen J. 2001. Focus on Focus Groups! *Health Promotion Practice*, *2*(1), 14–15.

Green, Lawrence, & Kreuter, Marshall. 2005. *Health Program Planning: An Ecological and Educational Approach* (4th ed.). New York: McGraw-Hill.

Hodges, Bonni C., Videto, Donna M., and Greeley, Aimee, E. 2011, October. *Working to Create Limitless Possibilities in Limited Environments.* Paper presented at 85th American School Health Association Conference, Louisville, KY.

Hodges, Bonni C., & Videto, Donna M. 2011. *Assessment and Planning in Health Programs* (2nd ed.). Sudbury, MA: Jones & Bartlett Learning.

Lohrmann, David K. 2010. *The Purpose of the Healthy School Report Card.* www.ascd.org/publications/books/110140/chapters/The-Purpose-of-the-Healthy-School-Report-Card.aspx

National Governors Association and State Education Chiefs. n.d. *The Common Core State Standards Initiative.* www.corestandards.org/html

Schwartz, Misty, & Laughlin, Ann. 2008. Partnering With Schools: A Win-Win Experience. *Journal of Nursing Education*, *47*(6), 279–282.

Torabi, Mohammad R., & Ding, Kele. 1998. Selected Critical Measurements and Statistical Issues in Health Education Evaluation and Research. *International Electronic Journal of Health Education*, *1*(1), 26–38.

United States Department of Education. n.d. *Race to the Top.* www2ed.gov/programs/racetothetop/html

Videto, Donna M., & Hodges, Bonni C. 2009. Use of University/School Partnerships for the Institutionalization of the Coordinated School Health Program. *American Journal of Health Education*, *40*(4), 212–219.

World Health Organization (WHO). 2000. *Reproductive Health During Conflict and Displacement: A Guide for Programme Managers.* Geneva, Switzerland: World Health Organization. www.who.int/reproductivehealth/publications/RHR_00_13_RH_conflict_and_displacement/PDF_RHR_00_13/chapter10.en.pdf

Yale Rudd Center. 2013. *Wellness School Assessment Tool* (WellSAT). http://wellsat.org

10

Implementing WSCC

DONNA M. VIDETO • DAVID A. BIRCH

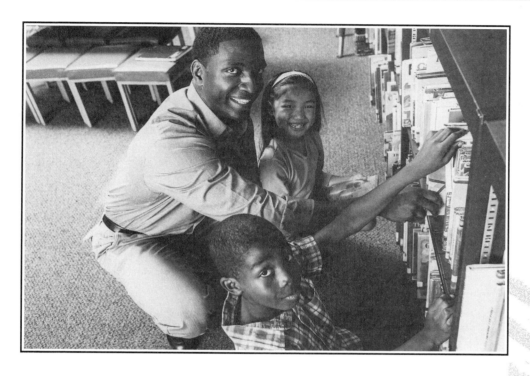

ASCD and CDC have identified the Whole School, Whole Community, Whole Child (WSCC) approach as an important avenue for improving education performance and the well-being of our youth (ASCD, 2014a) Similar to Coordinated School Health (CSH), WSCC is underpinned by the linkage of health and academics. To implement the WSCC approach, school districts need to establish the necessary infrastructure, analyze the initial WSCC assessment data, formulate action plans, and use the resulting plans to provide direction in the development of actual programs and policies designed to promote health and academic success (CDC, 2013a).

Implementation of CSH or WSCC is more likely to be successful if it is guided by a planned process. CDC provides a framework to implement or improve CSH in an effective and efficient way. In addition to the CDC strategies, ASCD has published *Nine Levers of School Change* to assist school districts in taking steps toward planning, implementing, or improving CSH or WSCC (Valois, 2011).

Program implementation involves carrying out the activities that make up an intervention while working toward the program objectives and ultimately the program goal or goals (Hodges & Videto, 2011). CDC has identified eight steps for consideration by schools and school districts for planning, implementation, and evaluation of CSH and now the WSCC approach.

1. Secure and maintain administrative support and commitment.
2. Establish a **school health council or team**.
3. Identify a **school health coordinator**.
4. Develop a plan (see planning process presented in chapter 9).
5. Implement multiple strategies through multiple components.
6. Focus on students.
7. Address priority **health-enhancing** and **health-risk behaviors**.
8. Provide professional development for staff (CDC, 2013b).

ASCD envisions WSCC as a strategy for achieving healthy school communities. According to ASCD, healthy school communities are those communities that "focus on making schools healthier and more efficient places for teaching and learning. It provides opportunities for school communities in all parts of the world to network and share best practices" (ASCD, n.d.a, para. 1). To address this concept, ASCD has identified strategies called the nine levers of school change that are designed to assist schools or school districts in their actions to plan, implement, and improve CSH (Valois, 2011).

To promote quality implementation of CSH/WSCC, Hodges (2013) has developed a combined list of both the CDC's eight steps and the ASCD's nine levers of change (figure 10.1) (ASCD, n.d.a.;

FIGURE 10.1

Integrated Steps for Implementing WSCC

Creating District Infrastructure and Preparing for Program Implementation

1. Secure and maintain administrative support and commitment.
   - School planning teams should be principal led.
   - Include health and wellness in the district mission statement.
2. Establish a district health council and school teams.
   - Create a districtwide council and teams for each school.
   - Team leaders ensure that stakeholders understand the value of their involvement.
3. Identify a school health coordinator.
   - Coordinator collects data and oversees planning and implementation processes.
   - Coordinator organizes the components, policies, programs, activities, and resources.

Program Implementation

1. Set goals and objectives and then develop a plan.
   - Develop goals and objectives from data and include systematic issues.
   - Prioritize the area or areas with the most need.
   - Action plans should align with and be part of the school improvement process.
   - Good planning includes identification of resources, collaborators, and strategies.
   - Collaboration begins from the start.

Evaluation

1. Implement the plan and strategies.
   - Focus on students.
   - Implement multiple strategies through multiple components.
   - Address priority health-enhancing and health-risk behaviors.
   - Develop ongoing, purposeful professional development integrated to support the process.
2. Monitor progress and impact; adjust as necessary.
3. Evaluate results and celebrate successes.
4. Communicate findings to district and community.

Reprinted, by permission, from B.C. Hodges. 2013, *The changing nature of school health.*

CDC, 2013b). In Hodges' list, steps 1 through 3 address the process of creating the district infrastructure and preparing for program implementation, step 4 is what is generally considered program implementation, and steps 5 through 7 address evaluation.

Some of the content in this chapter presents efforts conducted during the initial planning stages that can be considered as planning steps that take place before implementation. They are included here in chapter 10 because they are considered important stage-setting strategies for successful WSCC implementation. Figure 10.2 depicts the ASCD and CDC combined strategies in steps 1 through 5 in a way that might help to visualize how they fit into creating infrastructure for the implementation of CSH as well as the WSCC approach.

SECURE AND MAINTAIN ADMINISTRATIVE SUPPORT AND COMMITMENT

In chapter 9, strategies and specific examples for data collection used in planning are presented. Hodges' combined list of suggestions is presented in this chapter in the context of setting the stage for and moving forward with implementation of WSCC.

The first pre-implementation strategy for a school district is to secure and maintain administrative support and commitment. Critical strategies for CSH implementation and program maintenance include the superintendent's support at the district level and the principal's support at the school level. CDC suggests that school administrators can support a coordinated approach to school health by engaging in the following efforts:

- Incorporating health in the district's or school's vision and mission statements, including health goals in the school's improvement plan
- Appointing someone to oversee school health
- Allocating resources
- Modeling healthy behaviors
- Regularly communicating the importance of wellness to students, staff, and parents (CDC, 2013b)

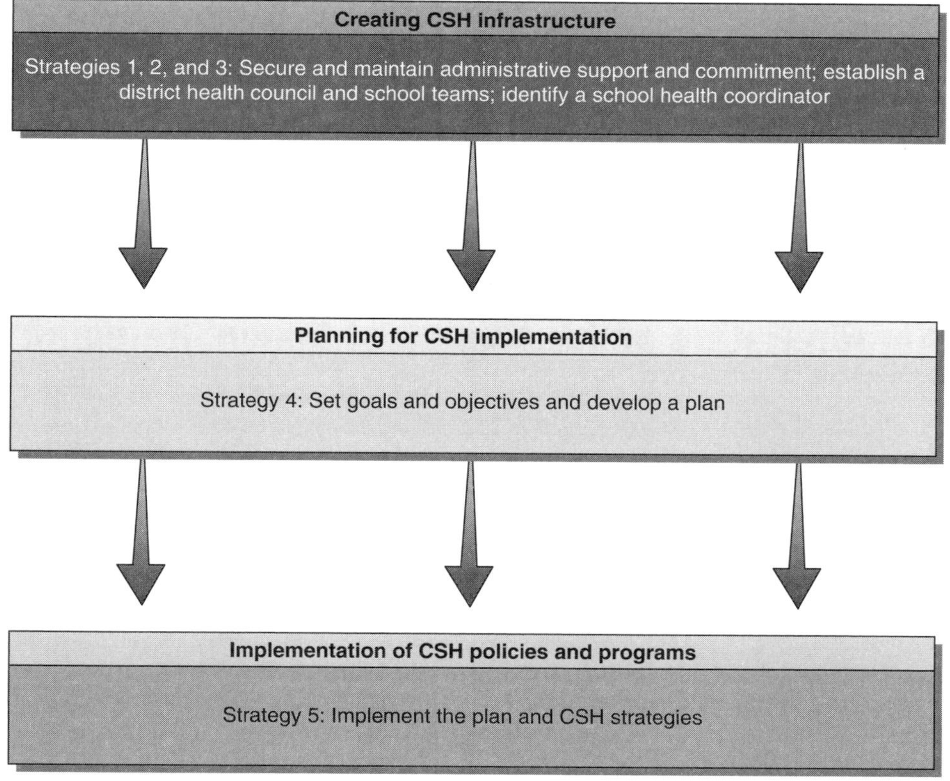

Figure 10.2 Visualizing steps 1 through 5 of WSCC implementation.

As a first step in this process, the team or committee should develop a vision statement based on the guiding principles of CSH and WSCC. This activity might have the team or committee defining the terms that could go into developing a vision, terms such as a *healthy school environment* or an *active lifestyle* (California School Boards Association [CSBA], 2009). The CSBA report *Building Healthy Communities: A School Leader's Guide to Collaboration and Community Engagement* (2009) suggests that the planning team develop a vision aligned with common values and community priorities. In the University of Kansas' *Community Toolbox*, an organization's vision is described as "your dream . . . the ideal conditions for your community." The vision statement is further described as the "hopes for the future." Characteristics and examples from *Community Toolbox* are presented in figure 10.3 (University of Kansas, 2013). The American School Health Association (2010) provides the recommendation that the vision include information about the importance of the health and well-being of students and staff as a foundation for school improvement and academic success.

After a vision statement has been established, the school health council or committee should develop a **mission statement**. Including health in a district's mission statement has been encouraged as a way to help move the actions of a district toward implementation of health-enhancing policies and programs. The mission of Namaste Charter School near Chicago is directly founded on many CSH principles. The school's motto is "Educating Children From the Inside Out." To support that motto, the following mission statement is provided:

> Namaste Charter School's fundamental belief is that all children possess the attributes necessary to become healthy, literate, and life-long lovers of learning. Children's learning is facilitated through investigations, interactions, and instruction that are intellectually challenging and developmentally appropriate. We provide support and opportunities for children to acquire the skills, knowledge, and understanding to thrive academically and socially, find personal health and fulfillment, and take responsibility as productive members of their community. Our curriculum is aligned to the Illinois State Learning Standards that goes beyond the standards through the development of a comprehensive framework which ensures that children make connections in their learning, develop the confidence necessary to think critically and independently, gain an interest in seeking solutions to their own problems, and realize a love of learning. All of this is encompassed by a daily focus on health, nutrition, and physical fitness. (Namaste Charter School, n.d.)

This statement makes clear to the school community the value of a healthy child and the role that being healthy plays in the school and in the academic success of that child.

FIGURE 10.3

Characteristics and Examples of Vision Statements

Characteristics of Vision Statements

- Understood and shared by members of the community
- Broad enough to include a diverse variety of local perspectives
- Inspiring and uplifting to everyone involved in the effort
- Easy to communicate, generally short enough to fit on a T-shirt

Examples of Vision Statements

- Caring communities
- Healthy children
- Safe streets, safe neighborhoods
- Every house a home
- Education for all
- Peace on earth

ESTABLISH A DISTRICT HEALTH COUNCIL AND SCHOOL TEAMS

Dilley (2011) suggests that successful CSH implementation involves the convening of a school health advisory committee as well as the designation of school coordinators to oversee the school health process, programs, and policies. Reinforcing what was written by Dilley (2011), CDC states the need for a district to establish a school health council or school health team as an important strategy for implementation (CDC, 2013b) and as a critical part of the CSH infrastructure.

Ideally, the district-level school health council includes at least one representative from each of the 10 WSCC components. It should also include school administrators, parents, students, and community representatives involved and supportive of the health and well-being of students (CDC, 2013b). Table 10.1 provides a list of potential or possible representatives of the 10 components of WSCC for a school health council. Note that individuals may be representing more than one component and that some components may have multiple representatives, such as one from the district and one from the community. At the school level the school health teams usually include an administrator, an identified school health leader, teachers,

Table 10.1 District School Health Council Possible Representatives

CSH component	Possible representatives
Health education	Health coordinator, health teacher, director of curriculum and instruction, student health club representative, family and consumer sciences teacher, district health education consultant, health department health educator
Physical education and physical activity	Physical education coordinator, physical education teacher, district physical therapist, student teachers from local colleges and universities, grant-funded physical activity program investigators
Nutrition environment and services	District dietician, food services manager or other personnel (business administrator), cafeteria support staff, healthy heart representative from health department
Health services	District medical consultant, school nurse, health department representative, speech therapists, special services personnel for students with special needs
Counseling, psychological, and social services	School psychologist, guidance counselor, social worker, teacher support aide
Social and emotional climate	Administrators such as a principal or vice principal, student representatives, school psychologists, guidance counselors, social workers
Physical environment	Administrators, buildings and grounds administrator, custodian, local law enforcement
Employee wellness	Elementary and secondary-level teacher, staff wellness coordinator, faculty or staff with a passion for wellness, community representative from worksite health
Family engagement	Representatives from parent groups (parents guild, PTO, PTA, representatives from issue-related parent groups), youth groups
Community involvement	Chamber of commerce, rotary club, health agencies, government agencies

other staff, parents, and student representatives reflective of the components at the district level (CDC, 2013b). Representatives of the council need to reflect the demographic composition of the school community.

After councils and teams are established, time should be devoted to making sure that all representatives understand the goals of WSCC and the evidence in the professional literature on the relationship between academic success and healthy youth (Basch, 2011). CSBA (2009) describes the importance of addressing values that the members share because this effort will help establish group cohesiveness. Gottlieb and colleagues (1999) recommend that these councils or teams allow the development of a common

School Health *in Action*

Tips for Implementation at District Level

The Cortland City (New York) school district was highlighted on the CDC website of success stories (CDC, 2013c) for the work conducted at Cortland City Schools in the CSH component of nutrition services. District initiatives included limiting student access to competitive foods, adopting marketing techniques to promote healthful choices, setting nutrition policies and standards, establishing nutrition standards for competitive foods, and making more healthy foods and beverages available. Six factors were reported as keys to the success of Cortland City Schools. The first factor was having a vision of being committed to a Coordinated School Health program. The second factor was leadership as demonstrated by administrative support from the board of education, superintendent, and the principals from the schools in the district. The third factor, collaboration, was shown through partnerships that were established with community agencies, staff, parents, and students. Teamwork in each building as well as districtwide provided a demonstration of the fourth factor. The fifth factor, data driven, was demonstrated by collecting baseline data to demonstrate improvements after repeated assessments, which were then conducted every two to three years. Finally, the sixth factor recognized was the issue of financial support, which was apparent in the use of minigrants such as one through the Healthy Heart Coalition.

Jeannette Dippo, former Health Education and Wellness coordinator with Cortland City Schools, offered five suggestions for the implementation of CSH programs and policies:

- Districts need to get administrative support for the CSH activities and to send out consistent messages.
- Broad involvement is needed, including support from parents, school staff, and community members. This support is necessary for strong advocates to assist in getting the CSH vision and goals converted into actual programs and policy. Administrators may respond more positivity to general staff and parents than to the typical school health champion, who is generally the health educator or health coordinator.
- The most critical CSH priorities need to be converted into policy. Such a policy will help ensure that work or effort in that area will continue. A policy will help to establish the priority after the champions leave or have moved on to other initiatives because the policy will still exist.
- Each school needs to have a health coordinator to drive and pull the work of the team together. The schools and the district need someone with real passion for CSH. CSH functions best when someone with continuity who believes in what is being done is there to oversee the actions. A health coordinator is someone to help develop the structure for the work to happen.
- A healthy school team is needed for every school building, along with a separate district team. The accomplishments that were made in individual schools happened because each school building had its own team to work with, and someone to take the program or initiative and make it happen at the school level. It is critical that school principals be members of each school team. This network needs to be in place to share ideas and develop and implement districtwide policies.

awareness, review how CSH was implemented in other districts, and come to an understanding of what the WSCC approach means and its potential effect on students. A common understanding of CSH has been identified as important to successful implementation (Deschesnes, Martin, & Jompe Hill, 2003). Therefore resources like *The Learning Connection: What You Need to Know to Ensure Your Kids are Healthy and Ready to Learn* by the Action for Healthy Kids (2014) and *Health and Academic Achievement* by CDC (2014a) are useful to help with the development of that educational process.

IDENTIFY A SCHOOL HEALTH COORDINATOR

The third strategy is to identify a school health coordinator to round out the necessary infrastructure (CDC, 2013b). A full-time or part-time school health coordinator is a critical factor for the successful implementation of a coordinated approach to school health. Before program implementation, data need to be collected to develop a clear picture of the needs and assets of the WSCC policies and programming efforts currently in place or lacking (see chapter 9 for more on data collection for identification of needs and assets). One role of the coordinator is to oversee the baseline and initial data collection process. To conduct the assessment, districts can use a number of possible tools. In chapter 9, and in the appendix, a variety of tools are identified and described that can be used to assess the CSH framework and the WSCC model. The school health coordinator helps maintain active school health councils and facilitates health programming between schools in the district and with the community (CDC, 2013b). The coordinator would also oversee the 10 (versus the traditional 8) components of school health and would facilitate the actions to achieve a successful WSCC approach, including policies, practices, activities, and resources.

Videto and Hodges (2009) assessed the level of **institutionalization** of action plans resulting from a School Health Index (SHI) assessment in school districts throughout upstate and central New York along with those factors that assisted in that process. Findings from this study reinforced the importance of health coordinators to ensure successful institutionalization of CSH plans. A school district may identify a school health educator, school administrator, education administrator, school nurse, food service coordinator, physical educator, or other school health stakeholder as a possible candidate for the role of a school health coordinator. In some cases, a community consultant or a university partner may serve in that position.

SET GOALS AND OBJECTIVES AND DEVELOP A PLAN

The results of the assessment strategies tools used in the baseline assessment will help to provide a district or school with guidance for identifying the priority areas for setting goals and objectives and for developing an action plan for addressing the priorities. School or district teams need to develop their own action plans based on what is important as well as what is achievable in their school or community (Alliance for a Healthier Generation, 2014). An assessment of the community assets and needs during this initial phase will enhance the process by helping to identify resources or potential collaborations that could address existing district gaps and needs.

Dilly (2011) recommends that after the assessment is conducted and data are reviewed, the council and teams go on to develop and implement a plan. Many of the available tools include the facilitation of steps whereby the people conducting the assessment develop action or implementation plans that include establishing priorities and determining implementation steps (CDC, 2013d; ASCD, 2014b).

In developing action plans, CDC suggests that they be based on realistic goals and measurable objectives. Following the format of CDC SMART (SMART represents specific, measurable, attainable, relevant, and time-based), a timeline for achievement of the goals and objectives would be established (CDC, 2011). CDC uses the acronym SMART to help refine short-term and long-term goals and define what is intended to be achieved through a program or policy (CDC, 2011). A short-term goal might be to implement an anti-bullying policy in all seven schools in the district by January 2016. A long-term goal might be to reduce the number of reported incidences of bullying throughout the district by 25 percent by September 2017.

Schools need to identify sufficient resources to help their plans succeed. These resources might include assessment tools such as the SHI and the Healthy Schools Report Card (HSRC), as well as funding for activities, shared resources, and

School Health *in Action*

Positive Effects of School Health Coordinators

School health coordinators are an important aspect of promoting quality implementation of CSH or WSCC. A study in Maine showed clear differences between schools with school health coordinators and those without one. In January 2001, the Maine Centers for Disease Control and Prevention formed a network of school and community partnerships called Healthy Maine Partnerships (HMP). Every part of the state belonged to an HMP. Some but not all HMPs hired at least one school health coordinator. But not all schools in all HMPs could be covered by a coordinator. The role of the coordinators was to implement CSH in the schools that they served and support it through grant writing, convening wellness councils, engaging in fund-raising, and making presentations to school boards.

In 2006 an evaluation was conducted to compare the schools that had a school health coordinator (intervention schools) with those that did not have a coordinator (nonintervention schools). The evaluation addressed two research questions:

- Were more physical activity, nutrition, and tobacco-related policies and programs associated with intervention schools than with nonintervention schools in 2006?
- Were school policies and programs associated with lower student risk behavior in intervention school than in nonintervention schools in 2006?

The results of the evaluation indicated that the intervention schools with coordinators were more likely to have physical activity intramural offerings, improved nutrition offerings, and tobacco cessation programs. School policies in intervention schools were associated with decreased soda consumption, decreased inactivity, and decreased tobacco use. In addition, required school health curricula in intervention schools were more predictive of decreased risk behaviors than in nonintervention schools. The results appear to demonstrate the positive effect of a school health coordinator in the Maine initiative.

Reference

O'Brien, L.M., Placsek, M., MacDonald P.B., Ellis, J., Berry, S., & Martin, M. 2010. Impact of a School Health Coordinator Intervention on Health-Related School Policies and Student Behavior. *Journal of School Health, 80*(4), 176–185.

experience and expertise needed for the successful implementation and maintenance of programs and systems (Dilley, 2011).

After a WSCC assessment of the components of school health is completed, the results are often channeled into a series of action steps that the district can take to improve or expand their efforts (CDC, 2014b). Four action steps are recommended after an assessment with the SHI:

1. Completing the overall scorecard
2. Completing the school health improvement plan
3. Implementing recommendations
4. Reassessing annually to strive for continuous improvement (CDC, 2014b)

The school health improvement plan (step 2) is a plan focused on improving some aspect of CSH. In the SHI assessment the school health improvement plan comes in the form of a worksheet. The SHI version was developed for writing down actions agreed on by the assessment team, a description of the steps that could be taken to achieve those actions, identification of who will be responsible for implementation, and the target date for achieving the desired outcome (CDC, 2014b).

Figure 10.4 shows an example of part of the SHI school health improvement plan completed for one action that could have resulted from a question in SHI Module 1, School Health and Safety Policies and Environment, in the area of nutrition outside regular school hours (CDC, 2014b). Note that although the SHI was developed to assess CSH, the WSCC approach reorganizes the content of the 8 components into 10 components. Thus, with some modification, the SHI can be adapted for use with the WSCC approach. In addition, other assessment tools include similar steps that result in a school health improvement plan.

Often appearing on school health improvement plans is the need to develop or to revise existing health-related policies. Implementing policies has the potential to affect multiple WSCC components because the outreach tends to be broader. Policy review and development often appears on a school improvement plan (not to be confused with the school health improvement plan). School improvement plans (SIPs) are required by law and are locally developed documents that keep a school on track as school staff work throughout the school year toward overall improvement and academic success for every student (U.S. Department of Education, 2010). The Alliance for a Healthier Generation (2014) defines SIPs as comprehensive plans that describes the long-range improvement goals for the school, which include improving academic performance, professional development, and school facilities. SIPs can also include specific goals that pertain to staff and student health and wellness (Alliance for a Healthier Generation, 2014).

When developing SIPs, Dilley (2011) offers the recommendation that all policies or efforts being described should support school health and the development of healthy student behaviors. A review of existing policies might uncover opportunities for revision where new wording can be introduced that would create opportunities for an environment conducive to healthy and successful youth (Dilley, 2011).

In a review of recommended policies, the following Jennings Public Schools policy to promote respect in schools was identified:

> Respect denotes both a positive feeling of esteem for a person and also specific actions and conduct representative of that esteem. Respect can be defined as allowing yourself and others to do and be their best. It is the goal of Jennings Public Schools to create a mutual respectful atmosphere between all individuals involved within our school including administrators, teachers, staff members, students, parents, and visitors (About.com, 2014).

The Jennings Public Schools policy to promote respect in schools can be rewritten to place a stronger focus on health promotion by using language clearly linked to healthy development and the whole child. It might then look like this:

> An environment supportive of the mental, emotional, physical, intellectual, and social health of the whole child includes showing respect for each other. Respect can be defined as allowing yourself and others to do and be their best. It is the goal of Jennings Public Schools to create a healthy, safe, challenging, supportive, and engaging environment based on mutual respect between all individuals involved within our school including administrators, teachers, staff members, students, parents, and visitors.

IMPLEMENT THE PLAN AND STRATEGIES

Putting the action plan into place consists of implementing the plan and strategies, which usu-

FIGURE 10.4

School Health Improvement Plan Example

Actions	Steps	By whom and when
1. Develop healthier fund-raising options	a. Revise wellness policy to address fund-raising b. Seek out healthier options to share with groups c. Meet with parent and student groups to address fund-raising options and revised wellness policy d. Communicate on school website revised wellness policy and highlight fund-raising changes	a. District health council under leadership of health coordinator Meg D., September 2015 b. Subcommittee of district health council under leadership of health coordinator, September and October 2015 c. Principals at each school along with coordinator and health teachers, October and November 2015 d. Technology representative Shelia G., September and November 2015

Adapted from Centers for Disease Control and Prevention 2013.

ally consists of adopting policies or programs. When implementing the plan, districts need to direct the focus of school health efforts on meeting the education and health needs of students (CDC, 2013b). In addition, providing opportunities for students to be meaningfully involved in the school and the community will help the team to focus on students. School health efforts in programming and policies should give youth the chance to develop and exercise leadership abilities, build skills, form positive relationships with caring adults, and contribute to their school and greater community (CDC, 2013a).

CDC suggests that students can promote a healthy and safe school and community through opportunities such as involvement in peer education, peer advocacy, or cross-age mentoring programs. Other opportunities include involving young people in service learning avenues and participation on school health teams' advisory committees and boards that address health and wellness, education, and youth-related issues (CDC, 2013b).

Moving into the taking-action phase of program and policy implementation, CDC suggests that school districts implement multiple strategies through multiple components. To address one school health component, a variety of efforts are needed to have an effect in that area. Because the components are often overlapping and dependent on each other, addressing multiple if not all of the components is recommended for achieving the positive health and learning outcomes desired (CDC, 2013b). Many possibilities exist for advancing each of the WSCC components, and examples of possible policies and programming efforts can be discovered in any of the CSH assessment tools or criteria (see table 10.2 for possible strategies for improvement). Tools such as the CDC School Health Index, ASCD Healthy Schools Report Card, and ASCD School Improvement Tool are some of the more well-known and commonly used tools. Any strategies pursued by a school or district should be based on an assessment conducted at the school or district.

Schools should consider implementing policies and programs to help students avoid or reduce health-risk behaviors that contribute to the leading causes of death and disability among young people as well as among adults (CDC, 2014d). CDC has identified six categories of priority health-risk behaviors as being linked to the leading causes of death and disability in the United States:

- Behaviors that contribute to unintentional injuries and violence
- Tobacco use
- Alcohol and other drug use
- Sexual behaviors that contribute to unintended pregnancy and STDs, including HIV infection
- Unhealthy eating
- Physical inactivity (CDC, 2014d)

Schools can assess health-risk behaviors among young people in these six categories as well as in general health status, overweight, and asthma through formal surveys such as the Youth Risk Behavior Survey (YRBS) (CDC, 2014d). The YRBS, available through CDC, is a national school-based survey that can provide the school and district with behavioral data for 9th through 12th graders (CDC, 2014d). Data resulting from the survey can be used to track behavioral trends at the local level for establishing priorities and for monitoring program and policy success. In addition, the local data can be used to make comparisons to state, regional, and national levels with the data available on the CDC YRBS website. For example if a school district discovers that the proportion of students who participated in at least 60 minutes of physical activity per day was lower than the proportion for students in the state and nation, the district may decide that they need to address the issue. The action could mean changing the academic schedule and requirements to include daily physical education, training teachers to incorporate physical activity into the classroom, allowing fit breaks throughout the day, or instituting a walk-to-school program. This example demonstrates how data from the YRBS system can be used to inform programming and policies as a district tries to improve the health and well-being of students and staff.

After a health-risk behavior or behaviors have been identified as a priority, the school or district faces the challenge of identifying or developing relevant policies or programs. Research-based programming that can reduce risk behaviors has been identified, and information is available through *Registries of Programs Effective in Reducing Youth Risk Behaviors* on the CDC website as well as through other similar sites (CDC, 2013d).

Besides selecting programming options, districts need to work to bring faculty and staff onboard with WSCC efforts. Education is

Table 10.2 WSCC Components and Possible Strategies for Improvement

WSCC component	Strategies
Health education	The district requires that all elementary schools teach health education in grades K through 5. After an extensive review, an elementary health curriculum was selected and teacher training for implementation was conducted.
Physical education and physical activity	All students would be required to participate in a minimum of 150 minutes of physical education per week by a new district mandate.
Nutrition environment and services	The breakfast program at the junior high and high school will now include offering at least one fruit other than juice at breakfast.
Health services	Each school is now required to have at least one full-time registered school nurse responsible for health services all day, every day.
Counseling, psychological, and social services	The counseling staff will now provide small group and classroom-based health promotion and prevention activities in each classroom on a regular basis in addition to one-on-one counseling sessions.
Social and emotional environment	Staff receive training on how to foster the emotional growth and development of the elementary-level child through guided social skill instruction.
Physical environment	Each school is required to make drinking water available to students free of charge throughout the day by installing additional water coolers when possible, making water available, and providing opportunities to take water breaks as needed.
Employee wellness	Each school is required to evaluate the employee wellness program annually and provide the district wellness coordinator with a report of the findings. These findings will be used to establish yearly staff wellness goals and help to shape programming efforts.
Family engagement	People are available during parent meetings and events to help translate into the language understood by a recent group of refugees that have relocated into the district.
Community involvement	The district allows a community agency access to school facilities to provide services to students and their families (mental health services, preventive care).

Strategies were adapted from Alliance for a Healthier Generation, 2013, *Healthy schools program framework; Centers for Disease Control and Prevention, 2012, School health index: Middle/high school: A self-assessment and planning guide.*

important to help faculty and staff see the value of a coordinated approach and the relationship between health and academics. With proper training, teachers and school leaders can become important health champions to support and reinforce efforts of the school health education coordinator or administrator (Healthy Schools Campaign, 2012). Education is also essential for teachers, administrators, and other school employees committed to improving the health, academic success, and well-being of students. CDC stated,

> Professional development can provide opportunities for school employees to identify areas for improvement, learn about and use proven practices, solve problems, develop skills, and reflect on and practice new strategies. In order to promote a Coordinated School Health approach, professional development should focus on the development of skills such as leadership, communication, and collaboration. (CDC, 2013b, para. 8)

In the 2013 document *A Framework for Safe and Successful Schools*, the recommendation was provided to conduct professional development for school staff and community partners that would address school climate and safety; positive behavior; and crisis prevention, preparedness, and response (NASP, 2013). As part of the professional development training, teachers and school leaders need to be provided with the information and resources they need to address student health issues and support a healthy school environment (Healthy Schools Campaign, 2012). Training might involve helping teachers to become aware of state-level health education regulations and requirements for health instruction so that those issues can be addressed outside the health education classroom and integrated into other subjects as a way to reinforce health-promoting concepts (Healthy Schools Campaign, 2012). Having more teachers and school leaders take on the role of health champion and work to support health concepts and health policies facilitates moving the district toward a more unified WSCC effort. Table 10.3 provides examples of how all teachers, not just health and physical education teachers, and school leaders can support WSCC though examples in each of the 10 components.

ASCD AND CDC COMBINED STRATEGIES 5, 6, AND 7

When programs and policies have been identified and put into place and implementation is underway, all efforts must be monitored to determine the level of impact. Monitoring the progress and effect of the policies and programming toward achieving the objectives also provides opportunities to give needed adjustments as a way to make continuous improvements (Dilly, 2011). After the evaluation results are in and the determination is made about whether the program or policy has achieved its goal, the celebration of any successes and communication of findings to the district and the greater community should occur (Alliance for a Healthier Generation, 2013). Chapter 11, Evaluating WSCC, provides details about the various types of evaluation that can be conducted and the strategies for conducting those evaluations.

SUMMARY

Implementation, or carrying out the WSCC activities in order to achieve the objectives and ultimately the goal as identified by the school district and community partners, was the focus of this chapter. WSCC program implementation, like any other process, requires the program planner whenever possible to follow evidence-based practices for creating program and policy success. The current literature includes a great deal of information about planning and implementation steps for school districts and their partners to follow. ASCD and CDC have provided strategies to assist in creating CSH infrastructure, planning for CSH implementation, and implementing CSH policies and programs. Although these resources were originally developed for CSH, with minor adaptation the resources and strategies can be useful with the WSCC approach. These strategies include securing and maintaining administrative support and commitment, establishing a district health council and school teams, identifying a school health coordinator, setting goals and objectives, developing a plan, and then implementing the plan and strategies (ASCD, 2014b; CDC, 2013b). Following program implementation, ASCD and CDC recommend that the progress of the policy and the programs be monitored, results assessed, and the results communicated to the school district and community (ASCD, 2014b; CDC, 2013b).

Glossary

health-enhancing behaviors—Behaviors that people engage in that will protect their health and wellness and decrease their risk of developing chronic diseases, such as getting enough sleep, engaging in physical activity, and selecting a nutritional diet.

health-risk behaviors—Behaviors that put people at risk for death and disability. CDC has identified six categories of priority health-risk behaviors for youth in the United States: behaviors that contribute to unintentional

Table 10.3 Teachers and School Leaders as WSCC Champions

WSCC component	Role of teachers	Role of school leader
Health education	Reinforce messages and lessons from health education specialists and promote healthy classroom rewards and celebrations	Support regular health education and support healthy school fundraisers
Physical education and physical activity	Integrate physical activity into lesson plans and model behaviors that promote a healthy, active lifestyle	Support daily physical education and model behaviors that promote a healthy, active lifestyle
Nutrition environment and services	Model healthy behaviors by eating healthy meals and eating school lunches	Eat school lunch, provide students with adequate time to eat lunch, provide students with easy access to breakfast, and incorporate food service workers into the school wellness team
Health services	Provide school nurse with information about a student's health (e.g., vision or hearing issues or chronic illness symptoms) and provide the school nurse with information about a student's family situation (e.g., abuse)	Incorporate the school nurse into the school wellness team; develop a plan for meeting the needs of uninsured students; offer vision, oral, and hearing screenings
Counseling, psychological, and social services	Support student connectedness and learn how to identify depression and suicidal tendencies	Support school connectedness and develop a plan for students with mental health issues
Social and emotional climate	Create an atmosphere where all children can thrive and feel accepted by developing a classroom of respect for all	Support a bully-free school and policies that foster acceptance and addresses harassment of all kinds
Physical environment	Practice good indoor air quality management in the classroom and report classroom problems related to indoor air quality (e.g., mold)	Organize and support an indoor air quality team and implement a no-idling policy for buses and cars
Employee wellness	Participate in a staff wellness program and be a health role model	Encourage and support a staff wellness program and participate in the events
Family engagement	Encourage and support family participation in a healthy school environment	Encourage and support family participation in a healthy school environment (e.g., open school facilities for family health and wellness events)
Community involvement	Provide administration with information on needs of students that might hinder health and academic success	Identify opportunities to work with community agencies as a way to address student and family needs

Adapted from Healthy Schools Campaign, Trust for America's Health, 2012, *Health in mind: Improving education through wellness* (Washington, DC: Trust for America's Health).

injuries and violence; tobacco use; alcohol and other drug use; sexual behaviors that contribute to unintended pregnancy and STDs, including HIV infection; unhealthy eating; and physical inactivity.

infrastructure—Elements necessary for successful implementation of a system such as CSH or the WSCC approach. Elements such as a council at the district level, committees at each school, a coordinator to oversee the process, and administrator support are considered necessary infrastructure for a coordinated approach to school health.

institutionalization—Becoming embedded in the organization so that the program or policy continues after the initial effort.

mission statement—A statement used to present the idea, direction, and philosophy of a program. Often broad in nature, it may include the program vision and desired outcome.

school health coordinator—A person charged with overseeing all efforts toward the achievement of a CSH or WSCC approach. The coordinator maintains active school health committees and the districtwide council while facilitating health programming in the district and school and between the school and community. The coordinator organizes the components of school health and facilitates actions to achieve a successful, Coordinated School Health system, including policies, programs, activities, and resources.

school health council—An organized group of professionals at the district level who represent the component areas of the CSH or WSCC model, along with a district administrator; community representatives involved in the health and well-being of students, such as a representative from the local health department and the school district's medical consultant; and teachers and parents who facilitate collaboration and guide programming across the district in a process of continuous improvement between the school and the community.

school health improvement plans—Comprehensive and specific plans that include goals to be achieved and actions to be taken that will move a school district toward improvement of CSH or WSCC. Generally included is a desired outcome, a description of steps to be taken, a timeline of when those steps will be conducted, and a list of those who are responsible for taking and overseeing those steps.

school health team—A school-level team that is charged with supporting the CSH or WSCC at the school level and reports to the school health council. School health teams generally include a site administrator, an identified school health leader, teachers and other staff representing the CSH or WSCC components, parents, students, and community representatives, when appropriate.

Application Activities

1. Develop a presentation for a school board meeting that includes a description of the value of creating a district health council and school health teams for each school in the district. Provide a list of the suggested representatives for the district-level and school-level groups along with the purpose and possible responsibilities of the council and the teams.
2. Explore several school district websites to locate their district mission statements. Revise the districts' mission statements that you have located to reflect both the Whole Child and WSCC approach.
3. Create an ideal vision and mission statement for a school district that has at its core the support of the whole child and the health and wellness of students, staff, and the community and emphasizes the link between a healthy student and academic success (overall, the WSCC approach).

Resources

American Academy of Pediatrics: www2.aap.org/sections/schoolhealth/

CDC School Health Profiles: www.cdc.gov/healthyyouth/profiles/index.htm

Dilley, Julia. 2011. *Research Review: School-Based Health Interventions and Academic Achievement.* Healthy Students, Successful Students Partnership Committee, Washington State Board of Health, Washington State Office of Superintendent of Public Instruction, Washington State Department of Health.

Hodges, Bonni C., & Videto, Donna M. 2011. *Assessment and Planning in Health Programs* (2nd ed.). Sudbury, MA: Jones and Bartlett Learning.

Effective Programs and Policies for Addressing Health-Risk Behaviors

Blueprints for Healthy Youth Development

http://blueprintsprograms.com/
Reviews and identifies prevention and intervention programs as well as education, emotional well-being, physical health, and positive relationships that have been demonstrated to be effective. In partnership with the Annie E. Casey Foundation and the University of Colorado Boulder.
CDC, *Registries of Programs Effective in Reducing Youth Risk Behaviors* www.cdc.gov/healthyyouth/AdolescentHealth/registries.htm
List of federal agencies and the youth-related programs that have been recommended (based on criteria that may differ from one agency to the next).

ETR Associates Evidence-Based Prevention Programs

http://pub.etr.org/docpages.aspx?pagename=evidence%20based
Two of the criteria for programs to be placed on the ETR list are that the programs must target health behavior outcomes and must include training and support for teachers (ETR website).

The Guide to Community Preventive Services, The Community Guide: What Works to Promote Health

www.thecommunityguide.org/index.html
The Guide to Community Preventive Services is a free resource to help select programs and policies to improve health and prevent disease in a community. Systematic reviews of programs and policies are used to answer these questions:

- Which program and policy interventions have been proven effective?
- Are there effective interventions that are right for my community?
- What might effective interventions cost; what is the likely return on investment?

Healthy People 2020 Evidence-Based Resources

Online tool with a searchable database providing access to evidence-based resources and information for the HP 2020 topic areas http://healthypeople.gov/2020/implement/EBR.aspx

Healthy People 2020 Adolescent Health Evidence-Based Resources (one of the topic areas)

www.healthypeople.gov/2020/topicsobjectives2020/ebr.aspx?topicid=2
An example is a link to School-Based Programs to Reduce Violence, a recommendation to reduce rates of violence among school-based violence prevention programs (Community Guide Recommendation, 2007)

What Works Clearinghouse, from the Institute of Education Sciences

http://ies.ed.gov/ncee/wwc/
Evidence for what works in education—programs, products, practices, and policies in education

References

ASCD. 2014a. *Whole School, Whole Community, Whole Child.* www.ascd.org/programs/learning-and-health/wscc-model.aspx

ASCD. 2014b. Healthy Schools Report Card Online Analysis Tool. www.healthyschoolcommunities.org/hsrc/pages/reportcard/Index.aspx

ASCD. n.d.a. *Developing Our Healthy School Communities.* www.ascd.org/ASCD/pdf/siteASCD/products/healthyschools/HSC_factsheet.pdf

About.com. 2014. *Policy to Promote Respect in Schools* (in School Policies, School Leadership and Administration, Teaching, About Education). http://teaching.about.com/od/SchoolPolicy/a/Respect-In-Schools.htm

Alliance for a Healthier Generation. 2014. *Healthy Schools Program Framework: Criteria for Developing a Healthier School Environment.* https://schools.healthiergeneration.org/_asset/l062yk/Healthy-Schools-Program-Framework.pdf

American School Health Association (ASHA). 2010. *What School Administrators Can Do to Enhance Student Learning by Supporting a Coordinated Approach to Health.* American School Health Association.

Basch, Charles E. 2011. Healthier Students Are Better Learner: High-Quality, Strategically

Planned, and Effectively Coordinated School Health Programs Must Be a Fundamental Mission of Schools to Help Close the Achievement Gap. *Journal of School Health, 81*(10), 650–662.

California School Boards Association (CSBA) and Cities Counties Schools Partnership. 2009. *Building Healthy Communities: A School Leader's Guide to Collaboration and Community Engagement*. West Sacramento, CA: California School Boards Association.

Centers for Disease Control and Prevention (CDC). 2011. *Define Your Goals*. www.cdc.gov/physicalactivity/growingstronger/motivation/define.html

Centers for Disease Control and Prevention (CDC). 2013a. *The Case for Coordinated School Health*. www.cdc.gov/healthyyouth/cshp/case.htm

Centers for Disease Control and Prevention (CDC). 2013b. *How Schools Can Implement Coordinated School Health*. www.cdc.gov/healthyyouth/cshp/schools.htm

Centers for Disease Control and Prevention (CDC). 2013c. *Cortland Enlarged City School District*. www.cdc.gov/healthyyouth/mih/stories/cortland.htm

Centers for Disease Control and Prevention (CDC). 2013d. *Registries of Programs Effective in Reducing Youth Risk Behaviors*. www.cdc.gov/healthyyouth/adolescenthealth/registries.htm

Centers for Disease Control and Prevention (CDC). 2014a. *Health and Academic Achievement*. www.cdc.gov/healthyyouth/health_and_academics

Centers for Disease Control and Prevention (CDC). 2014b. *School Health Index (SHI)*. www.cdc.gov/HealthyYouth/SHI/

Centers for Disease Control and Prevention (CDC). 2014c. *School Health Index Middle/High School: A Self-Assessment and Planning Guide*. www.cdc.gov/healthyyouth/shi/pdf/MiddleHigh.pdf

Centers for Disease Control and Prevention (CDC). 2014d. *Youth Risk Behavior Surveillance System (YRBSS)*. www.cdc.gov/HealthyYouth/yrbs/index.htm

Deschesnes, Marthe, Martin, Catherine, & Jomphe Hill, Adele. 2003. *Comprehensive Approaches to School Health Promotion: How to Achieve Broader Implementation. Health Promotion International, 18*(4), 387–396.

Dilley, Julia. 2011. *Research Review: School-Based Health Interventions and Academic Achievement*. Healthy Students, Successful Students Partnership Committee, Washington State Board of Health, Washington State Office of Superintendent of Public Instruction, Washington State Department of Health.

Gottlieb, Nell H., Keogh, Erin, F., Jonas, Judith, R. Grunbaum, Jo Anne, Walters, Susan R., Fee, Rebecca, Saunders, Ruth P., & Baldyga, William. 1999. Partnerships for Comprehensive School Health: Collaboration Among Colleges/Universities, State-Level Organizations, and Local School Districts. *Journal of School Health, 69*(8), 307–313.

Healthy Schools Campaign, Trust for America's Health. 2012. *Health in Mind: Improving Education Through Wellness, Preparing Teachers and School Leaders as Health Champions* (handout).

Hodges, Bonni C. 2013. *The Changing Nature of School Health* [Webinar].

Hodges, Bonni C., & Videto, Donna M. 2011. *Assessment and Planning in Health Programs* (2nd ed). Sudbury, MA: Jones & Bartlett Learning.

Namaste Charter School. n.d. www.namastecharterschool.org/academics.html

National Association of School Psychologist. 2013. *A Framework for Safe and Successful Schools*. www.nasponline.org/resources/handouts/Framework_for_Safe_and_Successful_School_Environments.pdf

University of Kansas. 2013. Proclaiming Your Dream: Developing Vision and Mission Statements in *Community Toolbox* (section 2 in chapter 8). http://ctb.ku.edu/en/table-of-contents/structure/strategic-planning/vision-mission-statements/main

U.S. Department of Education. 2010. *Laws and Guidance, Elementary and Secondary Education*. www2.ed.gov/policy/elsec/leg/esea02/index.html

Valois, Robert F. 2011. *The Healthy School Communities Model: Aligning Health and Education in the School Setting*. ASCD Healthy School Communities Information.

Videto, Donna M., & Hodges, Bonni C. 2009. Use of University/School Partnerships for the Institutionalization of the Coordinated School Health Program. *American Journal of Health Education, 40*(4), 212–219.

11

Evaluating WSCC

ROBERT F. VALOIS

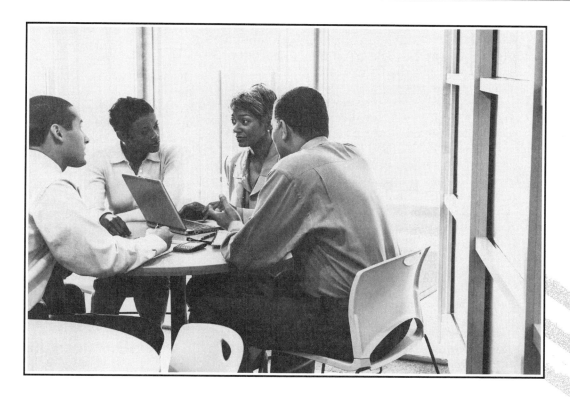

One critical reason for establishing a Whole School, Whole Community, Whole Child (WSCC) approach is that it will improve student academic performance and subsequently improve the employability, productivity, and quality of life of our future adults. An additional reason relates to the effect on public health; approximately one-third of the *Healthy People 2020* objectives can be attained or significantly influenced through intervention in the schools (DHHS, 2013). In turn, the WSCC approach can be perceived as a vehicle to cause a significant reduction in premature morbidity and mortality and to reduce the ever-increasing physical and mental health care expenditures. In addition, recent research strongly suggests that quality health promotion implementation can have positive effects on academic achievement over time (Basch, 2011; Murray et al., 2007; Rosas et al., 2009). It is reasonable to suggest that the prospect of implementing WSCC on a state, national, or international scale will be determined by the extent to which the approach can demonstrate a significant and sustained influence on academic and health status outcomes.

The planning, implementation, evaluation, and institutionalization of any health promotion program are strongly related, need to be ongoing, and must be coupled with school improvement efforts. The process of establishing CSH or WSCC policy, practice, and process is time and labor intensive and can be challenging (Valois & Hoyle, 2000; Hoyle & Valois, 1997). Evaluation of a health promotion program should be focused on the modification, maintenance, and change of health-related knowledge, attitudes, skills, intentions, self-efficacy, and behavior (among other measures). Effective evaluation of CSH or WSCC, however, is a complicated and challenging endeavor given the complexities embedded in each of the 10 components and the way in which personnel in each of the components coordinate their procedural efforts. When undergoing an evaluation, a variety of techniques and methodologies are needed and a number of factors need to be examined. Examples of policies, programs, services, or processes that are evaluated yet often overlooked include measuring results and subsequent judgments in regard to effective team collaboration; the commitment of school leadership to a collaborative approach; the influence of professional development; appropriate and effective use of people, time, and money; and effective communication for and about successes.

This chapter examines these and other issues, challenges, and methodologies related to the evaluation of the CSH or WSCC collaborative approach to health and learning. The purpose of this chapter is to examine the underlying philosophies, principles, methods, and procedures used to evaluate WSCC (or programs and policies related to the various components) in their developmental, implementation, and sustainability phases.

In health promotion the focus of evaluation efforts is usually on conducting **program evaluation**. Program evaluation can involve ongoing monitoring of programs, program processes, impacts, or outcomes. Program evaluation is considered a systematic method for collecting, analyzing, and using information to answer questions about projects, policies, and programs (ACF, 2010), particularly about their effectiveness and efficiency.

Imbedded in the word *evaluation* is the word *value*, which comes from the Latin word *valere*, meaning "to be strong" or "to have worth" (Gehlert & Browne, 2012, p. 43). The ability to determine the value, or worth, of a health promotion effort is essential to the process, impacts, outcomes, and sustainability of the WSCC approach.

RATIONALE FOR PROGRAM EVALUATION

In both the public and private sectors, stakeholders want to know whether the programs that they are funding, implementing, supporting, or receiving are having the intended effect (and at what cost). Equally important are questions such as how the program could be improved, whether the program is worthwhile, whether there are better alternatives, whether there are unintended outcomes, and whether the program goals are appropriate and useful (Shackman, 2013).

Evaluators, administrators, school health coordinators, and school health councils or teams need to recognize that the principal reasons for conducting a program evaluation will differ from situation to situation and from program to program. Expectations and demands from multiple stakeholders and audiences for the evaluation will significantly influence its purposes (Windsor, Clark, Boyd, & Goodman, 2004). But program evaluations are done for various reasons. Windsor, Baranowski, Clark, and Cutter (1994) outline these reasons for conducting evaluations of health promotion programs:

- Determining the rate and level of attainment of program goals and objectives
- Identifying strengths and weaknesses of program elements for making decisions in program planning
- Monitoring standards of performance and establishing quality assurance and control mechanisms
- Determining the generalizability of an overall program or program elements to other populations
- Contributing to the base of scientific knowledge
- Identifying hypotheses for future study
- Meeting the demand for public and fiscal accountability
- Improving the skill of the professional staff in the performance of program planning, implementation, and evaluation activities
- Promoting positive public relations and community awareness
- Fulfilling grant or contractual requirements

Evaluations can also help determine whether program materials are appropriate, help administrators improve services, and serve as an early warning system for potentially serious problems with the program (Thompson & McClintock, 2000). The W.K. Kellogg Foundation (1998) adds that conducting evaluation activities can serve to improve and increase the "skills, knowledge and perspectives" of the stakeholders involved in the evaluation, thus building the capacity of the institution or organization to continue the program and the evaluation process (p. 48).

According to Stuffelbeam (1971) and Creswell and Newman (1989), the purposes of evaluation are to improve rather than to prove, whereas Guba and Lincoln (1982) suggest that evaluation is the process of sharing accountability. These concepts are imperative for assisting stakeholders in understanding the rigors and benefits of program evaluation. Note as well that evaluation is a sociopolitical process (Guba & Lincoln, 1982). Social, cultural, and political considerations need to be considered when designing and implementing an evaluation. In turn, perspectives of the stakeholders, those affected by both the program and the evaluation, need to be considered by the evaluation team.

In general, program evaluation is essential to the knowledge base in health promotion program planning, implementation, sustainability, and institutionalization. Regardless of the size or scope of a health promotion program, evaluation is essential to the advancement of our field and to the people, programs, and services delivered.

PLANNING FOR PROGRAM EVALUATION

Note that a school health promotion action or intervention plan should be intimately related to the plan for the evaluation of the intervention. Planning and evaluation go hand in hand, and evaluation experts suggest that program evaluators should be involved early in the planning process. Evaluation needs to be an ongoing process that takes place on a continuous basis, beginning with program planning and implementation.

Health promotion program and policy planning usually begins in a general sense by gaining commitment from school- and district-based leadership, identifying key players, establishing a district council or a school health team with a school health coordinator, and conducting a **needs assessment and asset analysis** guided by a framework such as the CDC *School Health Index* (CDC, 2014), the Mariner Model needs assessment and planning guide (Hoyle, 2007; Valois & Hoyle, 2000), the ASCD *Creating a Healthy School Using the Healthy School Report Card* (Lohrmann,et al., 2005), or the PRECEDE and PROCEED planning and evaluation model (Green & Kreuter, 1991) (see the appendix for more on the available tools for conducting a needs assessment and asset analysis). From the needs assessment process, priority areas of concern and program objectives and goals are established with subsequent action planning and program implementation (see chapter 10 for more on implementation).

DEVELOPING AN EVALUATION PLAN: CDC'S FRAMEWORK FOR PROGRAM EVALUATION

Planning for evaluation should include a description or plan of how efforts will be monitored and evaluated, as well as how evaluation results will be used for development and continuous program improvement (Hoyle, Samek, & Valois, 2008). A clearly written group-facilitated evaluation plan can clarify the direction of the WSCC evaluation based on the program's priorities, objectives, goals, and resources (both human and financial), in addition to defining the time and skills needed to conduct the evaluation. CDC offers a framework for program evaluation in public health as a general guide to the evaluation planning process. The framework identifies the possible components for consideration in an evaluation plan (CDC, n.d.) and methods for using the resulting findings for capacity building, decision making, and continuous improvement (see figure 11.1).

Using the CDC framework to organize an evaluation will ensure the inclusion of concrete elements promoting transparent and insightful implementation of the evaluation. Although the CDC framework is stepwise, the actions are not always linear and are often cyclical in nature. The development of an evaluation is an ongoing process. Revisiting a step is not uncommon, and several steps may be completed in a concurrent fashion (CDC, n.d.).

Engage Stakeholders

An important feature of an evaluation is the identification, involvement, and acknowledgement of the role of the stakeholders in the evaluation team, which should include members of the school

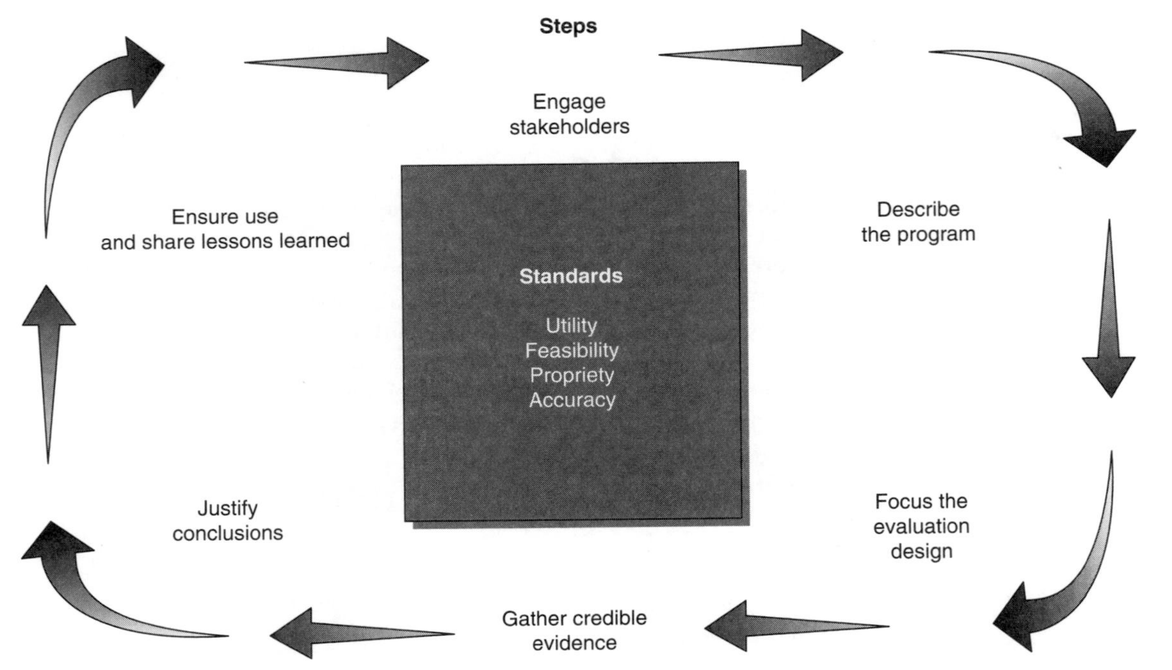

Figure 11.1 Recommended framework for program evaluation.

Adapted from Centers for Disease Control and Prevention, *Program performance and evaluation office (PPEO) - Program evaluation.* Available: http://www.cdc.gov/eval/framework/index.htm.

health council. People motivated to be involved in the evaluation are generally members who have a vested interest in the evaluation findings and those who are intended users of the evaluation results, such as school, community, and parent groups and other interested parties (Patton, 2011; Knowlton & Phillips, 2009). Engaging stakeholders enhances the understanding and acceptance of the utility of the evaluation information. Stakeholders are more likely to buy into and support the evaluation if they are involved in the evaluation process from the onset of program and policy development.

The process of developing a written evaluation plan in conjunction with the school health team or districtwide council will enhance collaboration; provide a sense of shared purpose with stakeholders; create transparency through the implementation process; and ensure that stakeholders have a common vision and understanding of the purpose, use, and consumers of the evaluation results (Lavinghouze & Snyder, 2013).

The intended use of the evaluation results needs to be planned, directed, and intentional and should be a component of the evaluation plan (Patton, 2011). Questions to address include the following: Who is going to need to see the evaluation results? And how will they be shared? Because schools and school districts are busy, complex entities, the WSCC approach and WSCC evaluations are also complicated endeavors. The stages of evaluation for a WSCC program, strategy, action, or policy will be cyclical in nature and seldom a one-shot process. In a multiyear and multilevel effort (for capacity building and continuous school improvement), the evaluation plan needs to consider baseline data collection and future data collection (analysis and reporting) as an ongoing process.

Describe the Program

A program description clarifies the purpose of the program, stage of WSCC development, program activities, capacity to improve health and academic performance, and implementation context (policy, practice, and process development and implementation). School and community personnel, program staff, school administrators, and the evaluators should have a shared understanding of the WSCC approach and what the evaluation can and cannot deliver. This point is crucial to the implementation of the evaluation activities and subsequent use of evaluation results.

A narrative description of the program in the evaluation plan is helpful for a complete and shared understanding of the program and serves as a ready reference for the stakeholders. The program description is also essential for focusing the evaluation design and selecting appropriate evaluation methods. The description will be based on objectives, goals, and factors such as the size of the district, school norms, and location (urban, suburban, small town, rural). Most program descriptions include the following:

- A statement of need to identify the academic or health issue being addressed
- Inputs or program resources needed to implement program or policy activities
- Activities linked to program outcomes via theory or best practice program logic
- Stage of program development to reflect program maturity
- Environmental context (social and environmental) within which the program is implemented

Focus the Evaluation Design

Articulating the purposes of the evaluation, its utilization, and the program description are conducted in this step of the evaluation plan. This process will assist in narrowing the evaluation questions and focusing the evaluation for continuous program improvement and subsequent program management decision making. The scope, sequence, and depth of program evaluation depend on stakeholder and program priorities and resources available for the evaluation. The evaluation team must work together to determine priority and feasibility of evaluation questions and identify uses of the evaluation results before designing the evaluation plan. Because it is a dynamic process, the focus of the evaluation design should be revisited annually (or more frequently as needed) to determine whether priorities and feasibility issues are sustained for planned evaluation activities. Note here that evaluation plans are cast in paper, not in stone. Evaluation plans need to be flexible and adaptive to possible changes to school and school district policies and procedures or new streams of funding. The evaluation plan enables the evaluators to document where the program has been and where it is going in the future in addition to why, when, and how changes were made to the plan.

Evaluation budget and resources, both human and financial, should be included in feasibility discussions. A general rule in the culture of evaluation is that 10 to 15 percent of total resources should be allocated to program evaluation. The evaluation questions and subsequent methodologies selected will have a direct effect on the financial resources available, the skills of evaluation team members, and environmental constraints. Stakeholder involvement may facilitate advocating for resources needed for evaluation implementation. But acquiring adequate resources can be a challenge, and evaluators sometimes do not have enough resources to answer all the evaluation questions identified in the planning process (see sample evaluation questions in figure 11.2).

Gather Credible Evidence

In a perfect world, evaluation questions inform the selection and utilization of evaluation methods. Following the steps in the CDC framework will lead to choosing the evaluation questions that

FIGURE 11.2

Sample WSCC Evaluation Questions

- Is the partnership with the health clinic resulting in fewer students being absent on a regular basis?
- Is a diverse group of families involved in school-related functions and activities?
- Is the new breakfast program meeting the needs of families in our community?
- Are we seeing improvements in faculty health because of the new wellness program being offered?
- Has the snack policy resulted in changes in the number of high-fat, high-sugar foods being eaten by elementary students?
- Does the health curriculum address students' physical, mental, emotional, and social dimensions of health?
- Are students and staff happier because of the new lunchroom policies focused on providing a more relaxing atmosphere?

will eventually provide information that can be used for continuous program improvement and decision making. The most appropriate method to answer evaluation questions should then be selected, and this process of selection should be outlined in the evaluation plan. A timeline and the roles and responsibilities of those managing the evaluation implementation, whether it is program staff, a stakeholder, an independent evaluation team, or an evaluator, should be defined early in the planning process. Six considerations for the process of choosing appropriate evaluation methods to answer the evaluation questions are as follows:

- Be mindful of the purpose, program description, and stage of development of the program evaluation questions, and what the evaluation can and cannot deliver.
- Determine the methods needed for the evaluation questions. Among the numerous options are **qualitative**, **quantitative**, **mixed methods**, multiple methods, **naturalistic inquiry**, and **experimental** and **quasi-experimental designs**.
- Consider what will constitute credible evidence for stakeholders or consumers (e.g., training and experience of people who collect and manage data, level of responsibility of people who authorize final documents, and use of a valid observation checklist by a trained person). Identify sources of evidence (e.g., people, documents, observations, administrative databases, and surveillance systems) and appropriate methods for obtaining quality (i.e., reliable and valid) data.
- Identify roles and responsibilities along with timelines to ensure that the program effort remains on track and on time.
- Stay flexible, adaptive, and be transparent.

One tool that CDC (n.d.) and Lavinghouze and Snyder (2013) suggest as particularly useful in program evaluation is an evaluation plan methods grid (see a sample in table 11.1). This tool is helpful for aligning evaluation questions with methods, indicators, performance measures, data sources, roles, and responsibilities and can facilitate a shared understanding of the overall evaluation plan with stakeholders. Such visualization of how the evaluation will be implemented enhances understanding and buy-in from stakeholders.

Justify Conclusions

Justifying evaluation conclusions includes analyzing the data collected, interpreting data, and drawing logical conclusions from the evaluation data. This step in the CDC framework is imperative for translating the data collected into meaningful, useful, and accessible program evaluation information. Procedures need to be outlined, and the timeline for this step in the evaluation plan needs to be defined. It can be incorrectly assumed that the school health teams or council are no longer needed in the decision-making process of formulating conclusions from the evaluation results. The tendency is to let the "evaluation experts" complete the analysis and interpret the program data. But continuous involvement of the team is critical to ensuring the meaningfulness, credibility, and acceptance of evaluation findings and conclusions. In turn, stakeholders often have unique perspectives and novel insights to guide interpretation, leading to more meaningful and thoughtful evaluation conclusions.

Allowing enough time and planning for data analysis and interpretation of data is anchored to the timeline initiated in the prior step to gather credible evidence. Mistakes or omissions in planning this step can create serious delays in producing evaluation reports (quarterly, biannual, annual, or others) and may result in missed opportunities (e.g., having data and results for a school board meeting or an end of academic year meeting) if

Table 11.1 Sample Evaluation Plan Methods Grid

Evaluation question	Indicators or performance measures	Methods	Data sources	Frequency	Responsibility
Is the district wellness policy being implemented as planned?	Description and update of activities	Key informant interviews and document reviews	Interview scripts and reports	Every three months	School principal and school teams

Adapted from Centers for Disease Control and Prevention, 2011, *Developing an effective evaluation plan* (Atlanta, GA), 27.

the report has not been timed to correspond with significant events (e.g., seasonal district, state, or national conference).

Overall, the evaluation plan must include time for interpretation and review of the conclusions by stakeholders to increase transparency and validity of the evaluation processes and conclusions. The important aspect here is to justify the logical conclusions, not just to analyze data. As a note of caution here, a dynamic in the stakeholder-driven process can be the subtle pressure to go beyond the data in interpreting the results and coming to conclusions. A reminder here is the old saying "Good results are sometimes never quite as good as they seem, and bad results are sometimes never quite as bad as they seem." The evaluators have a professional responsibility to ensure that findings and conclusions are drawn directly from the evaluation evidence. The issues of **reliability**, **validity**, and potential **biases** should be discussed in the planning stages and revisited as data and conclusions are considered and presented. Attention to detail and soundness of data collection, analysis, interpretation, and reporting on the front end usually result in quality data on the back end.

Ensure Use and Share Lessons Learned

Determining who should learn about the findings of the evaluation and how they should learn the information is an important aspect of the evaluation process. The impact and value of the evaluation results will increase if the program and the team take personal and professional responsibility for getting the results to the right people in a usable, appropriate, user friendly, and targeted format. This sharing of data through appropriate communication channels to the appropriate target groups is vital and needs to be determined early in the process. The audience for evaluation results is an important consideration.

Health staff and the evaluation team need to take personal and professional responsibility for ensuring the effective dissemination and subsequent application of WSCC results. Torres and Phillips' (2004) *Evaluation Strategies for Communicating and Reporting* is an excellent resource for creative techniques for reporting on evaluation results and conclusions.

Timmerick (1995), Dignan and Carr (1987), and Blum (1974) suggest a series of evaluation planning and implementation questions that can be altered for use in an ongoing evaluation of the WSCC approach:

- What is the original purpose of the evaluation, and what is to be achieved?
- Should the WSCC policy, practice, or process be continued in the same manner as it has been in the past?
- How can WSCC policies, practices, and processes be improved?
- Which policies, practices, and processes have resulted in the best impact and outcomes? Which have resulted in the worst impacts and outcomes?
- Could this policy, practice, or process be expanded and successful at other schools or in other districts?
- How well has the budgeting process functioned?
- How well have human resources functioned?
- Can the results of the evaluation process be used to make the policy, practice, or process better?
- Does the evaluation provide the information necessary to improve, make adjustments, or increase the functioning of the WSCC policy, practice, and process?
- What kind of results or change in the WSCC policy, practice, and process is desired?
- How are modifications to be made?
- How reliable are the measures of effectiveness and efficiency that are implied?
- Were there any unexpected occurrences or consequences?
- How effectively did the program planning, implementation, and management activities attain the objectives and goals?
- What desirable and undesirable side effects occurred?

In summary here, the old adage "If you fail to plan, you plan to fail" is appropriate for the complexities and evaluation of the WSCC.

INTERNAL OR EXTERNAL PROGRAM EVALUATION

Depending on the context, scale, funding source, and other aspects of the WSCC, a decision on an **internal** or **external evaluator** or evaluation team is an important one for the school health coordinator. Confidence in the evaluation process and

School Health *in Action*

Supporting CSH Goals

The Florida Coordinated School Health Program Pilot Schools Project (PSP) was designed to encourage innovative approaches to promote CSH in Florida schools. Each of eight pilot schools received $15,000 in project funding, three years of technical assistance including on-site and offsite assistance, a project office resource center, mailings of resource materials, needs assessment and evaluation assistance, and three PSP summer institutes. In return for the support provided, each pilot school agreed to collect baseline data on the status of CSH at their school, collect and provide additional data as requested, send the school CSH team to three summer institutes (1998, 1999, 2000), complete 16 to 20 hours of in-service training, and provide two days per year of CSH training for the staff at their schools.

The PSP posed two fundamental questions: Can financial resources, professional training, and technical assistance enable individual schools to create and sustain a Coordinated School Health program? What outcomes can one reasonably expect from a Coordinated School Health Program, assuming that programs receive adequate support over time?

Results at the eight schools confirmed that a CSH program can be established and sustained. Program strength and sustainability depended on long-term resources, qualified personnel, and administrative support. Second, although CSH may improve school performance indicators, the PSP yielded insufficient evidence to support that belief. Weiler, Pigg, and McDermott (2003) suggest that future CSH projects should include robust measurement and evaluation designs, thereby producing conclusive evidence about the influence of CSH on such outcomes.

validity of results may be greater when an outside source is used. Bringing in an outside evaluator, however, can bring unpredictable processes and results and possibly expose uncomfortable weakness while not being sensitive to the culture of an organization. Dignan and Carr (1987) suggest four critical issues to consider in deciding whether to use an inside or outside evaluator.

- What are the purposes and uses of the evaluation?
- Does anyone within the organization or program have the skills to evaluate a program according to the designated purposes and uses?
- Are sufficient funds available within the program to finance the evaluation?
- Does the funding source for the program include legal mandates regarding evaluation?

For internal evaluation the main question of concern is the obvious conflict of interest. An internal evaluator must be careful to remain as objective as possible. Objectivity is the obvious reason to use an outside evaluator. An outside evaluator should have no conflict of interest in the outcome of the evaluation and therefore is more concerned with evaluating the program based on an effective evaluation plan and a set of professional standards. Bringing in an evaluator from a local college or university to work with the team can be a win–win situation in which an evaluator may need to do community service and the school personnel needs evaluation expertise.

TYPES OF EVALUATION

Evaluation is not an action that happens by collecting baseline data at the onset of a program and again at the end of a program. Evaluation is a dynamic, complex, and ongoing process that produces meaningful information used by a variety of people to describe, improve, adapt, and make decisions regarding the efficacy and effectiveness of program components and efforts.

Evaluators can conduct a variety of program evaluations. The evaluation literature can vary in its use of evaluation terminology, but health promotion evaluations are generally defined with terms such as formative evaluation, summative evaluation, process evaluation, impact evaluation, and outcome evaluation. See table 11.2 for a diagram of the various types of evaluations to be addressed in this chapter and their placement in the evaluation process.

Table 11.2 Types of Evaluation and Placement in the Evaluation Process

Formative		Summative	
Developmental stage: Needs assessment and asset analysis	Process evaluation: Assessment of the process of program implementation	Impact evaluation: Assessment of attainment of program objectives	Outcome evaluation: Effect of program on morbidity, mortality and other indicators of health status of an individual or community

Based on Fetro 1998.

Formative Evaluation

Formative evaluation is an evaluation that produces information gathered during the planning and implementation stages of a health promotion program to modify and make improvements to the program (Windsor et al., 1984). During program planning, formative evaluation activities test program plans, messages, materials, procedures, and modifications of existing programs or material before they are implemented to verify the feasibility, appropriateness, and acceptability of their use in the program with a target population (CDC, n.d.). Pilot testing and a variety of process evaluation methodologies are components of formative evaluation. Formative evaluation activities are also conducted during and after initial program implementation to identify sources of and solutions to unanticipated challenges that may arise after a program has been initiated and implemented. WSCC efforts are in constant pursuit of continuous capacity building and continuous improvement in parallel with the overall school improvement process (Hoyle, Samek, & Valois, 2008; Valois, Slade, & Ashford, 2011). In turn, effective evaluations of WSCC efforts are in constant use of formative evaluation methodologies.

Needs Assessment and Asset Analysis

Conducting an assessment of the needs and assets associated with the healthy child tenets, the components of the WSCC, the schools, and the surrounding community provides an opportunity to gather the information needed for planning effective and efficient programming (Hodges & Videto, 2011). A review of existing assets that would help make the program implementation and delivery more successful is warranted here yet is often overlooked. An examination of existing policies, partnerships, communication avenues, and other resources that would help the process would be a good place to start.

Process Evaluation

Process evaluation is conducted to determine whether the CSH activity, action, component, or program is doing what it is supposed to be doing with adherence, or **fidelity**, to its written plan (CDC, 1997). Process evaluations monitor and document organizational and program-related factors to modify, maintain, or improve the effectiveness of the program; provide support for sustaining the program; help explain why goals and objectives may or may not have been attained; and help make decisions regarding the program and its various components (Kellogg [W.K.] Foundation, 1998). Questions to address during a process evaluation might look like these: Was the elementary school health curriculum taught as it was intended to be taught? Did the creation of a community dental clinic partnership between the school district and the community occur as planned? Is the new health and wellness policy being implemented as it was written? Did the group activity help you feel more comfortable demonstrating the skill?

Process evaluation data provide essential insight regarding what types of assessment and intervention methodologies can (and cannot) be routinely delivered for specific settings, behaviors, types of providers, and clients with fidelity to their established effectiveness. Program staff and evaluators should use process evaluation methods as a primary quality control mechanism to assess staff delivery of core health promotion procedures. Process evaluation should be conducted in all phases of an evaluation (Windsor et al., 1984).

Process evaluation activities should include a periodic and day-to-day review of program or project activities, staff performance, and performance of a system for monitoring participants. In a process evaluation, criteria for standards for determining acceptable performance are derived from independent professional judgment or available guidelines from procedural manuals, consultants, accrediting agencies, professional practice associations, and procedures proved effective and documented in the professional literature. Documents like the *School Health Index* (*SHI*) and the *Healthy School Report Card* (*HSRC*) may provide the ideal standards for school health programming and policies and may be useful for process evaluation, not just for the initial needs assessment and asset analysis (CDC, 2014; Lohrmann, Lewallen, & Karwasinski, 2005).

Effective process evaluation documents program feasibility and fidelity to a written program action plan (CDC, 1997). The process evaluation assesses the existence of a structure and the implementation by staff of process components and program content delivered to participants. A component of a process evaluation consists of directly observing (with a written checklist) the quality and quantity of procedures performed by program staff. This process evaluation component involves staff examination of the situation, events, challenges, people, and interactions during program development, implementation, and field testing. Evaluators assess components of the program for congruence between staff adherence to a written plan and the participants' responses to program delivery which can involve input from students on their perceptions regarding the quality of instruction and programs.

In addition, a resource review may be conducted as a component of the process evaluation. This review can involve a budget and retrospective record review (Windsor et al., 1984), an assessment of whether the staff was adequately trained, and an assessment of whether sufficient time to implement and conduct program activities within budget was allotted (Kellogg [W.K.] Foundation, 1998).

Summative Evaluation

Summative evaluation is a broad evaluation term that refers to an evaluation conducted to determine whether a program worked by meeting its objectives and goals over a specific period. Summative evaluation is focused on describing what level of **impact** and **outcome** was achieved (CDC, 2013).

Impact Evaluation

Impact evaluation is the measurement of the extent to which the program has caused short-term or intermediate changes in the target population or the program (CDC, 2013; Green & Kreuter, 1999; CDC, 1997). Changes in the program's objectives and short-term goals are assessed. Depending on the nature of the objectives and goals, an impact evaluation examines the improvement in behavioral, environmental, predisposing, reinforcing, and enabling factors. Typical impact evaluations examine changes in health-related knowledge and skills, attitudes, intentions, self-efficacy, and behaviors. In an impact evaluation of WSCC initiatives looking at changes in school attendance, the creation of a healthy school or community environment and the availability of student and staff drinking water throughout the day might be examined depending on initial program needs and the resulting objectives. In figure 11.3 objectives from *Healthy People 2020* for adolescent health

FIGURE 11.3

Healthy People 2020 Topics and Objectives for Adolescent Health

1 Increase the proportion of adolescents who have had a wellness checkup in the past 12 months

2 Increase the proportion of adolescents who participate in extracurricular and out-of-school activities

3 Increase the proportion of adolescents who are connected to a parent or other positive adult caregiver

3.1 Increase the proportion of adolescents who have an adult in their lives with whom they can talk about serious problems

3.2 Increase the proportion of parents who attend events and activities in which their adolescents participate

4 (Developmental) Increase the proportion of adolescents and young adults who transition to self-sufficiency from foster care

5 Increase educational achievement of adolescents and young adults

5.1 Increase the proportion of students who graduate with a regular diploma four years after starting 9th grade

5.2 Increase the proportion of students who are served under the Individuals with Disabilities Education Act who graduate high school with a diploma

5.3 Increase the proportion of students whose reading skills are at or above the proficient achievement level for their grade

5.3.1 Increase the proportion of 4th-grade students whose reading skills are at or above the proficient achievement level for their grade

5.3.2 Increase the proportion of 8th-grade students whose reading skills are at or above the proficient achievement level for their grade

5.3.3 Increase the proportion of 12th-grade students whose reading skills are at or above the proficient achievement level for their grade

5.4 Increase the proportion of students whose mathematics skills are at or above the proficient achievement level for their grade

5.4.1 Increase the proportion of 4th-grade students whose mathematics skills are at or above the proficient achievement level for their grade

5.4.2 Increase the proportion of 8th-grade students whose mathematics skills are at or above the proficient achievement level for their grade

5.4.3 Increase the proportion of 12th-grade students whose mathematics skills are at or above the proficient achievement level for their grade

5.5 Increase the proportion of adolescents who consider their schoolwork to be meaningful and important

5.6 Decrease school absenteeism among adolescents due to illness or injury

6 Increase the proportion of schools with a school breakfast program

7 Reduce the proportion of adolescents who have been offered, sold, or given an illegal drug on school property

8 Increase the proportion of adolescents whose parents consider them to be safe at school

9 (Developmental) Increase the proportion of middle and high schools that prohibit harassment based on a student's sexual orientation or gender identity

10 Reduce the proportion of public schools with a serious violent incident

11 Reduce adolescent and young adult perpetration of, and victimization by, crimes

11.1 Reduce the rate of minor and young adult perpetration of violent crimes

11.2 Reduce the rate of minor and young adult perpetration of serious property crimes

11.3 (Developmental) Reduce the proportion of counties and cities reporting youth gang activity

11.4 (Developmental) Reduce the rate of adolescent and young adult victimization from crimes of violence

Reprinted from Centers for Disease Control and Prevention, 2013, *Healthy people: Adolescent health* (Atlanta, GA). Available: http://healthypeople.gov/2020/topicsobjectives2020/objectiveslist.aspx?topicId=2

might have been similar to objectives identified in the needs assessment conducted at a school district and would be pursued during the impact evaluation.

Outcome Evaluation

Outcome evaluation focuses on changes in health status or quality of life indices (Green & Kreuter, 1999). Typical outcome evaluations examine reductions in premature morbidity and mortality rates such as reductions in a sexually transmitted infection rate, the rate of obesity, or traffic fatalities in a targeted population. In an outcome evaluation of the WSCC approach, increases in measures of academic performance and success, such as graduation rates and college enrollment, might be examined along with improved well-being of youth, measured by morbidity and mortality data as well as other health status and quality of life indicators.

QUANTITATIVE AND QUALITATIVE DATA COLLECTION

Both quantitative and qualitative data collection methods are possible approaches to collecting information about school health and the WSCC approach. Quantitative data is information that is in numeric form, whereas qualitative is narrative data that tends to provide more information and observations related to the subjects.

Quantitative Evaluation

Quantitative evaluation is focused on the testing of specific hypotheses or answering well-constructed research questions. It follows the traditional natural science model more closely than qualitative research does, emphasizing experimental design and statistical methods of data analysis. Quantitative evaluation is characterized by a focus not only on producing data but also on generating data that are suitable for statistical testing (Schofield & Anderson, 1984). Two questions of utmost importance in most program evaluations are (1) to what extent can the observed impacts and outcomes be attributed to the program that was implemented? and (2) to what extent can the results be generalized to other times, other settings, and other participants? Quantitative measures can be employed successfully to help answer these types of evaluation questions (McDermott & Sarvela, 1999). Surveys or questionnaires are generally used to collect this type of information or data. The collection of BMI data from children and questionnaires for knowledge, attitudes, self-efficacy, and behavior are used in a quantitative evaluation. Examples of some national surveys include the Youth Risk Behavior Surveillance System (YRBSS), the National Health and Nutrition Examination Survey (NHANES), the School Health Profiles, and the School Health Policies and Programs Studies (SHPPS).

Qualitative Evaluation

Qualitative evaluation is the type of evaluation that addresses the quality of relationships, activities, situations, or materials (resources) (Frankel, 1999). Qualitative evaluation methods differ from quantitative methods by their greater emphasis on holistic descriptions of various phenomena. It involves the minute details of what transpires with respect to a given activity or a given environment (McDermott & Sarvela, 1999). Qualitative methods usually include three general types of data collection: (1) in-depth, open-ended interviews (including focus groups); (2) direct observation; and (3) written documents (such as field notes and written records). Qualitative methods are often used in evaluations because they tell the program's story by capturing and communicating the stories of the participants and staff. These stories often explain how well program components worked or did not work. The three main questions in a qualitative program evaluation approach are (1) what is working and why?, (2) what is not working and why?, and (3) what needs to be done to fix what is not working?

A 10-component WSCC approach is, in many ways, larger than the sum of its parts. In turn, a variety of process and qualitative evaluation techniques should be used for various aspects of a WSCC formative and ongoing evaluation. The qualitative evaluation techniques used for WSCC initiatives are in-depth qualitative interviews, direct observations, and written documents such as field notes and program records.

In-Depth Qualitative Interview

The interview, conducted either in groups or individually, is considered the most important data-gathering technique in a qualitative evaluation (Coffey & Atkinson, 1996; Fetterman, 1989).

Evaluation in Healthy School Communities Project

In October 2006, ASCD selected 11 pilot school communities for the 2007 calendar year—three from Canada and eight from the United States. Two of the U.S. school communities were school districts that had multiple schools, adding a unique dimension to the HSC experiment. ASCD required that each site commit to the school improvement process outlined in *Creating a Healthy School Using the Healthy School Report Card: An ASCD Action Tool* (Lohrmann et al., 2005) and use the online data collection system. The process included engaging the community with a diverse HSC team, assessing the school health environment, developing HSC action plan, and integrating the HSC plan into the school improvement process. Each pilot school community received an initial (year 1) grant, and the year 2 grant was subject to renewal contingent on available funds and demonstrated school community progress toward projected goals through their application and the Healthy School Report Card process.

The evaluation of the HSC project relied heavily on qualitative evaluation methodologies but included some use of quantitative methods. Qualitative methods used primarily during site visits included

- a visual tour of each school community;
- face-to-face interviews with key personnel;
- small group question-and-answer meetings with students, parents, and small groups of other stakeholders;
- meal meetings with team members and community stakeholders;
- site progress reports and debrief notes;
- review of action plans; and
- stakeholder inventory reports.

In essence, the ASCD internal team determined that the HSC evaluation should answer this question: What are the levers of change in a school and community that support the initiation and implementation of best practice and policy for improving school health? This evaluation question was applied to the 11 school and community sites in the Healthy School Communities Project. For the HSC project a lever was considered an aspect of the project that caused a positive change to occur.

These qualitative methods assisted the evaluation team in answering the evaluation question about the levers of change. Nine levers of change were associated with the schools that had the most potential for sustaining their HSC efforts:

1. Principal as leader of the HSC efforts
2. The creation of, or modification in, school policy related to HSC
3. Authentic and mutually beneficial community collaborations for HSC
4. Integration of HSC process with the school improvement process
5. Effective use of the HSC and planning process for continuous improvement
6. Effective and distributive team leadership
7. Active and engaged leadership
8. Ongoing and embedded professional development
9. Stakeholder support of the local HSC effort

Four global findings were also flushed out:

1. Principal leadership (when the principal led the HSC effort at the school) and her or his distributive leadership were imperative for HSC project success.
2. For change to be meaningful, it needs to address school improvement at the systematic level rather than just the programmatic level.
3. Community collaboration needs to start at the beginning of the project, resources need to be shared, and the collaboration needs to be authentic.
4. The HSC health improvement process is directly related to and functions in tandem with the school improvement process (Valois, Slade, & Ashford, 2011).

The interview is distinct from other types of data collection in its open-endedness. According to Yin (2009), how and why questions predominate in eliciting the rich details and nuances of program dynamics as perceived by the interviewee. Chapter 10 includes descriptions of key informant interviews and focus groups conducted as a preassessment of a CSH, along with sample questions and instructions.

Direct Observation

When possible, observing various aspects of WSCC programming efforts can be an essential component of a qualitative evaluation. Observations of council or team meetings, activities within the 10 components such as students' selecting foods for their breakfast, or physical activities occurring during recess can provide insights that a recollection by interview cannot provide. An advantage of direct observation is that it combines "participation in the lives of the people under study with maintenance of a professional distance that allows adequate observation and recording of data" (Fetterman, 1989, p. 45). Observation activities may include observation of a skill being demonstrated, a windshield or walking tour of a neighborhood, and the use of photos to depict the effect of a program or policy (see chapter 10 for more on conducting direct observations).

Field Notes

The evaluator should either write down or verbally record various aspects of the encounters:

- A description of the people, school health events, or situations that were involved
- Impressions of participants' and WSCC staff members' demeanor
- Points of emphasis that emerged as most central to an observation session that just concluded
- Possible hunches, speculations, theories, or hypotheses that were developed or stimulated by an observation session
- Additional questions to be asked of contacts as follow-up procedures (Miles & Huberman, 1994)

The recording of field notes can be an important technique for rounding out the data collection after an observation session or an interview. Field notes should be jotted down unobtrusively. Alternatively, the observer could make an audio recording of observations after finishing. Jotting down short notes during the observation as cues and recording the details afterward is a useful combination of techniques. Where possible, field notes should be recorded immediately after interviews and observations so that fresh impressions are preserved. After they are compiled, field notes should become part of the written record, and can be coded during data analysis in the same manner as transcribed interviews (Windsor et al., 2004).

Program Records

Depending on what developmental or sustainability stage the WSCC approach might be in, most programs have written documents that provide a historical record. Yin (2009) distinguishes between documentation and archival records. Documentation includes agendas, minutes from meetings, letters, proposals, progress reports, newsletter and newspaper clippings, and other written documentation. Archival records include such things as organizational charts; participant records; budgets and expenditures; and personal staff records such as e-mails, telephone logs, and project calendars. Both forms of documentation have the following attributes for qualitative evaluation:

- Stability—they can be used repeatedly.
- Unobtrusive—they do not affect the evaluation process.
- Exacting—they provide names, dates, references, and details of events.
- Broad coverage—they can span the lifetime of the WSCC program or policy.

The major challenge to written records is the bias that can be present in the recording of written data, which can be subtle and difficult to discern. For example, the minutes from a school health team meeting or a board of education meeting might be influenced by the format used to record the minutes, by the person taking the minutes, by the time of day, or by the setting and tone of the meeting.

SUMMARY

School health evaluations have demonstrated that improving the delivery of quality programming in any of the eight components of the CSH framework can have positive effects on selected health behaviors and indicators of academic success.

Though defensible, the final list of evidence-based programs that affect academic performance is relatively small (Murray et al., 2007, p. 599). From a school heath evaluation perspective, it might be time to consider a variety of processes, philosophies, and frameworks for advancing the field of school health and the evaluation approaches needed to document future success.

Glossary

bias—To influence in a particular, typically unfair direction; also considered prejudice. Bias is often referred to as a preference that would inhibit a person from being impartial.

cost effectiveness—Economical in terms of the goods or services received for the money spent. Something that is a good value, in that the benefits and usage are worth at least what is paid for them, is considered cost effective.

efficacy—The ability or power to produce the desired effect or reach a specific goal.

experimental design—Considered the strongest research design, it is used to test cause-and-effect relationships between variables in a study in which the experimenter has interest in the effect of some process or intervention. The classic experimental design specifies an experimental group and a control group. True experiments must have control, randomization, and manipulation.

external evaluator—Someone carrying out the evaluation who is outside the focus of the evaluation or outside the agency or institution in which the evaluation is occurring.

fidelity—Accuracy in implementing a program or intervention as intended (follows the implementation protocol).

formative evaluation—Evaluation used to modify or improve programs, activities, or interventions based on feedback obtained during planning, development, and implementation of a health promotion program.

internal evaluator—Someone carrying out the evaluation who is inside the focus of the evaluation or inside the agency or institution in which the evaluation is occurring.

impact evaluation—A measurement of the extent to which a program or intervention has caused intended short-term changes in the group or community being addressed.

mixed methods—Research that combines both qualitative and quantitate methods in the collection and analysis of the data; considered to include the benefit of both approaches.

naturalistic inquiry—An investigation in which a researcher employs an observational method to study subjects in the field as they engage in daily life experiences.

needs assessment and asset analysis—The process of identifying needs and inventorying assets to move toward workable solutions that cause improvement in a group or community. A goal of a community assessment is to develop an informed understanding of the gaps or needs that exist within a community and their effect on the community's members.

outcome evaluation—A measurement of the extent to which a program has caused the intended long-term changes in a population.

process evaluation—An evaluation conducted to explain why a program or intervention may or may not have been effective. The evaluation often includes monitoring the implementation, measurement of progress toward goals and objectives, assessment of satisfaction levels, staff performance reviews, and resource reviews. In general, process evaluation looks at how the program activities were delivered.

program evaluation—A systematic method for collecting, analyzing, and using information to answer questions about projects, policies, and programs. CDC describes effective program evaluation as a systematic way to improve and account for public health actions.

qualitative evaluation—Evaluation methods that result in data that is descriptive and nonnumeric. Qualitative data are often in the form of narratives and descriptions that result from observations, key informant interviews, and focus groups.

quantitative evaluation—Used to collect data that are empirical and numerical (such as in the CDC YRBSS). Quantitative data can undergo mathematical and statistical operations.

quasi-experimental design—A research design that uses a treatment group and a nonequivalent or nonrandomized comparison group with measurements of both groups.

reliability—The overall consistency of a measure or instrument. An instrument is said to have a high reliability if it produces similar results under consistent conditions.

summative evaluation—A type of evaluation used to determine whether a program or policy was effective. Measures used to draw conclusions about the policy or program that was implemented. Often used to answer the question "Did it work?"

validity—The extent to which a test or instrument measures what it claims to measure.

Application Activities

1. As a member of a district health council, you are involved in developing an evaluation plan for your district. Fill in the missing pieces of the table to complete an evaluation plan methods grid for the following evaluation question: Are the school efforts to communicate with the school families working as planned?
2. For each of the following types of evaluation, develop an appropriate CSH evaluation question that could be investigated.
    - Needs assessment and asset analysis
    - Process evaluation
    - Impact evaluation
    - Outcome evaluation
3. Select a professional article that examines some aspect or component of the WSCC model. Compose a research paper that describes the type of evaluation methods used to collect the data. In addition, present a summary of the findings of the evaluation and your personal reaction.

Resources

Office of Coordinated School Health Monitoring Instrument: www.healthyschoolsms.org/ohs_main/documents/MonitoringtoolCSHP.doc.

Using Evaluation to Improve Programs Strategic Planning www.cdc.gov/healthyyouth/evaluation

Evaluation Handbook. W.K. Kellogg Foundation. January 1998. www.wkkf.org/Pubs/Tools/Evaluation/Pub770.pdf

Centers for Disease Control and Prevention: www.cdc.gov/eval/

Evaluation question	Indicators or performance measures	Methods	Data sources	Frequency	Responsibility
Are the school efforts to communicate with the school families working as planned?					

Adapted from Centers for Disease Control and Prevention, 2011, *Developing an effective evaluation plan* (Atlanta, GA), 27.

Community Tool Box, University of Kansas: http://ctb.ku.edu/

Harvard Family Research Project: www.gse.harvard.edu/hfrp/

The University of Wisconsin Extension: learningstore.uwex.edu/pdf/G3658-5.pdf

The Power of Proof: www.ttac.org/power-of-proof/data_coll/observation

Social Research Methods: www.socialresearchmethods.net

Key informant interviews by the University of Illinois Extension: ppa.aces.uiuc.edu/KeyInform.htm

Research Methods Knowledge Base: www.socialresearchmethods.net/kb/intrview.php

Performance Monitoring and Evaluation Tips: www.usaid.gov/pubs/usaid_eval/pdf_docs/pnaby233.pdf

SMART objectives: www.marchofdimes.com/files/HI_SMART_objectives.pdf

www.cdc.gov/healthyyouth/evaluation/pdf/brief3b.pdf

References

Administration for Children and Families (ACF). 2010. Chapter 2: What Is Program Evaluation? In *The Program Manager's Guide to Evaluation*. Washington, DC: U.S. Government Printing Office..

Basch, Charles E. 2011. Healthier Students Are Better Learners: High Quality, Strategically Planned, and Effectively Coordinated School Health Programs Must Be a Fundamental Mission of Schools to Help Close the Achievement Gap. *Journal of School Health*, 81(10), 650–662.

Blum, Henrick L. 1974. *Planning for Health: Development and Application of Social Change Theory*. New York: Human Sciences Press.

Centers for Disease Control and Prevention (CDC). n.d. *A Framework for Program Evaluation*. Office of the Associate Director for Program Evaluation. www.cdc.gov/eval/framework/index.htm

Centers for Disease Control and Prevention (CDC). 1997. *Coordinated School Health Program Infrastructure Development: Process Evaluation Manual*. Atlanta, GA: U.S. Department of Health and Human Services, Centers for Disease Control and Prevention.

Centers for Disease Control and Prevention (CDC). 2014. *School Health Index: A Self-Assessment and Planning Guide. Middle School/High School Version*. Atlanta, GA.

Centers for Disease Control and Prevention (CDC). 2013. *Hints for Conducting Strong Evaluations in Program Evaluation*. Office of the Associate Director for Programs, Program Evaluation. www.cdc.gov/eval/strongevaluations/

Coffey, Amanda, & Atkinson, Paul. 1996. *Making Sense of Qualitative Data: Contemporary Research Strategies*. Thousand Oaks CA: Sage.

Creswell, William H., & Newman, Ian M. 1989. *School Health Practice*. St. Louis, MO: Times Mirror/Mosby College.

Department of Health and Human Services (DHHS). 2013. *Healthy People 2020*. http://healthypeople.gov/2020/

Dignan, Mark B., & Carr, Patricia A. 1987. *Program Planning for Health Education and Health Promotion*. Philadelphia: Lea & Febiger.

Fetro, Joyce. 1998. *Step by Step to Health Promoting Schools: A Guide to Implementing Coordinated School Health Programs in Local Schools and Districts*. Santa Cruz, CA, ETR Associates.

Fetterman, David M. 1989. *Ethnography: Step by Step. Applied Social Research Methods Series*, Vol. 17. Newbury Park CA: Sage.

Frankel, Robert. 1999. Standards of Qualitative Research. In Benjamin F. Crabtree and William L. Miller (eds.), *Doing Qualitative Research* (2nd ed.) (pp. 333–346). Thousand Oaks, CA: Sage.

Gehlert, Sara, & Browne, Teri. 2012. *Handbook of Health Social Work* (2nd ed.). Hoboken, NJ: Wiley.

Green, Lawrence W., & Kreuter, Marshal W. 1991. *Health Promotion Planning: An Educational and Environmental Approach* (2nd ed.). Palo Alto, CA: Mayfield.

Green, Lawrence W., & Kreuter, Marshal W. 1999. *Health Promotion Planning: An Educational and Ecological Approach* (3rd ed.). Palo Alto, CA: Mayfield.

Guba, Egon G., & Lincoln, Y.S. 1982. *Effective Evaluation*. San Francisco: Jossey-Bass.

Hodges, Bonni C., & Videto, Donna, M. 2011. *Assessment and Planning in Health Programs* (2nd ed.). Sudbury, MA: Jones & Bartlett Learning.

Hoyle, Tena B. 2007. *The Mariner Model: Charting the Course for Health Promoting School Communities*. Kent, OH: American School Health Association.

Hoyle, Tena B., Samek, Beverly B., & Valois, Robert F. 2008. Building Capacity for the Continuous Improvement of Health-Promoting Schools. *Journal of School Health*, *78*(1), 1–8.

Hoyle, Tena B., & Valois, Robert. 1997, October. *Mariner Project Evaluation: Eleven Critical Elements*. Paper presented at Research

Consortium, 71st National School Health Conference of the American School Health Association, Daytona Beach, FL.

Kellogg (W.K.) Foundation. 1998. *Evaluation Handbook*. Battle Creek, MI: Collateral Management.

Knowlton, Lisa W., & Phillips, Cynthia C. 2009. *The Logic Model Guidebook: Better Strategies for Great Results*. Thousand Oaks CA: Sage.

Lavinghouze, S. Rene, & Snyder, Kimberly. 2013. Developing Your Evaluation Plans: A Critical Component of Public Health Infrastructure. *American Journal of Health Education*, *44*(4), 237–243.

Lohrmann, David K., Lewallen, Theresa, & Karwasinski, Pamela. 2005. *Creating a Healthy School Using the Healthy School Report Card: An ASCD Action Tool*. Alexandria VA: Association for Supervision and Curriculum Development.

McDermott, Robert J., & Sarvela, Paul D. 1999. *Health Education Evaluation and Measurement: A Practioner's Perspective* (2nd ed.). New York: McGraw-Hill.

Miles, Matthew B., & Huberman, Michael. 1994. *Qualitative Data Analysis: An Expanded Sourcebook*. Thousand Oaks, CA: Sage.

Murray, Nancy G., Low, Barbara J., Hollis, Christine, Cross, Alan W., & Davis, Sally M. 2007. Coordinated School Health Programs and Academic Achievement: A Systematic Review of the Literature. *Journal of School Health*, *77*, 589–600.

Patton, Michael Q. 2011. *Utilization-Focused Evaluation* (4th ed.). Thousand Oaks, CA: Sage.

Rosas, Scott, Case, Jane, & Tholstrup, Linda. 2009. A Retrospective Examination of the Relationship Between Implementation Quality of the Coordinated School Health Program Model and School-Level Academic Indicators Over Time. *Journal of School Health*, *79*(3), 108–115.

Schofield, Janet W., & Anderson, K.M. 1984. *Combining Quantitative and Qualitative Methods in Research on Ethnic Identity and Intergroup Relations*. Paper presented at the Society for Research on Child Development Study Group on Ethnic Socialization, Los Angeles, CA.

Shackman, Gene. *What Is Program Evaluation?: A Beginner's Guide*. The Global Social Change Research Project. http://gsociology.icaap.org/methods/Evaluationbeginnersguide_WhatIs Evaluation.pdf

Stufflebeam, David L. 1971. The Relevance of the CIPP Evaluation Model for Educational Accountability. *Journal of Research and Development in Education*, *5*, 19–25.

Timmerick, Thomas C. 1995. *Planning Program Development and Evaluation: A Handbook for Health Promotion, Aging and Health Services*. Boston: Jones and Bartlett.

Thompson, Nancy J., & McClintock, Helen O. 2000. *Demonstrating Your Program's Worth: A Primer on Evaluation on Programs to Prevent Unintentional Injury* (2nd ed.). Atlanta GA: Centers for Disease Control and Prevention, National Center for Injury Prevention and Control.

Torres, Rosaline, Knowlton, Lisa W., and Phillips, Cynthia C. 2004. *Evaluation Strategies for Communicating and Reporting* (2nd ed.). Thousand Oaks, CA: Sage.

Valois, Robert F., & Hoyle, Tena B. 2000. Formative Evaluation Results From the Mariner Project: A Coordinated School Health Pilot Program. *Journal of School Health*, *70*(3), 95–103.

Valois, Robert F., Slade, Sean, & Ashford, Ellie. 2011. *The Healthy School Communities Model: Aligning Health and Education in the School Setting*. Alexandria, VA: ASCD.

Yin, Robert K. 2009. *Case Study Research: Design and Methods*. Sage Publications, Thousand Oaks, 4th ed.

Weiler, Robert M., Pigg, Morgan Jr., & McDermott, Robert J. 2003. Evaluation of the Florida Coordinated School Health Program Pilot Schools Project. *Journal of School Health*, *73*(1), 3–8.

Windsor, Richard A., Baranowski, Thomas, Clark, Noreen, & Cutter, Gary. 1984. *Evaluation of Health Promotion and Education Programs*. Mountain View, CA: Mayfield.

Windsor, Richard A., Clark, Noreen, Boyd, Neal Richard, & Goodman, Robert M. 2004. *Evaluation of Health Promotion, Health Education and Disease Prevention Programs* (3rd ed.). Mountain View, CA: Mayfield.

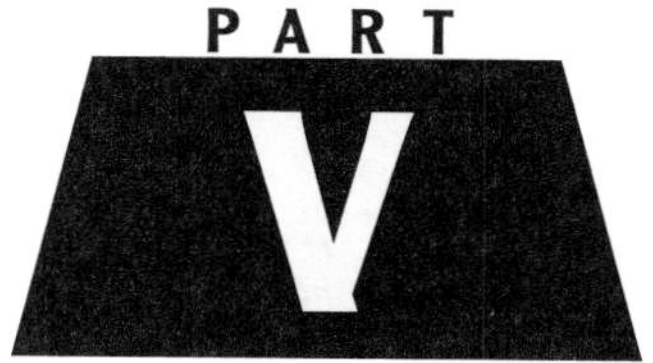

The Path Forward

12

Building on the Past and Moving Into the Future

SEAN SLADE

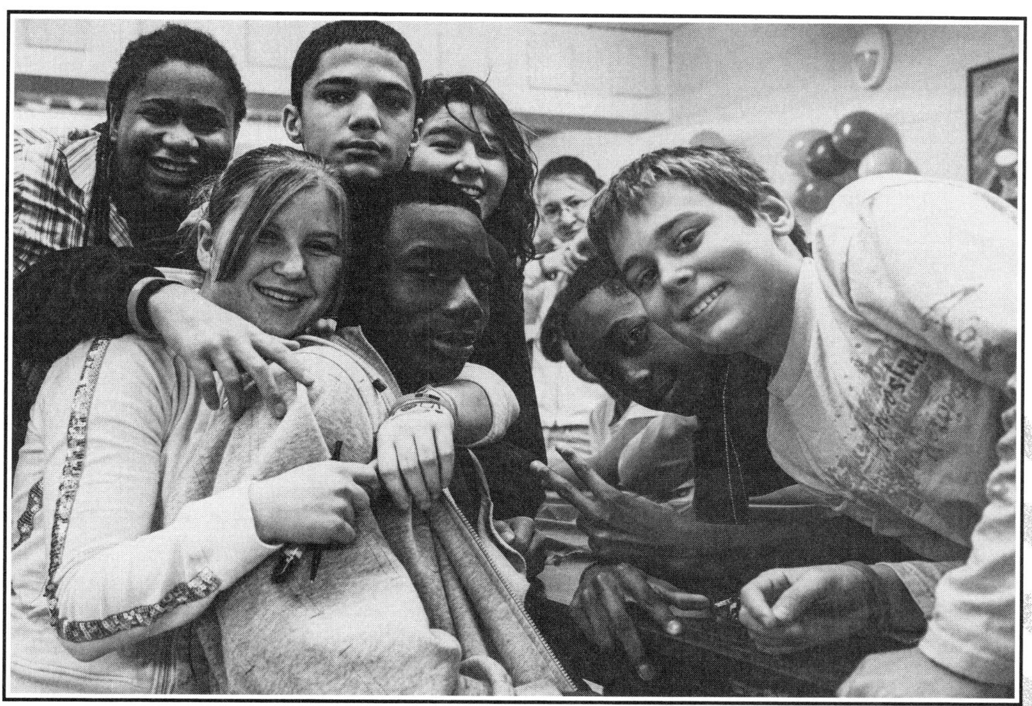

Coordinated School Health (CSH) was introduced in 1987 as a model for health promotion in the schools. In the years since its introduction, the quality and sustainability of implementation has been sporadic at best. Many CSH authorities, and some education leaders outside health education, attribute this lack of quality and commitment to the perception of school decision-makers that the CSH approach is a health model but not an education model. But research indicates the positive effect that initiatives, policies, and programs within some WSCC components have had on learning. Because of the unsuccessful history and the supportive research, the WSCC model has been developed and is being presented as an interrelated education and health approach (ASCD, n.d.). This chapter, presents a revisiting of key aspects of CSH history along with examples of the linkage between implementation and academic achievement, the importance of the alignment of WSCC with a school or school district's academic mission, and the trends in education that have the potential to affect WSCC. In addition, an overview of the benefits to both education and health resulting from quality implementation of WSCC is included in the chapter.

Coordinated School Health (CSH) has been implemented in numerous states and in at least four countries since 1987, when it was first introduced by Diane Allensworth and Lloyd Kolbe in their landmark publication in the *Journal of School Health*. Despite this national recognition, CSH has not been truly implemented nor adopted by the sector that is required for its sustainability, the sector of education. CSH has been viewed and implemented primarily as a health sector initiative and thus has been unable to gain widespread support and sustainability across school sites and districts. As Eva Marx, Susan Wooley, and Daphne Northrop stated in the landmark CSH publication *Health Is Academic* in 1998, "The promise of a Coordinated School Health program, thus far, outshines its practice" (p. 10). Unfortunately, this statement still holds true today. Charles E. Basch, in his 2010 research review *Healthier Students Are Better Learners: A Missing Link in School Reforms to Close the Achievement Gap* stated,

> Though rhetorical support is increasing, school health is currently not a central part of the fundamental mission of schools in America nor has it been well integrated into the broader national strategy to reduce the gaps in educational opportunity and outcomes. (p. 9)

Tena Hoyle, Todd Bartee, and Diane Allensworth in 2010 described their perception of this issue by stating,

> Insistence on alignment of programs under the "health" banner is detrimental to the purpose and mission of both school health and school improvement. Persistence in garnering support for health "programs" rather than finding the niche of the health-promotion process in ongoing school improvement efforts contributes to insurmountable language and organizational barriers that detract from the existent value of health in the school setting. (p. 165)

Research related to the relationship between health and learning includes recent reports such as Charles Basch's 2010 *Healthier Students Are Better Learners*; the CDC report *Association Between School-Based Physical Activity, Including Physical Education, and Academic Performance* (2010); *National School Climate Research* by the National School Climate Center (2013); and the California Department of Education reports *Getting Results: Student Health, Supportive Schools, and Academic Success* (2005) and *Getting Results: Developing Safe and Healthy Kids* (2008).

A broad swath of research has outlined the benefits of education to health both in the United States and across the globe. Whether it is because education is a way out of poverty (Iton, 2006; Freudenberg & Ruglis, 2009) or a vehicle to improve socioeconomic status, education has been linked to better health measures (Seith & Isakson, 2011). Education is the one social factor that is consistently linked to longer lives in every country where it has been studied, and it has been shown to be more important than race in obliterating the effects of income disparity (A Surprising Secret, 2007).

Even with this surplus of research that outlines the benefits for both education and health, the challenge has been to integrate it into a setting that has become increasingly outcome driven and time adverse. This challenge has been compounded, as highlighted by Valois et al (2011), by the temporary and programmatic nature of most health initiatives:

> [A]chieving that degree of support is difficult when school health is seen not as a systematic approach to addressing school improvement, but as a programmatic issue. Programmatic changes either tend to be tried and rolled back or tend to become the project of an individual staff member or department, which make them unsustainable if the staff member leaves or the department makeup changes and no one is willing or able to take charge (p. 3).

Benefits can be gained, but only if we introduce, integrate, and implement health initiatives effectively, given the context and culture of schools. Only by viewing CSH as a systemwide approach for improving the school and district environment and increasing the potential for reaching high academic standards, will we truly see the future of CSH.

CSH SUCCESS

Locations where CSH has made inroads and become part of the culture and practices of the school, such as Hays Consolidated Independent School District, Texas, and Charlotte–Mecklenburg Schools, North Carolina, are settings that have viewed school health as benefitting the education of their youth. Whether those results have occurred because improved health is related to higher academic achievement from students (Basch, 2010; Case & Paxson, 2006; Crosnoe, 2006; Haas & Fosse, 2008; Hass, 2006; Heckman, 2008; Koivusilta, Arja, & Andres, 2003; Palloni, 2006; Walker et al., 2010); increased **staff satisfaction** and decreased **staff turnover** (Byrne, 1994; Dorman, 2003; Grayson & Alvarez, 2008); greater efficiency (Bergeson, Heuschel, Hall, & Willhoft, 2005; Harris, Cohen, & Flaherty, 2008); increased attendance (Basch, 2010; Cura, 2010); or the development of a positive school climate that promotes and enhances student growth (Basch, 2010; Strolin-Goltzman, 2010) is debatable, but these localities and others have clearly experienced positive educational outcomes from focusing on health and well-being.

FOCUS ON STANDARDIZED TESTING

Education during this time also experienced a corresponding but unrelated change in how it was viewed and how it was being evaluated and assessed. The No Child Left Behind Act of 2001 refocused attention primarily onto **academic standardized testing** results in two subject areas—language arts and math. **Annual yearly progress** (AYP) in these two content areas was used to make decisions ranging from student retention through to school closures. The consequences for education in general were that test scores were held up as the only important target and all else was seen as potentially superfluous. Many schools and districts reduced or eliminated nonacademic subjects such as physical education, art, and music. Some schools even replaced recess and after-school activities with added instructional time in hopes of improving academic outcomes. Overall, this shift began to refocus teachers' attention away from what is required for a healthy learning environment and toward a myopic view of academic testing above all else.

In this environment of education being increasingly focused on academic outcomes and health initiatives being focused solely on specific health-related outcomes, the two sectors seem to have moved further apart. Yet they serve the same communities and the same populations, often in the same settings.

School Health *in Action*

CSH Vision in Action

Milwaukie High School, located in Milwaukie, Oregon, was the winner of ASCD's Vision in Action Award for 2013. The award recognizes schools that move beyond a vision for educating the whole child to actions that result in learners who are knowledgeable, emotionally and physically healthy, civically active, artistically engaged, prepared for economic self-sufficiency, and ready for the world beyond formal schooling. In 2012 Milwaukie High School opened a 2,800-square-foot (260 square meters) state-of-the-art health center on its campus to meet the health needs of students. Staff helped raise more than $600,000 to help fund the project and engage the local community and its partners to ensure that the physical, emotional, and dental health services were free and available to all students.

"The staff at Milwaukie High believes that there is more to education than just to teach a student how to read, write and think critically," said Mark Pinder, principal of Milwaukie High School. "The physical and emotional well-being of a student must be nurtured as a part of teaching and learning," he said. "When the whole child is educated at Milwaukie High, we are guaranteeing that we will produce a graduate ready to participate as an active, contributing community member" (ASCD, 2013, paragraph 8).

Ensuring the health, safety, and support of each student is paramount at Milwaukie, which blends both the health sector and the education sector seamlessly in the school setting. Combining the needs, resources, and roles available across the school and its community provides a sound basis for sustainability of efforts. This example of coordinating health, well-being, and educational success at Milwaukie provides us an example of where we would like to see CSH now and in the future (ASCD, 2013).

BEYOND COOPERATION: ALIGNMENT AND INTEGRATION

The question from here should therefore be not whether health and education should be linked, for the benefit of both and the benefit of youth, but what model, framework, or procedure is best for the future of CSH. Should we aim for cooperation, alignment, or integration of the two sectors?

It could be argued convincingly that the original CSH model and process were developed around the concept of cooperation. In fact, Allensworth and Kolbe used the term *sympathetic cooperation* in the opening paragraph of their 1987 article:

> Promoting the health of the school-age child is no easy task. It cannot effectively be accomplished through the singular efforts of an individual, a school, or an agency. Often these groups find themselves duplicating services and competing with each other while working toward a similar goal. What is needed to serve the public effectively is sympathetic cooperation . . . (p. 1)

But sympathetic cooperation has not proved to be the central focus of the CSH process. Too frequently, cooperation and coordination have been replaced in the school setting by marginalization and strategic selection. If we are to benefit from each sector, we should look beyond cooperation, which requires effort, time, and goodwill, and plan for alignment or, better still, integration.

Health and well-being should be integrated into what is already undertaken by the school by being incorporated into the fundamental procedures of the running and planning of the school. Ideally, any model or initiative developed around school health and well-being would become intertwined as part of the educational policies of the setting and into the school improvement process of the institution.

HEALTHY LEARNING ENVIRONMENT

Health must position itself as the best way to ensure a healthy learning environment—one that maximizes time, effort, and resources and allows teachers to teach and students to learn. Health initiatives can promote the development of healthy environments that are safe and supportive. The healthy school environment must address all dimensions of health—social, emotional, mental, and physical for both students and staff. Well-planned health initiatives can create environments where students can learn and teachers can teach. Any school that does not have a healthy learning environment must spend time and effort either combatting or trying to ameliorate its negative effects. The following healthy and safe tenets from the ASCD Whole Child initiative present important consideration for promoting health and learning in schools.

Each student enters school healthy and learns about and practices a healthy lifestyle.

1. Our school culture supports and reinforces the health and well-being of each student.
2. Our school collaborates with parents and the local community to promote the health and well-being of each student.
3. Our school health education curriculum and instruction supports and reinforces the health and well-being of each student by addressing the physical, mental, emotional, and social dimensions of health.
4. Our school integrates health and well-being into the school's ongoing activities, professional development, curriculum, and assessment practices.
5. Our school physical education schedule, curriculum, and instruction support and reinforce the health and well-being of each student by addressing lifetime fitness knowledge, attitudes, behaviors, and skills.
6. Our school sets realistic goals for student and staff health that are built on accurate data and sound science.
7. Our school facility and environment supports and reinforces the health and well-being of each student and staff member.
8. Our school facilitates student and staff access to health, mental health, and dental services.
9. Our school addresses the health and well-being of each staff member.
10. Our school supports, promotes, and reinforces healthy eating patterns and

food safety in routine food services and special programming and events for staff and students.

Each student learns in an environment that is physically and emotionally safe for students and adults.

1. Our school building, grounds, playground equipment, and vehicles are secure and meet all established safety and environmental standards.
2. Our school upholds social justice and equity concepts and practices mutual respect for individual differences at all levels of school interactions—student to student, adult to student, and adult to adult.
3. Our school provides our students, staff, and family members with regular opportunities for learning and support in teaching students how to manage their behavior and reinforcing expectations, rules, and routines.
4. Our school staff, students, and family members establish and maintain school and classroom behavioral expectations, rules, and routines that teach students how to manage their behavior and help students improve problem behavior.
5. Our school teaches, models, and provides opportunities to practice social and emotional skills, including effective listening, conflict resolution, problem solving, personal reflection and responsibility, and ethical decision making.
6. Our school climate, curriculum, and instruction reflect both high expectations and an understanding of child and adolescent growth and development.
7. Our students feel valued, respected, and cared for and are motivated to learn.
8. Our physical, emotional, academic, and social school climate is safe, friendly, and student centered.
9. Our school physical plant is attractive; is structurally sound; has good internal (hallways) and external (pedestrian, bicycle, and motor vehicle) traffic flow, including for those with special needs; and is free of defects.
10. Our teachers and staff develop and implement academic and behavioral interventions based on an understanding of child and adolescent development and learning theories (ASCD, n.d.).

RESPONDING TO TRENDS IN EDUCATION

According to many, education is about to enter a period of great change and adjustment. Daniel Pink (2010) describes this change as leaving the information age and entering the conceptual age—a period when less focus will be placed on content knowledge and more emphasis placed on individualized use of knowledge. This period will likely affect our ways of learning, our systems of support, and, of course, our schools. Change will occur in an educational sense based on several key concepts including greater personalization of learning; less control and ownership of education by schools; and greater integration of sectors and resources. Consequently, these changes will clearly have ramifications for health; school health; and the roles of educators, health professionals, and schools. The Organization for Economic Cooperation and Development (OECD), along with other key forecasting organizations such as KnowledgeWorks, see schools becoming hubs of a community where all sectors reside or are accessed—education, welfare, and, of course, health. KnowledgeWorks has described these hubs as "centers of resilience"—as "critical sites for promoting health, well-being, academic growth, environmental vitality, and connections across their communities" (KnowledgeWorks, 2011, paragraph 4).

But health may have another role, an expanded role, as the education sector enters a period of self-reflection, self-analysis, and change. KnowledgeWorks (2013a) recently released its *Glimpse Into the Future of Learning (Forecast 3.0).* This document identified five trends that will reshape learning over the next decade. These trends include greater **personalization**, less **standardization**, increased links into and out of the community, greater emphasis on **self-directed learning** and learning across various platforms and institutions, and decreased emphasis on a centralized system. KnowledgeWorks further describes this future by stating,

> Learning is seen as a shared community asset, with many people creating, preserving, and protecting critical resources.

School Health *in Action*

Community Learning Center Campus

Cincinnati Public Schools has created community learning center (CLC) campuses that strengthen the link between schools and communities. The campuses serve as hubs for community services, providing a system of integrated partnerships that promote student growth and development, including academic success, and at the same time provide links into recreational, educational, social, health, civic, and cultural opportunities for not only students but also families and members of the community. Over the past 10 years, this model has drawn national attention for successfully engaging community–school partnerships within school buildings.

Incorporated into these CLCs are health services, counseling, after-school programs, nutrition classes, parent and family engagement programs, early childhood education, career and college access services, youth development activities, mentoring, and arts programming. Each center employs a full-time resource coordinator.

Services valued at over $1 million have been provided to the program by over 600 CLC community partners. An important aspect of the project is that the CLC services are aligned to school goals and have resulted in improved academic outcomes in the participating schools (Cincinnati Public Schools, n.d.).

> Learners and learning agents need skills such as visual literacy, collaboration, networking, and flexibility to navigate the learning ecosystem effectively. (Knowledgeworks, 2011, paragraph 4)

In short, they are hypothesizing a change in how knowledge is acquired and how it is developed, transferred, and subsequently used. And with any major change in the process of education, a logical change would have to occur in the structures that provide services to support students. Just as we have seen a move away from learning that takes place only in a structured school classroom with desks arranged in rows, we will likely see a rapid expansion in who provides and delivers education services and services to support student growth. Such an expansion, if coordinated and collaborative, can be a unifier of communities in garnering services to help their youth.

One thing that is becoming clearer is that opportunities will arise to break down silos as the individual becomes the focus to be served by numerous sectors based on a geographical hub. Greater personalization and an expansion of where and how learning takes place can at the same time promote the use of services provided by noneducation sectors located at that same hub (KnowledgeWorks, 2011). Greater freedom for people to chart their own learning course also increases the need for schools to provide access to supports and structures that fundamentally aid learning and growth, including what we currently call health services.

If this educational forecasting is correct, it may force the alignment and greater integration of the health and education sectors. In fact, the community school models that we currently see around the United States are likely to become much more the norm. Services will be located together and available to community members and students alike to aid their growth and development.

ASCD AND CDC

In 2014 ASCD and the Centers for Disease Control (CDC) launched an update and revision of the Coordinated School Health model. The new model was developed by a consultation and review group of notable school health, public health, and education experts as a response to many of the issues outlined in this book and in particular in this chapter—greater collaboration between sectors, common understanding of symbiotic nature of learning and health, need to align policies and practices, and appreciation of the ecological effect on the child.

The model, the Whole School, Whole Community, Whole Child (WSCC) model, presented in chapter 1, combines and builds on elements of the traditional Coordinated School Health (CSH) model and the Whole Child tenets. WSCC responds to the call for greater alignment, integration, and collaboration between health and education to improve each child's cognitive, physical, social, and emotional development.

The most noticeable aspects of the new model are the following:

- Positioning of the components of a Coordinated School Health program and the tenets of a Whole Child approach to education
- Expanded components, in particular the emphasis placed on the social and emotional climate in addition to the physical environment, and community involvement along with family engagement
- Call for greater coordination in developing joint policy, processes, and practices
- Placement of the model inside the greater community

The focus of the model is an ecological approach directed at the whole school; the school draws its resources and influences from the whole community and serves to address the needs of the whole child. Students who suffer economically are disproportionately served by underfunded, underresourced schools and have less access to social services, including the vast range of health services (SOPHE–ASCD, 2012).

These factors include a lack of early childhood education for students living in poverty, inequitable distribution of master teachers and K through 12 funding, lower parent involvement in the education of poor students, and chronic absenteeism among some students. A major barrier to the achievement of poor students that is often overlooked is their physical and mental health status (SOPHE–ASCD, 2012). A framework that aligns or even integrates school health components with the tenets of a Whole Child approach to education has potential to move the policies, processes, and practices of each sector closer together. Both sectors serve the same youth, often in the same location and frequently for the same or similar issues. It is time to stop dividing the child and see him or her as a whole individual requiring a holistic, coordinated, and integrated approach.

WHAT'S IN IT FOR EDUCATION?

Education has been undergoing a period of reduced resources and a period of redefinition of what constitutes an effective education. Communities should be a source of resources for their schools and school systems as they refocus on holistic approaches that require the integration of the local community. If the predictions of organizations such as KnowledgeWorks play out, schools will increasingly become learning hubs where resources are drawn together. In addition, these learning hubs will likely become locations where students are provided support and assistance beyond academics. These centers of resilience will likely also be required to become "critical sites for promoting health, well-being, academic growth, environmental vitality, and connections across their communities" (KnowledgeWorks, 2011, paragraph 4).

Similar forecasts have been made by the Organization for Economic Cooperation and Development (OECD) arising from the 2001 publication *What Schools for the Future?* and the work of their Centre for Educational Research and Innovation (CERI) (n.d.). Based on this work the OECD predicted three varying scenarios including:

- Status quo extrapolated—An approach that proposes an expansion and continuation of the current functions of schools.
- Deschooling—A prediction that forecasts a break up of schools as institutions.
- Reschooling—A proposal for scenarios that see schools transformed into core social centers and learning organizations with greater responsibility for providing and addressing the widespread, not just educational, needs of the child. It "describes a strengthened, creative school institution available to all communities, meeting critical social responsibilities" in which "greater priority is accorded to the social/community role of schools, with more explicit sharing of programmes and responsibilities."

Regardless of how accurate these forecasts are regarding future structures we are likely to see both a change in what constitutes an effective education and also a corresponding change in how schools operate. These changes would require bridging the gap between education and health systems and create what was originally envisioned in regard to real cooperation within the CSH framework.

WHAT'S IN IT FOR HEALTH?

A more holistic or **Whole Child approach** to education will in turn focus increased attention onto the development of the child socially, emotionally, mentally, and physically. Health, the broad understanding of health, becomes an embedded and integral part of not only what students learn but also how they learn. The same benefits that exist for health currently in working closely with schools and school systems would continue. Schools are one of the most efficient locations for reaching children and youth to provide health services and programs because approximately 95 percent of all U.S. children and youth are in school. It is also true that establishing healthy behaviors during childhood means that these behaviors will likely continue into adulthood and throughout a person's life. Teaching healthy behaviors is far easier and more effective than trying to change unhealthy ones later during adulthood (CDC, 2011).

The more that education can see its role as expanding beyond mere academic achievement to include social, emotional, mental, and physical development and the more that health can see how it plays a critical role in aiding the functions of education, the greater the benefit will be for the development and growth of our youth. Each sector, along with the critical roles of individual community members and organizations, serves the same youth and in the same location. The Whole School, Whole Community, Whole Child approach can be the catalyst of the integration, but to do so it must see its role as spanning both sectors.

SUMMARY

We are entering a time when change will be a constant in our lives. This circumstance will apply not only to people but also to communities and the sectors, institutions, and locations, including schools and the school districts that serve them. Change will require health and education to collaborate, align, and integrate.

The new framework for the way that health and education work together in the school setting is needed to ensure that both sectors realize full potential for each child. We have had a growing separation of the two entities for too long, and it is time for a more concerted, collaborative approach.

But one caveat applies here. For health to be truly integrated into the processes of the school and education, it must present itself and align itself to the policies, practices, and outcomes of education.

Glossary

academic standardized testing—A testing system administered and scored in a consistent or standard manner. Standardized testing was a hallmark of the No Child Left Behind (NCLB) Act.

annual yearly progress—A measurement defined by the No Child Left Behind Act that determines how each public school and school district in the country is performing academically according to results on standardized tests from one year to the next.

personalization—Adjusting the teaching and the content to suit the level of the learner. Personalization can also refer to adjusting the learning to suit how a person learns (kinesthetically, visually, interpersonally, and so on)

self-directed learning—A process of student learning that is led by the student or is based on his or her interests.

staff satisfaction—The degree to which school staff feel valued and important at their school and in their roles.

staff turnover—The degree to which teachers are removed or replaced in a school, often because of resignation or transfer.

standardization—Education that is similar or standard across a system, which can include standardization of goals, curriculum, or teaching methods.

Whole Child approach—An approach to education that aims to focus attention on each child's social, emotional, mental, and physical development as well as her or his cognitive development.

Application Activities

1. Interview a school administrator, teacher, parent, or student regarding his or her perceptions of the future of education. What will be the same? What will be different? How can schools promote health and academic success in the future? Write a summary of the interviews; in addition include your personal reaction to the information you have gained in the report.

2. Write an opinion article (op-ed) for a newspaper on your vision for education in the future. Include your findings from your interviews in the preceding application activity. Remember, however, to report your own opinion, not just the opinion of others. Include your thoughts on the schools' role in promoting both academic success and health.
3. As a member of your school health team, you believe that your school is slow to consider possible changes in school health and the potential effect of those changes on education. Identify one specific group of school stakeholders (administrators, teachers, parents, students, or community members) and develop an agenda for a meeting with two purposes: (1) to inform participants of potential changes and (2) to generate discussion about these changes, specifically their potential effect on education. The discussion should also generate possible actions that your school can consider now to prepare for possible change. In addition to establishing the agenda for this meeting, provide PowerPoint slides for the presentation on the potential changes and a description of the questions and activities that you will use to generate discussion.

Resources

ASCD www.ascd.org. ASCD information on the WSCC model is available at www.ascd.org/programs /learning-and-health/wscc-model.aspx.

Charles Basch's 2010 publication *Healthier Students Are Better Learners*, www.equitycampaign.org/i/a/document/12557_EquityMattersVol6_Web03082010.pdf

Centers for Disease Control and Prevention, Coordinated School Health, www.cdc.gov/HealthyYouth/cshp/

CDC report, *The Association Between School-Based Physical Activity, Including Physical Education, and Academic Performance*, 2010, www.cdc.gov/healthyyouth/health_and_academics/pdf/pa-pe_paper.pdf

Whole Child Education, www.wholechildeducation.org

The Healthy School Communities Model: Aligning Health and Education in the School Setting, www.ascd.org/ASCD/pdf/siteASCD/publications/Aligning-Health-Education.pdf School Climate Research, National School Climate Center, 2013, https://schoolclimate.org/climate/research .php

References

A Surprising Secret to a Long Life: Stay in School. 2007, January 3. *New York Times*. www.nytimes.com/2007/01/03/health/03aging.html

Allensworth, Diane D., & Kolbe, Lloyd J. 1987. The Comprehensive School Health Program: Exploring an Expanded Concept. *Journal of School Health*, *57*(10), 409–412.

ASCD. n.d. *The Whole Child*. www.ascd.org/programs /The-Whole-Child/Healthy.aspx

ASCD. 2013. The ASCD Whole Child Award Winner. Press release. www.ascd.org/news-media/Press-Room/News-Releases/Oregon-Milwaukie-High-School-ASCD-2013-Vision-in-Action-Whole-Child-Award-Winner.aspx

Basch, Charles E. 2010. *Healthier Students Are Better Learners: A Missing Link in School Reforms to Close the Achievement Gap*. Equity Matters, Research Review No. 6. www.equitycampaign.org/i/a/document/12557_EquityMattersVol6_Web03082010.pdf

Bergeson, Terry, Heuschel, Mary Alice, Hall, Greg, & Willhoft, Joe. 2005. *Guidelines for Participation and Testing Accommodations for Special Populations in State Assessment Programs*. Olympia, WA: Washington Office of Superintendent of Public Education.

Byrne, Barbara M. 1994. Burnout: Testing for the Validity, Replication, and Invariance of Causal Structure Across Elementary, Intermediate, and Secondary Teachers. *American Educational Research Journal*, *31*(3), 645–673.

California Department of Education. 2005. *Getting Results: Student Health, Supportive Schools, and Academic Success*.

California Department of Education. 2008. *Getting Results: Developing Safe and Healthy Kids*. www.cde.ca.gov/ls/he/at/gettingresults.asp

Case, Anne, & Paxson, Christina. 2006. Children's Health and Social Mobility. *Future of Children*, *16*, 151–173.

Centers for Disease Control and Prevention (CDC). 2010. *The Association Between School-Based Physical Activity, Including Physical Education, and Academic Performance*. http://www.cdc.gov/healthyyouth/health_and_academics/pdf/pa-pe_paper.pdf

Centers for Disease Control and Prevention (CDC). 2011. *School Health Programs: Improving the Health of Our Nation's Youth*. www.cdc.gov/chronicdisease

/resources/publications/aag/pdf/2011/school_health_aag_web_pdf.pdf

Centre for Educational Research and Innovation (CERI). n.d. *The OECD Schooling Scenarios in Brief.* www.oecd.org/fr/edu/scolaire/centreforeducationalresearchandinnovationceri-theoecdschoolingscenariosinbrief.htm

Cincinnati Public Schools. n.d. *Community Learning Centers.* www.cincinnaticlc.org and www.cps-k12.org/community/clc

Crosnoe, Robert. 2006. Health and the Education of Children From Racial/Ethnic Minority and Immigrant Families. *Journal of Health and Social Behavior, 47,* 77–93.

Cura, Maureen Van. 2010. The Relationship Between School-Based Health Centers, Rates of Early Dismissal From School, and Loss of Seat Time. *Journal of School Health, 80*(8), 371–377.

Dorman, Jeffrey P. 2003. Relationship Between School and Classroom Environment and Teacher Burnout: A LISREL Analysis. *Social Psychology of Education, 6*(2), 107–127.

Freudenberg, Nicholas, & Ruglis, Jessica. 2007. Reframing School Dropout as a Public Health Issue. *Preventing Chronic Disease, 4*(4). www.cdc.gov/pcd/issues/2007/oct/07_0063.htm

Grayson, Jessica L., & Alvarez, Heather K. (2008, July). School Climate Factors Relating to Teacher Burnout: A Mediator Model. *Teaching and Teacher Education: An International Journal of Research and Studies, 24*(5), 1349–1363.

Haas, Steven A., & Fosse, Nathan E. 2008. Health and the Educational Attainment of Adolescents: Evidence From the NLSY97. *Journal of Health and Social Behavior,* 49(2), 178–192.

Harris, Joseph R., Cohen, Phyllis L., & Flaherty, Todd D. 2008. *Eight Elements of High School Improvement: A Mapping Framework.* Washington, DC: National High School Center, American Institutes of Research. www.betterhighschools.com/pubs/documents/NHSCEightElements7-25-08.pdf

Hass, Steven A. 2006. Health Selection and the Process of Social Stratification: The Effect of Childhood Health on Socioeconomic Attainment. *Journal of Health and Social Behavior, 47,* 339–354.

Heckman, James J. 2008. Role of Income and Family Influence on Child Outcomes. *Annals of the New York Academy of Sciences, 1136,* 307–323.

Hoyle, Tena B., Bartee, R. Todd, & Allensworth, Diane D. 2010. Applying the Process of Health Promotion in Schools: A Commentary. *Journal of School Health, 80*(4), 163–166.

Iton, Anthony. 2006. Tackling the Root Causes of Health Disparities through Community Capacity Building. In R. Hofrichter (ed.), *Tackling Health Inequities Through Public Health Practice: A Handbook for Action* (pp. 115–136). Washington DC: NACCHO.

KnowledgeWorks. 2011. Schools as Centers of Resilience in *2020 Forecast: Creating the Future of Learning.* http://knowledgeworks.org/sites/default/files/u1/Scenario%20Overview%2011x17.pdf

KnowledgeWorks. 2013a. *Glimpse Into the Future of Learning (Forecast 3.0).* www.knowledgeworks.org/sites/default/files/A-Glimpse-into-the-Future-of-Learning-Infographic_0.pdf

Koivusilta, Leena., Arja, Rimpelä, & Andres, Vikat. 2003. Health Behaviors and Health in Adolescence as Predictors of Educational Level in Adulthood: A Follow-Up Study From Finland. *Social Science and Medicine, 57,* 577–593.

Marx, Eva, Wooley, Susan, & Northrop, Daphne (Eds.). 1998. *Health Is Academic: A Guide to Coordinated School Health Programs.* New York: Teachers College Press.

No Child Left Behind (NCLB) Act of 2001. Pub. L. No. 107-110, § 115, Stat. 1425.

National School Climate Center. 2013. *National School Climate Research.* OECD, Education Indicators in Focus. www.oecd-ilibrary.org/docserver/download/5k4ddxnl39vk.pdf?expires=1376576246&id=id&accname=guest&checksum=0AB30FD90ED892F56F99B68726FC781D)

Palloni, Alberto. 2006. Reproducing Inequalities: Luck, Wallets, and the Enduring Effects of Childhood Health. *Demography, 43,* 587–615.

Pink, Daniel. 2010. Daniel Pink in Conversation With Prof. Yong Zhao, Schools Network Conference. www.youtube.com/watch?v=wrk3vfEE8i4

Seith, David, & Isakson, Elizabeth. 2011. *Who Are America's Poor Children? Examining Health Disparities Among Children in the United States.* New York: National Center for Children in Poverty. www.nccp.org/publications/pdf/text_995.pdf

SOPHE–ASCD. 2012. *Expert Panel on Reducing Youth Health Disparities—Overview.* Washington, DC: SOPHE. www.sophe.org/SchoolHealth/Disparities.cfm

Strolin-Goltzman, Jessica. 2010. The Relationship Between School-Based Health Centers and the Learning Environment. *Journal of School Health, 80*(3), 153–159.

Valois, Robert, Slade, Sean, & Ashford, Ellie. 2011. *The Healthy School Communities Model: Aligning Health and Education in the School Setting.* Alexandria, VA: ASCD.

Walker, Sarah Cusworth, Kerns, Suzanne, Lyon, Aaron R., Brun, Eric J., Cosgrove, T.J. 2010. Impact of School-Based Health Center Use on Academic Outcomes. *Journal of Adolescent Health, 46*(3), 251–257.

13

Perspectives From the Field

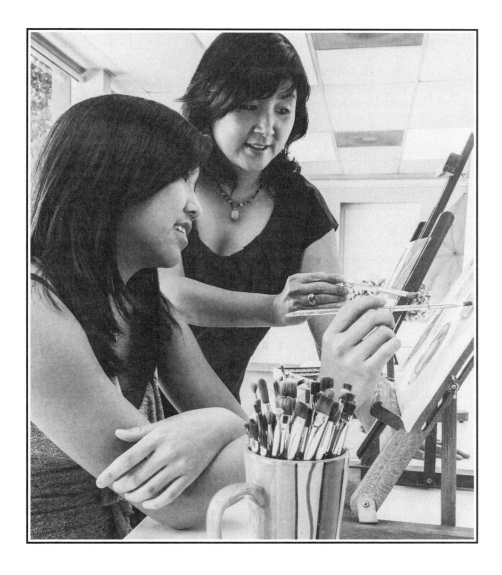

Chapter 13 presents the perspectives of school health and education in relationship to the Whole School, Whole Community, Whole Child (WSCC) model. The contributors include teachers, school nurses, school administrators, agency directors, and university faculty members. They are the people who will be ultimately responsible for supporting and implementing the WSCC model. Their perspectives can be used to provide direction for helping our communities and schools become bastions for better health and improved academic achievement.

CREATING SUPPORT FOR EDUCATION AND HEALTH

Sharon Murray,
President, RMC Health, Colorado

Several years ago, I was presenting to school administrators on the impact that Coordinated School Health could have on student academic achievement. A comment from a high school assistant principal has stayed with me ever since: "I've been in education for over 30 years. When I first started out, I felt like I was an educator who sometimes did social services. Now, I feel like I am a social worker who sometimes educates."

This administrator understood how negative health and social issues could hinder a student's ability to be successful in school. But his sense of frustration was palpable—schools are being asked to be all things to all students, and they simply do not have the resources or expertise to address the myriad challenges facing our nation's young people.

Having an expanded, articulated role of the broader school community is a significant step forward with the Whole School, Whole Community, Whole Child model. Although family and community involvement has always been a key component of Coordinated School Health, implementing this component has proven elusive. I hope that the Whole School, Whole Community, Whole Child initiative will lead to concrete guidance and resources that will effectively engage community leaders in meeting the needs of each student within those communities. Moreover, the initiative offers an opportunity to help schools and districts create meaningful partnerships with community members and agencies to bring needed resources and services to students and families. I believe that it must be a two-way street, in which community partners are invited early and often to participate in a community input process.

Another important aspect of the Whole School, Whole Community, Whole Child model is the stated relationship between health and learning. Over the last two decades, more evidence of the link between student health and academic achievement has been identified. In spite of this, Coordinated School Health has often been seen as an add-on. The expanded model recognizes and explicitly states the integral relationship between student health and learning.

Promoting the expanded model and making it accessible to local schools will take time. We need federal and state leadership and funding to enable local implementation. We need to build school and district accountability systems to include the components and tenets of the model. As a nation, we must expect partnerships at every level to support schools. We need the U.S. Department of Education to embrace the Whole School, Whole Community, Whole Child model and foster innovative partnerships and alliances at the federal level that will serve as a model for state and local education agencies.

In short, we need a sea change. Our colleges of education and teacher preparation programs must start preparing future teachers and administrators to understand and be part of the Whole School, Whole Community, Whole Child initiative. We must create an expectation for each education professional that this strategy is vital to meeting the education mission of schools. We must help families be empowered to collaborate with schools. And we must eliminate silo thinking that this issue is strictly about health. Frankly, this issue is about the future.

PROMOTING A SENSE OF COMMUNITY

Karen Cottrell, Former Health Educator for Lakota School District, Ohio

The Whole School, Whole Community, Whole Child (WSCC model) takes me back to thoughts of *Little House on the Prairie*, the TV show in which families within the community all had a vested interest in the education of their children. In today's society with larger communities and larger school districts, we seem to have lost the sense of community. The former Coordinated School Health model provided a template of how the resources of a school district could cooperatively work together to plan programs to improve the health of students. Community and family involvement was considered one aspect of the model. From my experience in public schools, community and family involvement was often more of an afterthought and was used primarily to support programs developed by the schools. The new WSCC model broadens the scope of what is needed to improve the health and academic success of all students. The family and community need to take a leadership role in making this happen.

Experience over the past 26 years has shown the difficulty of establishing and maintaining a coordinated approach to focus on the health and well-being of students, school staff, and community. Health education teachers and school nurses were typically the springboard to initiate a comprehensive school health model. They needed to seek support from the school administration and school board as well as from the other component areas of the Coordinated School Health model. It was often an uphill battle. Administrators were more concerned about the "core" areas, such as math and science, than they were about health. Families and communities often participated in the random health fair, community walk, or nutrition committee, but they played more of a participant or support role than a leadership role.

Success in improving the health and ultimately the academic achievement of students must come from a broad array of community and school leaders. Administrators, school boards, and community leaders must see the value in implementing this model, vest their time and resources into it, and then recruit key participants. Equal participation needs to come from all sectors of the schools and community, not one small group of leaders. Public health agencies, health educators, administrators, city or town council members, police, PTA, youth sport programs, school board members, teachers, and nutritionists must all advocate for and participate in the WSCC model. The more engaged that family and community become, the more likely that programs are to succeed. Mandates or incentives from state or federal governments would help drive the WSCC model forward. Having a high-profile spokesperson such as Michelle Obama endorse and advocate for the model would be helpful. A large-scale public relations campaign using television, radio, and social media to make the population at large aware of the model would also be important to moving the model forward.

SUPPORTING HEALTHY STUDENTS AND LEARNING ENVIRONMENT

Richard A. Lyons, Superintendent of Schools, Maine Regional School Unit 22, Hampden, Maine

The Coordinated School Health model defines and strengthens the partnership among school, community, and child. The Whole School, Whole Community, Whole Child collaborative efforts will undeniably enhance all aspects associated with effective teaching and learning. The national and state initiatives associated with Common Core and other standards that drive curricula are gaining the limelight, but the desired student outcomes will not be attained if we do not enhance research practices associated with the healthy child.

I encourage national organizations and state legislatures to support funding associated with the Coordinated School Health model. Each state has embraced educational standards and learning outcomes to raise the academic status of American students. The desired outcomes will only be attained when all support a healthy learning environment and healthy students.

ENHANCING THE DEVELOPMENT OF THE WHOLE CHILD

Barb McDowell, Middle School Health Teacher and School Nurse Special Assignment, Bath Central School District, Bath, New York

I think the Whole School, Whole Community, Whole Child (WSCC) model picks up where the Coordinated School Health (CSH) model leaves off. It takes the shared implementation of the eight components and gives it a framework that makes sense and is focused, not just kind of connected. It gives it a clearer sense of how the interactions can work to improve learning and health in a cooperative effort and affect both at the same time. This model clarifies the bigger picture of what school health is. It shows a multidisciplinary, shared responsibility like the CSH model, but it links those components to community and families as well. I think this model will serve as an avenue to implement school health with more involvement and with a clear focus of both learning and health for the child. The inclusive nature of the model will help to bring the support required for a balanced approach.

The WSCC has far-reaching potential in terms of preparing our children (pre K–12) not only in college and career readiness but also in being healthy, well-rounded citizens. The child is central in this model, and public education must seek to equip each child with the support, opportunities, and resources needed for healthy development.

With the ever-changing, fast-paced nature of our culture, we need to reevaluate our efforts and work collaboratively to serve our communities, schools, and children. In strengthening these relationships, programs can be assessed and fostered to meet current and future needs, for any of the 10 components in the model. The economic challenges that many districts face may need community support to find creative and cooperative ways to resolve concerns or meet new needs. Grant opportunities from the public and private sector may be possible with a coordinated effort. Even how we define community may need to be broadened.

This model makes perfect sense to me as a connector to community agencies and resources. To become literate, people needs support, safety, challenge, engagement, and health. Literacy and health go hand in hand. In terms of global health, we know that literacy is an important health indicator among nations, but for literacy to happen, the quality of life must support health and well-being. For true "health literacy" to occur, we need health and literacy coupled with health education. With the increasing stress, demands, and needs of families and children, health literacy needs to become a reality for the child, school, and community.

As the school and community recognize that the model already has successful elements in place and see the benefits of these collaborative interactions, then viewing, valuing, and implementing school health as an integral part of education will become natural. It can become how we do business.

The 10 components of the WSCC model help to broaden the circle. The model expands the base of support and draws more resources to the table to serve the child, school, and community. Expanding the healthy school environment into two components, the physical environment and the social and emotional climate, gives clarity and allows specific identification of the area of the environment that needs to be implemented or addressed. Defining these two entities helps to involve those working there to see their role clearly and to connect. I think that our district is already implementing this aspect.

IMPROVING HEALTH EDUCATION THROUGH WSCC

Vanessa Booth, National Board-Certified Health Educator, Half Hollow Hills CSD, Dix Hills, New York

Health education is not an extra. Instead, it must be the central piece of our educational system, its most essential component. Unfortunately, health programs in schools have been marginalized philosophically, socially, and economically. They are shrunk down to bare state mandates, and rarely are they a topic of serious pedagogical discussions. Therefore, the release of the WSCC model is both timely and much needed.

Although school leaders are making tough decisions to balance budgets, health education programs need to be supported by a clear advocacy message, namely, that health is essential to learners' success. WSCC provides that message. Its framework supports and validates school-based health education. This framework revolves around the basic idea that healthy students learn better and achieve more. If this simple premise is accepted as true, then a radical overhauling of our entire approach to education must ensue. The WSCC model provides the framework for such an approach. The learner, education's most basic entity, must be viewed as a complex whole. The whole child—rather than the math child, or the English child, or the athlete child, or the special education child—must be examined, assisted, and guided on a daily basis. A student must be given the tools to assure that what matters most, his or her health, is addressed. Of course, the tools will vary in accordance with the specific needs of a community.

Health education should be a central part of school reform, not an item on the chopping block when budgets get tight. Although professional meeting time is often devoted to pending budget cuts, new curriculum, and other housekeeping items, this new framework is worthy of the deepest consideration of every school district's work force and of every community's residents. School wellness needs to be an ongoing, top priority agenda item.

What's really missing is a nationwide acknowledgement of the central role of health education. More than ever, this is the time for advocacy and organization. The WSCC framework validates the central place of health in education. Today, 95 percent of our youth are in schools, and health education, as implemented by the WSCC model, is the perfect vehicle for delivering the message that it must not be marginalized by "core" subjects. Indeed, health must be seen as the most core subject.

This framework is a call to action for educational leaders to prioritize students' health.

Next, what is needed is widespread buy-in from key stakeholders, which should foster action. Funding must be made available to support efforts in all districts, focused on the areas of highest need. School heath education programs and the overall quality of education will benefit greatly from the implementation of this framework. The message must be delivered feverishly and consistently to community leaders, school officials, and politicians for consideration until they begin to listen. Wellness is the foundation for academic success, and school health educators are already poised to have great influence. But they need the class time and the collaborative support to do so.

School health policies need teeth. If a policy is adopted but is merely full of suggestions, the action will likely not materialize within the classrooms and school communities. Policy should be carefully drafted to set expectations and should use definitive language. Many initiatives are thrown at educators today, and WSCC could be interpreted as just one more. But WSCC is the foundation on which all educational programs should sit. It's about making each school a healthier place by making health education both central in the community and responsive to the community's needs.

Health and wellness are the headliners of the show, not the encore or extra takes. I look forward to sharing this framework with colleagues and leaders in my area, and I hope for emphatic consensus on the importance of action as soon as possible. We can always do better for our students. The WSCC framework considers the whole picture, the whole child, and the whole community. Its real value is in pointing us all in the right direction.

PROMOTING THE COMMUNITY'S ROLE IN EDUCATION AND HEALTH

Rochelle Davis, President and CEO, Healthy Schools Campaign, Chicago, IL

The new Whole School, Whole Community, Whole Child (WSCC) model is a key strategy for ensuring that students across the country are healthy and ready to learn. The model's emphasis on alignment, integration, and collaboration between education and health provides an important foundation for ensuring that schools support the conditions of health.

The model's recognition of the key role that communities can play in supporting student health and wellness is especially important. Schools are not positioned to transform their health and wellness environment on their own, so they must collaborate with communities to meet their dual goals of supporting the education and health needs of their population. We have seen the importance of this collaboration firsthand in Chicago, where Healthy Schools Campaign has worked with schools and dozens of other nonprofits and community organizations to increase access to healthy food, nutrition education, and opportunities for physical activity in schools across the city. The WSCC model can help ensure schools and communities understand the need to and importance of working together and leverage key resources to support student health.

In addition to recognizing the importance of collaborating with surrounding communities, Healthy Schools Campaign, in collaboration with over 100 stakeholders across the country, has identified key strategies for improving school health and wellness, which aligns closely with the core components of the WSCC model. These strategies, which are highlighted in Healthy Schools Campaign's and Trust for America's Health's report, *Health in Mind: Improving Education Through Wellness*, include integrating health and wellness into professional development programs for teachers and principals, increasing access to school health services, engaging parents in school health and academic improvement efforts, integrating health and wellness into school data and transparency systems, and building the capacity of the U.S. Department of Education to support student health.

The WSCC model aligns closely with these recommendations and can help ensure key decision makers at the federal, state, and local levels understand the importance of supporting health and wellness and recognize the need to engage the entire school community in creating healthier school environments for students. We commend ASCD and CDC for developing this new model and look forward to working with them and advocates across the country to ensure that all students are able to learn in environments that support the conditions of health.

EMBRACING WSCC: PROFESSIONAL PREPARATION

Beth H. Chaney, Assistant Professor, Department of Health Education and Promotion, East Caroline University

Despite the best efforts of researchers and practitioners in school health education, school health has not been a central focus in the education of

America's children. For too long, our complex education system has separated learning from health, even though research findings indicate a relationship between health, learning, and academic achievement. As a result, as described by the Children's Defense Fund in their 2014 report *The State of America's Children*, our nation's education system is failing to prepare our children to compete in the 21st century by not recognizing that when a child's health suffers or when health needs go unmet, learning and academic achievement are also affected.

Fortunately, with the recent acknowledgement of the interconnectedness of health and education and the release of ASCD's and the Centers for Disease Control and Prevention's (CDC) Whole School, Whole Community, Whole Child (WSCC) model for coordinated school health, we are seeing a shift toward a more collaborative approach to learning and health. This new, ecological approach to improving the overall health and well-being of students for long-term student success provides a framework that combines years of research and practice in school health and student education. This approach to health and education is long overdue. The WSCC model views the school, and therefore the students, as a vital part of the community. This model, unlike any other, focuses on improving the whole child (by addressing the comprehensive needs of students), the whole school (by acknowledging that health and education must be a schoolwide endeavor), and the local community (by acknowledging that the school is reflection of the community).

I hope that school administrators, educators, and community members will embrace the new WSCC model and incorporate it into existing school structures. The model calls for a collaboration of schools and communities to meet the needs of students and improve their long-term success. Obviously, that job is easier said than done, because policies and practices will need to be established to ensure effective implementation of the model. But it is worth the effort, because every child deserves an opportunity to be healthy and excel academically. One place to start is with training of our future teachers, school administrators, and key community decision makers. Our professional preparation programs need to align curricula with the new model to train future educators and community members on the importance of the collaborative approach. Children are truly our future, and the Whole Child approach will ensure that we are providing every opportunity for each child to succeed.

UNDERSTANDING THE HEALTH AND LEARNING RELATIONSHIP

Linda Morse,
American School Health Association,
President, 2012–2014

Although the 1987 Coordinated School Health model generated discussion in public health circles, it was largely unknown in education circles. Because I spent most of my career with one foot in each pond, I can attest to the lack of brand identity for the Coordinated School Health model. It was not an easy sell in education circles. But when ASCD released its Whole Child initiative in 2007, "nonhealth people" said that students should be healthy, safe, and supported. What a revelation! Suddenly, ASCD discovered that physical, social, and emotional health actually affects student achievement. When ASCD spoke, educators listened.

The updated WSCC model itself is not revolutionary; frankly, the changes to the Coordinated School Health model were logical and expected. But is the new model enough to facilitate real change? Will the WSCC model really make an impact in schools? Will this model have a direct effect on student health and achievement, and if so, how will we know? What will it take to make the WSCC model the norm in every school?

- First, all school personnel must understand the relationship between health and academic achievement. Teacher preparation programs must educate all future teachers and administrators about Whole Child issues that affect teaching, learning, and lifetime success. Ongoing professional learning for all school personnel should reinforce the connections between health and learning.
- Second, because school board members play a pivotal role in policy development and school funding, they too must become cognizant of the relationship between health and achievement. They are a direct link to the community.
- Third, parents and family members must be educated about the relationship between health and academic achievement. This

process must begin in early childhood education programs and continue from kindergarten through grade 12. Many factors that affect learning (e.g., healthy eating, sleep patterns, and control of health conditions like diabetes or asthma) rest with the family. We need to provide families with support and education, too.

- Fourth, agencies such as the Departments of Education, Agriculture, Environmental Protection, Health and Human Services, and Justice should adopt the WSCC model and provide state and local education agencies with consistent language, support, and funding to support implementation. We must all begin to speak the same language.
- Finally, we need to acknowledge that all students are at risk. Yes, some students need more individualized services and supports, but our job as educators is to do whatever it takes to ensure that every child has the opportunity
- to learn. We need to build on the basic WSCC model to reflect a tiered system of support that ensures that all students are healthy, safe, supported, challenged, and engaged.

Every school can be a safe and supportive place to learn, work, and play; a place that nurtures both health and a love of learning; a place where every child and every family has the support to improve their health and subsequently the health of the community. Healthy schools embrace the challenge of the whole child and find innovative ways to promote health and learning. They see health and learning as inextricably linked. We cannot wait another 25 years to deliver this for every child. The WSCC model is a new beginning for school health.

BUILDING HEALTHY SCHOOL COMMUNITIES

Denise M. Seabert,
Professor and Chair, Department of Physiology and Health Science,
Ball State University

I started my career in school health over 20 years ago—a time when the concept of Coordinated School Health was just taking off. My state was seen as forward thinking because teams of K through 12 educators had the opportunity to participate in a weeklong professional development conference focused on creating an employee wellness culture within the district. As a team, we focused on improving our personal health as well as developing a plan for improving the health of those in our district—including faculty, staff, bus drivers, custodians, and students. We were ahead of our time!

Today I am encouraged about the progress that has been made to make schools healthier environments for nurturing learning. The Coordinated School Health model has helped us transform policies and programs to address major health concerns in school communities and in turn influence the learning of our students. The new Whole School, Whole Community, Whole Child model will further guide us in the process of improving school communities. Because this model was introduced by an educational organization and supported by health organizations, the potential influence is tremendous.

Education of our youth continues to be a challenge because of standardized test requirements, significant health and learning challenges for our students, and state and federal demands for student learning outcomes, so we must use the best practice evidence we have to improve our schools for the health of the community. The new Whole School, Whole Community, Whole Child model reminds us that we must take care of our entire school and community. By doing so, our children will be healthier learners.

Years from now, when schools have fully embraced a collaborative approach, we will have healthy school communities where our young people feel safe, cared for, supported, and challenged to meet their potential. I believe that reaching this goal will require a grassroots effort from communities that have experienced success with implementing the Coordinated School Health approach to addressing health programs and policies. We need these communities to share their stories and inspire other communities so that we are all able to walk to school or work safely, select healthy foods every day, engage in physical activity throughout the day, and do the right thing within an environment that allows us to have our learning needs met, be healthy, and achieve our potential!

MEETING THE NEEDS OF ALL YOUTH

Deborah A. Fortune, Associate Professor, Department of Public Health Education, North Carolina Central University

WSCC is a necessary evolution to address the health and education needs of 21st-century learners. As the needs of youth have expanded, so has the model for school health, going from a 3-component model to an 8-component model and now to a 10-component model. If implemented as planned, WSCC will have a vast influence, especially for students from economically disadvantaged rural and urban school districts. The health and education challenges in these school districts are enormous, whether it is childhood obesity, food insecurities, homicides, drive-by shootings, or sexual risk-taking behaviors. If fully actualized, WSCC could help close the education and health disparity gap for racial and ethnic minority children, adolescents, and their families. Lastly, the new expanded model seems to embrace the concept "It takes a village to raise a child."

The issue with this model is how it will be implemented in all school districts. What resources (human, financial, policy, and so on) are needed to implement WSCC? What will be required to get buy-in and support from state and local education agencies? How will WSCC be actualized in economically disadvantaged school districts? Will the model close the education and health disparity gaps among school districts or widen it? Although the WSCC model is a collaborative approach designed to enhance the education and health of all children, how will it be put into practice in all school districts?

In summary, WSCC is needed to address the education and health needs of all school-age youth. The model is well thought out and considers all aspects of the lives of children and adolescents. The WSCC model encourages schools, in collaboration with the community and families, to function fully to prepare all young people to be healthy, well-educated, and responsible citizens.

INCORPORATING WSCC INTO SCHOOL CULTURE

Jill Deuink Pace, Health and Wellness Coordinator, Cortland Enlarged City School District`, Cortland, New York

Through our experience in our local school district, we learned that health education can make a significant difference in the daily lives of students when it is fully supported and integrated into their total academic program. The WSCC model will encourage collaboration by seeking input from the people making the decisions that affect students.

Recently, during a professional development day with the theme "Lifestyle Impacts Learning," we introduced the WSCC model to staff and explored health outcomes that can be fostered with our students to improve their health and academic success. First, in a general session, participants were introduced to the WSCC model in a brief presentation that included the video from the ASCD website. An expert in the field of health education reinforced the need for the new model and discussed how to make the shift to refocus our school community. As a health educator, I was excited to have this presentation in a forum in which all academic disciplines in grades K through 12 were represented and health was viewed as the means to tie together all aspects of students' lives for their health and academic success. A community physician followed by offering a practical application of the model titled "Better Choices = Better Grades," which discussed how lifestyle choices of students affect learning. This presentation explained how posture, exercise, and nutrition influence student learning. The participants immediately recognized the relationship between student learning and health.

After the general presentation, participants engaged in workshops led by community providers focused on mindfulness, health literacy, nutrition, physical activity, energy in the classroom, local foods, social media, and communication skills. Each workshop explored how a person's personal practice or habits can be incorporated into the classroom to affect how each student can learn while continuing to explore topics of how health, wellness, and a healthy lifestyle affect achievement. By using reflection questions at the conclusion of the workshop, we were able to gain information about practicing and educating our students in a safe, healthy school community that encourages academic success while keeping the focus of the whole child. Through discussion, staff transitioned from applying what they learned to how to use it to improve the social, emotional, physical, and cognitive health of students. They worked collaboratively to connect healthy lifestyle behaviors to academic achievement. When adults working in our school can make that connection, they can then model in their respective classrooms to help students make the connections. Students will see that health and well-being are not separate entities but an integral part of their daily academic life.

Currently, our district is developing a plan to incorporate this model into our school culture. The WSCC will be reflected in our updated wellness policy, school theme, and individual classrooms for the upcoming school year. Outreach is ongoing to all community players to join our efforts, precipitating a detailed resource list to provide to staff. The WSCC model will create a closer connection between school and community agencies on a consistent basis, thus integrating their resources into the academic day and beyond.

We believe that our district can improve a child's health and academic success by adopting and integrating the Whole School, Whole Community, Whole Child model in our school district. The model will help us set realistic goals for our staff and students while supporting and promoting healthy connections for healthy behaviors. The model will also increase collaboration between the school and our community to provide education and resources that support the health and well-being of each student.

EXTENDING WSCC BEYOND THE SCHOOL

Laurence Spring, Superintendent, Schenectady School District, Schenectady, New York

The new model of Coordinated School Health, the WSCC model, is a better way of looking at how we can all work together more effectively for our children. For too long, bureaucracies have been about compartmentalizing our objectives and jobs. We know that children are whole beings and are best treated as such. The WSCC model provides the framing necessary to have common conversations about all the dimensions of children that require our careful and calculated attention.

This model can become the common language spoken between agencies that have responsibility for all aspects of health and health education. By incorporating an ecological approach, all service providers can find themselves in the model because it lends itself to the natural next steps of common principles of practice and collaboration. These should have the effect of bringing more providers to the table and helping to minimize the parochialism that often gets in the way of multiagency collaboration. This process will help to ensure that families and students are receiving coordinated care that is provided in a thoughtful way that honors and respects them as they transition between home, community, and school.

This model seems to reflect best practices that are already in existence. I plan to bring this model to our regular multiagency meetings and ask people to engage in conversation about where their agency has responsibility and how they see that role assisting with other objectives in the model. Bringing all our team members to the table, not just our school health team, is the critical element to ensuring that this model has an effect that extends beyond the school walls and the school day.

SUPPORTING WSCC: ADMINISTRATIVE LEADERSHIP

Caroline Eberle, Master Teacher (instructional coach) and Health and Wellness Instructor, UNO Charter School Network, Maj Hector P. Garcia, MD Charter High School, Chicago

I have taught health education for six years in the urban high schools of Chicago. Developing whole school health initiatives falls on the health coordinator (if a school has one) or more often on the physical education and health education teachers. The new model, WSCC, puts more emphasis on the administration and leadership to help ensure that these programs are developed and maintained.

After reading about the new model, I was happy to see that health initiatives should be derived primarily from the principal (or director in charter schools). The model puts the pressure on the principal to get health programs started by using leadership abilities and emotional intelligence to bring other staff members on board. But the model specifically states that the principal is not the only person responsible for health programs and systems. I believe that a helpful modification would be to require specific action items for a principal and specific action items for other members of the school body, staff, and faculty. Being in an urban school district, I have noticed that turnover is constant. To maintain the healthy initiatives, a specific road map should be in place for the next principal to pick up and use to makes sure that a year isn't lost in the leadership transition. For the leadership of any school to give their time, energy, and push for a health-conscious school, the initiative needs to be part of the mission and vision of the school itself. If a director is judged or graded by some aspect of the health and wellness initiatives that he or she created or maintained, effort and accountability in this direction may increase.

Educators have known forever about the connection between academic achievement and student health. Just last week, our school made a huge push for the juniors to eat breakfast before their ACT testing. Why just one day? More pressure needs to be applied on a constant basis to push for healthier habits in the school system.

I hope that this new model will be introduced not only to health educators but also in school administration courses throughout the United States. The model makes health programs not just a segmented addition to the school but a major focal point of education. The healthier the students are, the more engaged they are in school and the more likely they are to succeed in the classroom. With whole school initiatives, the parents and community will be involved after expectations are set for family involvement. Communication with students and family to be health conscious is extremely important. Direction from the school should come first; involvement from the student body and community will then likely follow.

For a school looking to implement more health education events and participation, I would align programs with national awareness months. For example, in October a tradition around homecoming could be that all players wear pink for breast cancer awareness month. Health agencies could help give doctor referrals at the game while parents are there watching their children. The same goes for heart health month. Each month a school can tie in activities and events around nationally recognized health-enhancing events. By using recognized awareness months, more collaboration could occur with established organizations in the community.

Being a health educator is a rewarding profession. The more help we have with leadership, administration, and our colleagues, the more comprehensive our health programs will be. They say it takes a village to raise a child; it takes the whole community to raise a healthy one.

These perspectives support the vision of WSCC as an essential strategy for improving health and academic achievement for students in our schools. These views also illuminate the need for all stakeholders to understand the connection between health and student success; the necessity for advocacy, leadership, support, and policy development; and the importance of quality professional preparation and development for educators. Beyond these needs, WSCC presents a framework not only for educators but also for parents, community members, and organizations to become active participants in promoting success for all children.

Appendix

Assessment Instruments and Tools

LISA C. BARRIOS • SARAH M. LEE

The United States government and national nongovernmental organizations have created these assessment tools based on scientific evidence, behavior change and education theory, and best practices from the field. These tools are used extensively to address key aspects of CSH. Some can be used to address multiple health topics because they focus on CSH components such as policy, environment, and health education. Most recently, many tools specifically addressing nutrition and physical activity have been developed. The tools described here are organized to some extent by the components of CSH being assessed. For each tool, we describe its purpose, potential audience, and ways to access and apply it in practice. As the WSCC collaborative approach to health and learning replaces the CSH framework, the tools themselves may be revised at some point to reflect those changes. In the meantime the tools can be used to address school health and school health programming and those traditional components of the CSH framework now present in the WSCC model.

ASSESSING THE OVERALL SCHOOL HEALTH PROGRAM

School Health Index (SHI): Self-Assessment and Planning Guide

Purpose: *School Health Index: Self-Assessment and Planning Guide* is a self-assessment and planning tool that schools can use to improve their health and safety policies and programs (Centers for Disease Control and Prevention, 2014a, 2014b). The SHI was developed by the U.S. Centers for Disease Control and Prevention (CDC) in partnership with school administrators and staff, school health experts, parents, and national nongovernmental health and education agencies to

- enable schools to identify strengths and weaknesses of health and safety policies and programs;
- enable schools to develop an action plan for improving student health; and
- engage teachers, parents, students, and the community in promoting health-enhancing behaviors and better health.

The SHI contains eight modules, one for each component of CSH. The SHI addresses cross-cutting policies and practices as well as the following six specific health topic areas: physical activity; healthy eating; tobacco-use prevention; unintentional injury and violence prevention (safety); asthma; and sexual health, including HIV, other STDs, and pregnancy prevention. The SHI is based on CDC's research-based guidelines for school health programs (CDC 2011, 2001, 1994), which identify the policies and practices most likely to be effective in reducing youth health-risk behaviors.

Audience: The SHI is designed to be completed by school health teams. This approach gives teachers, administrators, students, parents, and community members a means of contributing to school health promotion by involving them in the assessment process and inviting them to help shape plans to improve school programs. Multiple people can access the same SHI online, allowing the appropriate representatives to answer relevant questions.

Use: The SHI has two activities to be completed by teams from a school: the eight self-assessment modules and a planning for improvement process. The self-assessment process involves members of a school community coming together to discuss what the school is already doing to promote good health and to identify strengths and weaknesses. The planning for improvement process guides teams to identify and prioritize recommended

The findings and conclusions in this report are those of the authors and do not necessarily represent the views of the Centers for Disease Control and Prevention.

actions that their school can take to improve its performance in areas that received low scores in the self-assessment. Several articles have been published in scientific journals that have evaluated the SHI implementation process and described the results of the process (Austin et al., 2006; Pearlman et al., 2005; Staten et al., 2005). Other studies have used the items from the SHI as indicators of best practices (Brener et al., 2006, 2011).

Access: *School Health Index: Self-Assessment and Planning Guide* (and related materials) is available as an interactive, customizable online tool or a downloadable, printable version. It is available in elementary school and middle school and high school versions. In 2014, new editions of both versions of the SHI were released to the public. The School Health Index can be found at www.cdc.gov/healthyyouth/shi/index.htm. (See figure 1 for examples of questions from different SHI modules.) The Alliance for a Healthier Generation's Healthy Schools Program has adopted CDC's School Health Index as its assessment tool to help schools assess their current policies and practices as well as track progress over time. To compete the SHI for the Alliance's Healthy Schools Program, users may go to http://schools.healthiergeneration.org/dashboard/about_assessment/.

Healthy School Report Card (HSRC)

Purpose: The HSRC was developed by ASCD to help schools become more efficient, effective, and healthy by improving classrooms, staff rooms, cafeterias, and playgrounds. The HSRC helps schools organize their school wellness plan, track progress, score their current school wellness plan, and set goals for improvement (ASCD, 2010).

Audience: The HSRC uses a coordinated approach that involves staff, agencies, and programs—both in and out of the school. It can be used by schools with or without a well-functioning school health team or council.

Use: The HSRC process begins by gaining approval to engage in the process, establishing a wellness team and work groups, and planning for implementation of the process. It includes assessment questions and a spreadsheet for collecting and analyzing data. A section on reporting describes how to interpret and share results of data analyses. The HSRC also discusses how to use the results to plan short- and long-term actions and how to incorporate results into a healthy school improvement plan.

The HSRC assesses healthy school characteristics in the following areas:

- School health program policy and strategic planning
- Coordination of school health programs
- Social and emotional climate
- Family and community involvement
- School facilities and transportation
- Health education
- Physical education and physical activity
- Food and nutrition services
- School health services
- Counseling, psychological, and social services
- School site health promotion for staff

Access: The HSRC is available for purchase at http://www.healthyschoolcommunities.org/hsrc/pages/reportcard/Index.aspx.

School Improvement Tool (SIT)

Purpose: Also from ASCD, the school improvement tool is a free, online tool based on the Whole Child approach to education, which is at the core of the WSCC collaborative approach to health and learning. It can be used to identify important schoolwide improvements and ensure that all learners are healthy, safe, engaged, supported, and challenged (ASCD, 2012).

Audience: Individual school administrators or teacher–leaders can use the SIT. Additionally, teams from within a school can use this tool, and a district can use it to look across schools.

Use: This online tool consists of a 15-minute survey that can be completed by individuals or school teams to evaluate their school's strengths and weaknesses in the following areas:

- School climate and culture
- Curriculum and instruction
- Leadership
- Family and community engagement
- Professional development and staff capacity
- Assessment
- Ability to provide and sustain a Whole Child approach to education across all aspects of the school experience

FIGURE 1

Sample School Health Index Discussion Questions from the Assessment for Middle and High School Students

MODULE 1
School Health and Safety Policies and Environment

Does your school have a representative committee or team that meets at least four times a year and oversees school health and safety policies and programs?

Possible Reponses:

3 = Yes.

2 = A committee or team does this, but it could be more representative.

1 = A committee or team does this, but it is not representative or it meets less often than four times a year.

0 = No.

MODULE 2
Health Education

Do all teachers of health education provide opportunities for students to practice or rehearse the skills needed to maintain and improve their health?

Possible Responses:

3 = Yes; all do.

2 = Most do.

1 = Some do.

0 = None do, or no one teaches health education.

MODULE 3
Physical Education and Other Physical Activity Programs

Do teachers keep students moderately to vigorously active for at least 50 percent of the time during most or all physical education class sessions?

Possible Responses:

3 = Yes, during most or all classes.

2 = During about half the classes.

1 = During fewer than half the classes.

0 = During none of the classes, or there are no physical education classes.

MODULE 4
Nutrition Services

Do students have at least 10 minutes to eat breakfast and at least 20 minutes to eat lunch, counting from the time they are seated?

(continued)

Figure 1 *(continued)*

Possible Responses:

3 = Yes. (Note: If the school does not have a breakfast program but does provide at least 20 minutes for lunch, you can select 3.)

2 = Have adequate time for breakfast or lunch but not for both.

1 = No, but there are plans to increase the time.

0 = No.

MODULE 5
School Health Services

Does your school facilitate or provide case management for students with poorly controlled asthma?

Possible Responses:

3 = Yes; case management is facilitated or provided to all students with poorly controlled asthma.

2 = Case management is facilitated or provided to most students with poorly controlled asthma.

1 = Case management is facilitated or provided to some students with poorly controlled asthma.

0 = No; case management is not facilitated or provided to students with asthma.

MODULE 6
School Counseling, Psychological, and Social Services

Does your school aid students during school and life transitions (such as changing schools or changes in family structure) in the following ways?

- Matching new students with another student or buddy
- Opportunities for students to check-in with a trusted adult
- Orientation programs that focus on adapting to transitions

Possible Responses:

3 = Yes; our school aids students during school and life transitions in all three of these ways.

2 = Our school aids students during school and life transitions in two of these ways.

1 = Our school aids students during school and life transitions in one of these ways.

0 = No; our school does not aid students during school and life transitions in these ways.

MODULE 7
Health Promotion for Staff

Does the school or district offer staff members training on conflict resolution that is accessible and free or low cost?

Possible Responses:

3 = Yes.

2 = Offers training on conflict resolution, but some staff members find it inaccessible or expensive.

1 = Offers training on conflict resolution, but many staff members find it inaccessible or expensive.

0 = Does not offer training on conflict resolution.

MODULE 8
Family and Community Involvement

Do families and other community members help with school decision making?

Possible Responses:

3 = Yes; families and community members are actively engaged in most school decision-making processes.

2 = Families and community members are actively engaged in some school decision-making processes.

1 = Families and community members are offered opportunities to provide input into school decision making but are not otherwise engaged.

0 = No; families and community members are not engaged in school decision-making processes.

Adapted from Centers for Disease Control and Prevention. 2012, *School health index: A self-assessment and planning guide.* Middle School/High School Version. (Atlanta, GA). Available: http://www.cdc.gov/healthyyouth/shi/pdf/MiddleHigh.pdf.

Upon completion of the survey, the tool generates a summary of strengths and areas for improvement. These can be compiled for individual survey takers, a school, or a district. Based on these summary results, the SIT suggests additional resources that might help address identified challenges.

Access: The SIT is available at http://sitool.ascd.org.

ASSESSING SCHOOL HEALTH POLICY

Policies—including laws, mandates, regulations, standards, resolutions, and guidelines—provide a foundation for school district practices and procedures. CDC and national nongovernmental organizations provide information, tools, and resources to help audiences from state education agency staff, school board members, and school practitioners to parents understand, implement, and evaluate school health policy. Three policy-related tools are highlighted here.

State School Health Policy Database

Purpose: The National Association of State Boards of Education's (NASBE) State School Health Policy Database is a comprehensive set of laws and policies from all 50 states on more than 40 school health topics. It was designed to facilitate sharing of policies across states and to allow tracking of policy changes as they occur across the country. The database contains descriptions of a wide range of policies authorized at the state level such as laws, legal codes, rules, regulations, administrative orders, mandates, standards, and resolutions. It also includes links to the full policies where possible as well as supplemental materials that provide more detail related to the policies.

Audience: The database can be used by policy makers and educational staff to explore policies enacted in other states for applicability in their own situations. It also can help state, district, and school staff access the full set of their own state school health policies. Researchers and policy evaluators can use the database to analyze school health policies across the nation.

Use: The database is organized into six categories: (1) curriculum and instruction, (2) staff, (3) health-promoting environment, (4) student services, (5) accommodation, and (6) coordination and implementation. Most of the collected policies govern the education system, but some health department, transportation, and social services policies are included. The database can be searched by state, topic (e.g., "health education" or "bullying, harassment, and hazing"), and keyword.

Access: The NASBE State School Health Policy Database can be accessed at http://www.nasbe.org/healthy_schools/hs/index.php.

Fit, Healthy, and Ready to Learn

Purpose: NASBE's *Fit, Healthy, and Ready to Learn* was first published in 2000, and chapters have been updated and added in the years since. The most recent update was in 2012 (Bogden et al., 2012a, 2012b; Meyer and Chang, 2012). During the 1990s, education policy makers were beginning to become aware of the effect of health and safety on academic achievement as well as the role that schools could play in ameliorating the high societal costs associated with poor health and safety. The purpose of *Fit, Healthy, and Ready to Learn* is to generate awareness of the importance of addressing health and safety through schools and to provide the resources needed to support policy approaches that address this need.

Audience: *Fit, Healthy, and Ready to Learn* is intended for state and local education policymakers, administrators, and school health professionals.

Use: *Fit, Healthy, and Ready to Learn* includes chapters on healthy eating, physical activity, safety and violence prevention, and asthma. Each chapter provides a rationale for why education leaders should support efforts to address that health topic as well as data on the health issue, examples of best practices, and model policies.

Access: NASBE's *Fit, Healthy, Ready to Learn* can be downloaded or ordered in hard copy at www.nasbe.org/project/nutrition-and-physical-activity/fit-healthy-ready-to-learn-updated-release/.

Wellness School Assessment Tool (WellSAT)

Purpose: Developed by leading school health experts at Yale University's Rudd Center for Food Policy and Obesity, the WellSAT is an assessment tool to analyze school district local wellness policies, a requirement of each district participating in federal school meal programs. The WellSAT is a **quantitative assessment tool** that provides an analysis of both the comprehensiveness and the strength of local wellness policies (Schwartz et al., 2009). Users are provided with personalized guidance, resources, and assistance for addressing gaps or weaknesses in the local wellness policy, based on the results of the WellSAT.

Audience: WellSAT is aimed primarily at public health and education professionals who work directly with school districts and schools. Additionally, school administrators, district wellness council members, school board members, and researchers can use the tool.

Use: The WellSAT consists of five main areas of assessment, based on the local wellness policy requirements: (1) nutrition education and wellness promotion, (2) standards for USDA school meals, (3) nutrition standards, (4) physical education and physical activity, and (5) evaluation. Users should complete the entire WellSAT to have a full picture of the comprehensiveness and strength of the wellness policy. After all five areas of assessment are complete, a scorecard is generated. The scorecard helps users identify where gaps exist in the wellness policy.

Access: The WellSAT is available online at no cost and includes a complete description of the tool, instructions for use, and details about how to interpret the comprehensiveness and strength scores. It is located at www.wellsat.org/default.aspx (see figure 2 for sample WellSAT discussion questions).

ASSESSING HEALTH EDUCATION

Health Education Curriculum Analysis Tool (HECAT)

Purpose: Selecting and using the best possible health education curriculum is a critical step in ensuring that health education effectively promotes healthy behaviors. CDC's HECAT supports a clear, complete, and consistent approach to curriculum selection and development (CDC, 2012c). The HECAT is aligned with the National Health Education Standards (Joint Committee on National Health Education Standards, 2007) and is based on *Characteristics of an Effective Health Education Curricula* (CDC, n.d.), which help

FIGURE 2

WellSAT Assessment Tool Sample Discussion Questions

SECTION 1

Nutrition Education and Wellness Promotion

Does the school wellness policy encourage staff to be role models for healthy behaviors?

Possible Responses:

0 = The item is not included in the text of the policy.
1 = Weak statement.
2 = Meets or exceeds expectations.

SECTION 2

Standards for USDA School Meals

Does the school wellness policy address access to or promotion of the School Breakfast Program?

Possible Responses:

0 = The item is not included in the text of the policy.
1 = Weak statement.
2 = Meets or exceeds expectations.

SECTION 3

Nutrition Standards for Competitive and Other Foods and Beverages

Does the school wellness policy address limiting sugar content of foods sold or served outside USDA meals?

Possible responses:

0 = The item is not included in the text of the policy.
1 = Weak statement.
2 = Meets or exceeds expectations.
3 = Meets Institute of Medicine (IOM) standards.
4 = District has a competitive food ban.

SECTION 4

Physical Education and Physical Activity

Does the school wellness policy address time per week of physical education for elementary school students?

(continued)

Figure 2 *(continued)*

Possible Responses:

0 = The item is not included in the text of the policy.
1 = Weak statement.
2 = Meets or exceeds expectations.

SECTION 5
Evaluation

Does the school wellness policy identify a plan for revising the policy?

Possible Responses:

0 = The item is not included in the text of the policy.
1 = Weak statement.
2 = Meets or exceeds expectations.

Adapted from WellSAT, 2013, *Wellness school assessment tool.* Available: http://www.wellsat.org/evaluation.aspx.

young people adopt and maintain health-enhancing behaviors. The National Health Education Standards are a widely accepted framework of written expectations of what students should know about health education and what they should be able to do because of this education. *Characteristics of an Effective Health Education Curricula* is a synthesis of the professional literature based on research evidence on the types of information and learning experiences that help young people adopt and maintain health-enhancing behaviors.

Audience: The HECAT is designed to be used by those who select, develop, or use school health education curricula and those who are interested in improving school health education curricula.

Use: The HECAT contains process guidance, appraisal tools, and resources for carrying out an analysis of commercially packaged or locally developed school-based health education curricula. Process guidance includes directions for establishing coordination and organization for carrying out a complete examination of a health education curriculum using the HECAT. The process includes the following steps to be completed before the curriculum appraisal:

1. Identify a health education curriculum coordinator.
2. Form a health education curriculum review team and identify the roles and responsibilities of each member.
3. Obtain curriculum for review and assessment and determine the HECAT items that are essential for analyzing the curriculum.
4. Finalize the curriculum analysis tool for use by the reviewers and provide an orientation and direction for team members.
5. Determine curriculum review assignments for team members and develop a timeline for the review process.

The HECAT can also be customized to meet local community needs and conform to the curriculum requirements of the state or school district. Analysis results can help schools select or develop appropriate and effective health education curricula, revise and improve locally developed curricula, strengthen the delivery of health education, and improve the ability of school health educators to influence healthy behaviors and healthy outcomes among school-age youth.

The HECAT addresses major health risk areas for children and adolescents through separate modules on the following topics:

- Alcohol and other drugs
- Healthy eating
- Mental and emotional health
- Personal health and wellness
- Physical activity
- Safety

- Sexual health
- Tobacco
- Violence prevention

The HECAT also includes a module for analyzing comprehensive health education curricula. For each health topic, the HECAT systematizes the review of specific health topic content and skills. In addition, the HECAT includes templates for recording important descriptive curriculum information for use in the curriculum review process and analysis tools for considering curriculum characteristics such as accuracy, acceptability, feasibility, affordability, quality and completeness of teacher materials, instructional design, and instructional strategies and materials. Summary score forms are included for consolidating scores from the review of a single curriculum and for comparing scores across multiple curricula. After the curriculum analysis is completed, the HECAT provides the following recommendations to guide the curriculum selection or revision process:

1. Convene a meeting with health education curriculum review team members to discuss the completed HECAT analysis.
2. Review the score and comments and reach a consensus on final scores.
3. Identify items that the team believes are substantially more important and then rank the curricula.
4. Make curricula analysis available for public comment and then consider whether the review team should revise ranking based on input received.
5. Make curriculum recommendations and assignments for selection or improvement.

Access: The HECAT and supporting materials can be downloaded from www.cdc.gov/healthyyouth/HECAT/index.htm.

ASSESSING PHYSICAL EDUCATION

Physical Education Curriculum Analysis Tool (PECAT)

Purpose: The Physical Education Curriculum Analysis Tool is a self-assessment and planning guide developed by CDC (2006). It is designed to help school districts and schools conduct clear, complete, and consistent analyses of physical education curricula, based on national physical education standards. The PECAT specifically helps users assess how close a physical education curriculum aligns with national standards for physical education. The PECAT is organized as follows:

- Introduction and instructions
- Preliminary curriculum considerations: accuracy, acceptability, feasibility, and affordability analyses
- Content and student assessment analyses
- Appendices, including an example of a completed PECAT scoring sheet, the National Standards for Physical Education (National Association for Sport and Physical Education, 2004), a glossary of terms, and a comprehensive list of resources

Audience: The PECAT is designed to be used by school district physical education coordinators as well as curriculum coordinators. These people are in positions that guide overall curriculum development and implementation and are suited to lead the PECAT process. Additional PECAT users include school health council members, including physical education teachers, school administrators, and parents; state education agency staff; institutions of higher education; and curricula developers.

Use: PECAT users are guided through a five-step process:

1. Select a PECAT coordinator, form a PECAT committee, and identify roles and responsibilities of each member. The PECAT coordinator should lead the committee's efforts and the committee can be formed from an existing school health group. If a school health council does not exist, a committee should be formed that is representative of the school and community. People for the PECAT committee can include members from an existing curriculum review committee, physical education coordinators and teachers, curriculum specialists, college professionals, parents, students, and public health practitioners.
2. Review existing curriculum materials (e.g., the existing written physical education curriculum, scope, and sequence), the

PECAT itself, and any state or local physical education standards that might exist.

3. Complete the curriculum description form and the preliminary analyses for accuracy, acceptability, feasibility, and affordability of the curriculum.
4. Review the instructions for scoring and then complete the content and student assessment analyses. These analyses determine whether the content described in the curriculum matches the national physical education standards and whether there are protocols matched with each national physical education standard to guide the assessment of student skills and abilities.
5. Create a plan for improvement.

Access: The PECAT is available online at www.cdc.gov/healthyyouth/PECAT. Hard copies also can be requested by e-mail at cdc-info@cdc.gov or by phone at 800-CDC-INFO.

Comprehensive School Physical Activity Programs: A Guide for Schools

Purpose: This guide, developed by CDC and the American Alliance for Health, Physical Education, Recreation, and Dance (now known as SHAPE America), provides schools and school districts with a step-by-step process to develop, implement, and evaluate comprehensive school physical activity programs (CSPAP) (CDC, 2013). The guide has three main sections: (1) an overview and introduction of youth physical activity; (2) an overview and introduction to CSPAP; and (3) a step-by-step process for developing, implementing, and evaluating a CSPAP.

Audience: The CSPAP guide can be used by school health councils or CSPAP teams or committees made up of physical education teachers, classroom teachers, health education teachers, administrators, parents, students, and other stakeholders who have an interest in increasing physical activity opportunities for students.

Use: The CSPAP guide should be used by the school health council or CSPAP team. The step-by-step process outlined in the CSPAP guide is as follows:

1. Establish a team or committee and designate a physical activity leader.
2. Assess existing physical activity opportunities.
3. Create a vision statement, goals, and objectives for your CSPAP.
4. Identify the outcomes or specific changes that will be direct results of program implementation.
5. Identify and plan the activities for your CSPAP.
6. Implement your CSPAP.
7. Evaluate your CSPAP.

Going through each step of the process is important in ensuring that a needs assessment is conducted, clear vision and goals and objectives are developed, and the planning of actual physical activities is done in a comprehensive fashion before implementation and evaluation. Teams can use the tools and templates within the guide to document each step of their process.

Access: The CSPAP guide can be found online at www.cdc.gov/healthyyouth/physicalactivity.

School Physical Activity Policy Assessment (S-PAPA)

Purpose: The S-PAPA is a three-module assessment tool that enables schools to assess policies regarding recess; physical education; and other activities before, during, and after school (e.g., walk or bike to school, classroom physical activity). Each module contains a combination of open-ended, dichotomous, multichotomous, and checklist questions. The S-PAPA provides a comprehensive overview of the status of these policies, enabling schools to identify strengths, weaknesses, and opportunities for policy change (Lounsbery, 2013).

Audience: The S-PAPA can be used by school health councils, physical education teachers, classroom teachers, parents, and other stakeholders within elementary schools.

Use: The S-PAPA should be completed by a team and can be completed at one time or over the course of a few days. The S-PAPA developers estimate that it will take users approximately 23 minutes to complete all three modules of the tool. Users are encouraged to complete all three modules to gather information about all physical activity policies and practices that exist for physical education; recess; and other activities before, during, and after school. Results of the S-PAPA can be compiled and summarized, followed by the development of a plan of action for addressing weaknesses and opportunities.

Access: The S-PAPA is available online at http://activelivingresearch.org/files/S-PAPA_Instrument_1.pdf.

School Physical Education Program Checklist

Purpose: Based on national standards and guidelines developed by the American Alliance for Health, Physical Education, Recreation and Dance (SHAPE America), the School Physical Education Program Checklist is designed to help schools conduct a brief assessment of their whole physical education program, identify strengths and weaknesses, and develop a plan for improvement. Specific questions within the checklist focus on teacher qualifications and training, time requirements for physical education, equipment and facilities for physical education, student assessment, and communication strategies used by administrators and physical education teachers (National Association for Sport and Physical Education, 2013).

Audience: The checklist is designed for use by principals, physical education teachers, and parents.

Use: The 15-item checklist provides users with a question and a corresponding yes or no response option. The checklist should be completed at one time and should be followed by the identification of strengths and weaknesses. The checklist provides a template for users to develop an action plan for high-quality physical education. The action plan encourages users to identify the following: the action to be conducted, short-term goals and objectives, long-term goals and objectives, and the date that the criteria are met.

Access: The School Physical Education Program Checklist can be found online at www.aahperd.org/naspe/publications/teachingTools/upload/School-PE-Program-Checklist-Web-9-14-09.pdf.

ASSESSING SCHOOL ENVIRONMENTAL SAFETY

Healthy School Environments Assessment Tool (HealthySEATv2)

Purpose: The U.S. Environmental Protection Agency (EPA) developed the HealthySEATv2 to help school districts assess their school facilities for key environmental, safety, and health issues. EPA, states, and districts generate environmental health and safety standards and requirements. Many states and districts require regular environmental assessment to identify health and safety hazards such as chemical releases, pesticide exposures, flaking lead paint, mold, and other indoor air quality problems. HealthySEATv2 allows districts to incorporate district-specific requirements into customized checklists that include only the hazards that the district chooses to track.

Audience: HealthySEATv2 is designed for use at the district level by collecting and analyzing information from any number of school facilities. Districts may conduct the assessments using district staff, school-based staff, contractors, or a combination, depending on their circumstances and available resources.

Use: The HealthySEATv2 software comes loaded with critical elements from all of EPA's regulatory and voluntary programs for schools to which districts can add their own assessment standards. The software builds custom checklists organized by the physical areas of the school to be assessed, the issue-specific topics and subtopics for each area of the school, and specific assessment standards. In addition to tailoring the content to district policies, programs, and priorities, this tool allows districts to add local information (e.g., district name and logo, names of specific facilities, names of assessors, and contacts for remediation) as well as store and track information on the status of assessments and remediation at individual schools. Based on the information selected for the checklists, the HealthySEATv2 software creates a detailed customized guidebook for use by the assessor and other district staff that provides additional guidance on the hazards that the district selected. The software also can generate customized letters and reports.

Access: EPA's HealthySEATv2 and supporting materials can be downloaded at no cost from www.epa.gov/schools/healthyseat/index.html.

ASSESSING NUTRITION SERVICES

Discover School Breakfast Toolkit

Purpose: This toolkit, from the Food and Nutrition Service of the U.S. Department of Agriculture, was developed to help schools assess current breakfast patterns and programs, calculate costs of implementing or changing breakfast programs, identify the type of meal service to provide to students, and create a marketing plan to engage and sustain a customer base. The toolkit includes the following sections:

- Introduction
- Successful use of the toolkit, which guides users through the toolkit
- An initial assessment, which provides surveys that schools can use to evaluate the interest levels of parents and students
- Cost calculator, which includes worksheets to help schools calculate the costs of implementing the School Breakfast Program
- Description of multiple methods for serving breakfast, which can help schools determine the best method for their needs
- Roadmaps to success
- Marketing efforts, which includes a marketing plan for schools to market the School Breakfast Program
- Resources
- Program evaluation, which provides information about how and what to evaluate specific to the School Breakfast Program

Audience: The toolkit is targeted toward individuals interested in increasing access to the School Breakfast Program. That might include school health councils, school nutrition staff, school administrators, parents, and community members.

Use: Toolkit users should first become familiar with the items in the toolkit and the steps to take. The next step is to use the student, parent, and administrator surveys to identify current knowledge, attitudes, and behaviors of these audiences as it relates to eating breakfast and breakfast programs. The third step is to use the tools to calculate a variety of cost-related items, such as breakfast profit/loss, revenue per reimbursable breakfast, daily revenue breakfast, and annual expenses to revenue comparisons. The remaining components of the toolkit guides users through identifying the best method for serving breakfast and developing and implementing a marketing plan to increase access and participation in the School Breakfast Program.

Access: The toolkit is found online at www.fns.usda.gov/cnd/breakfast/toolkit/.

ASSESSING HEALTH SERVICES

Body Mass Index Measurement (BMI) in Schools

Purpose: Developed by CDC researchers, with extensive input from experts from the field of school health, the BMI Measurement in Schools document, published in both full journal article (Nihiser, 2007) and executive summary formats, provides schools with an overview of what BMI is, the differences between BMI surveillance and screening, and a list of safeguards for schools choosing to implement a BMI measurement program.

Audience: The document can be used by school health councils, school nurses, and physical education and health education teachers. Any school interested in conducting BMI measurement can use the document to learn more about options for such a strategy and to identify the best option for the school.

Use: The BMI Measurement in Schools document presents both a synthesis of the science on measuring BMI in schools and safeguards to have in place when developing and implementing such a program or initiative. Leaders within the school who are interested in BMI measurement use the document to determine whether the school prefers surveillance or screening and to identify how the safeguards can be put in place.

Access: Both the full journal article and the executive summary can be found online at www.cdc.gov/healthyyouth/npao/publications.htm#10.

Safe at School and Ready to Learn: A Comprehensive Policy Guide for Protecting Students With Life-Threatening Food Allergies

Purpose: Developed by the National School Boards Association (NSBA), the *Safe at School and Ready to Learn* policy guide provides school boards with an overview of the prevalence of food allergies, policy guidance for school boards to consider when developing food allergy policies, and a policy checklist (National School Boards Association, 2012). The policy checklist guides the user through a process of identifying policy areas that need attention and actions that can be taken towards improvement.

Audience: The policy guide is to be used primarily by school board members. Secondary users can be school administrators, school health services staff, physical and health education teachers, parents, and school nutrition staff.

Use: In addition to providing policy guidance to school boards and other stakeholders, the guide's checklist is to be completed by identifying whether a specific policy element is included or not included and whether it is implemented or not implemented. When policy gaps are determined, a section for identifying action steps is provided. Results of the policy checklist can be used to inform and develop food allergy policies for schools.

Access: The guide is available online at www.nsba.org/foodallergyguide.pdf.

ASSESSING SCHOOL EMPLOYEE WELLNESS

School Employee Wellness— A Guide for Protecting the Assets of Our Nation's Schools

Purpose: The Directors of Health Promotion and Education (DHPE) developed *School Employee Wellness—A Guide for Protecting the Assets of Our Nation's Schools* to promote the benefits of school employee wellness programs, describe a model for implementing a school employee wellness program, and provide information and tools schools can use to implement or improve wellness programs (Directors of Health Promotion and Education, n.d.).

The guide was developed based on a literature review and interviews with school and district administrators and staff, insurance providers, and state health and education agency staff. It was reviewed by several national education and health organizations and pilot tested in 25 sites.

The guide takes a comprehensive approach to school employee wellness programs, addressing health education and health promotion, individual behavior change interventions, and worksite screening activities. It also addresses the need for longer-term and integrative actions such as linking the employee wellness programs with related programs in the school or district (e.g., employee assistance programs) and with outside sources for follow-up, treatment, and health care decision making; formalizing the place of employee wellness programs in the school or district structure; and conducting evaluation and improvement activities.

Audience: The guide identifies four key target audiences as critical players in developing, implementing, and sustaining school employee wellness programs: (1) the school staff who implement wellness programs, (2) decision makers, (3) school employees, and (4) community stakeholders.

Use: *School Employee Wellness—A Guide for Protecting the Assets of Our Nation's Schools* is structured around nine steps to creating or strengthening a school employee wellness program.

1. Obtain administrative support.
2. Identify resources.
3. Identify a leader.
4. Organize a committee.
5. Gather and analyze data.
6. Develop a plan.
7. Implement the plan.
8. Evaluate and adapt the program.
9. Sustain the program.

For each step, the guide provides tips, stories, questions to consider, and tools. It also includes nearly 20 pages of appendices with sample letters, surveys, checklists, and other useful resources for planning and implementing school employee wellness programs.

Access: *School Employee Wellness—A Guide for Protecting the Assets of Our Nation's Schools* is available for download at https://dhpe.site-ym.com/members/group_content_view.asp?group=87568&id=124831.

ASSESSING FAMILY AND COMMUNITY INVOLVEMENT

Parent Engagement: Strategies for Involving Parents in School Health

Purpose: *Parent Engagement: Strategies for Involving Parents in School Health* was developed by CDC to help parents and school staff come together to support and improve the learning, development, and health of children and adolescents (CDC, 2012d). The strategies and actions recommended in this publication are based on a synthesis of parent engagement and involvement research and guidance from the fields of education, health, psychology, and sociology. Materials in the review include peer-reviewed journal articles, books, reports from government agencies and nongovernmental organizations, and websites. Information from these sources was summarized to identify parent engagement practices in school that demonstrated an influence on students' academic and health behaviors. In addition, recommendations were informed by the opinions of expert researchers, public health practitioners, and educators who identified **evidence-based strategies** and specific actions that can be taken to increase parent engagement in school health activities.

Audience: The audience for the strategies document is school administrators, teachers, nurses, support staff, parents, and others interested in promoting parent engagement. In addition to the strategies document, CDC has fact sheets on promoting parent engagement tailored for district and school administrators, teachers and other school staff, and parents.

Use: *Parent Engagement: Strategies for Involving Parents in School Health* gives tips for all three aspects of parent engagement: (1) connecting with parents, (2) engaging parents in school health activities by providing a variety of activities and frequent opportunities to fully involve parents, and (3) sustaining parent engagement by addressing common challenges to getting and keeping parents engaged. The strategies document can be tailored to focus on the actions that are most feasible and appropriate, based on the needs of the school and parents, school level (elementary, middle, or high school), and available resources.

Promoting Parent Engagement in School Health: A Facilitator's Guide for Staff Development

Purpose: Staff development is critical to enhance the ability of school staff to involve parents. CDC developed *Promoting Parent Engagement in School Health: A Facilitator's Guide for Staff Development* to help school staff

- generate enthusiasm and interest in improving parent engagement in school health;
- understand the essential aspects of parent engagement, including how to connect positively with parents, engage parents in meaningful school health activities, and address challenges of engaging parents in school health activities;
- share information with other staff not attending the program; and
- initiate steps to implement a parent engagement action plan.

Audience: District and school staff that provides staff development activities can use this guide to expand the degree to which schools engage parents in school health.

Use: This guide provides the step-by-step procedures, activities and exercises, promotional and handout materials, resources, and PowerPoint presentation (with facilitator narrative and notes) needed to implement this staff development program.

Access: *Parent Engagement: Strategies for Involving Parents in School Health, Promoting Parent Engagement in School Health: A Facilitator's Guide for Staff Development* and related materials are available at no cost from www.cdc.gov/healthyyouth/adolescenthealth/parent_engagement.htm.

REFERENCES

ASCD. 2010. *The Purpose of the Healthy School Report Card*. Alexandria, VA. www.ascd.org/publications/books/110140/chapters/The-Purpose-of-the-Healthy-School-Report-Card.aspx.

ASCD. 2012. ASCD Launches Free Online Needs Assessment and School Improvement Tool.

Alexandria, VA. Press release. www.ascd.org/news-media/Press-Room/News-Releases/ASCD-Releases-Free-Online-School-Improvement-Tool.aspx.

Austin, S.B., Fung, T., Cohen-Bearak, A., Wardle, K., & Cheung L.W.Y. 2006. Facilitating Change in School Health: A Qualitative Study of Schools' Experiences Using the School Health Index. *Preventing Chronic Disease*, *3*(2) [serial online]. www.cdc.gov/pcd/issues/2006/apr/05_0116.htm

Bogden, J.F., Brizius, M., & Walker, E.M. 2012a. *Fit, Healthy, Ready to Learn: A School Health Policy Guide*. Chapter D: Policies to Promote Physical Activity and Physical Education (2nd ed.). Arlington, VA: National Association of State Boards of Education.

Bogden, J.F., Brizius, M., & Walker, E.M.. 2012b. *Fit, Healthy, Ready to Learn: A School Health Policy Guide*. Chapter E: Policies to Promote Healthy Eating (Second Edition). Arlington, VA: National Association of State Boards of Education.

Brener, N.D., Pejavara, A, Barrios, L.C., Crossett, L., Lee, S.M., McKenna. M., Michael, S., & Wechsler, H. 2006. Applying the School Health Index to a Nationally Representative Sample of Schools. *Journal of School Health*, *76*(2), 57–66.

Brener, N.D., Pejavara, A., McManus, T. 2011. Applying the School Health Index to a Nationally Representative Sample of Schools: Update for 2006. *Journal of School Health*, *81*(2), 81–90.

Centers for Disease Control and Prevention. 1994. Guidelines for School Health Programs to Prevent Tobacco Use and Addiction. *MMWR, 43*(RR-2), 1–18.

Centers for Disease Control and Prevention. 2001. School Health Guidelines to Prevent Unintentional Injuries and Violence. *MMWR*, *50*(RR-22), 1–73.

Centers for Disease Control and Prevention. 2006. *Physical Education Curriculum Analysis Tool (PECAT)*. Atlanta, GA: Centers for Disease Control and Prevention.

Centers for Disease Control and Prevention. 2011. School Health Guidelines to Promote Healthy Eating and Physical Activity. *MMWR,* 60(RR-5), 1–76.

Centers for Disease Control and Prevention. 2012a. *Health Education Curriculum Analysis Tool, 2012*. Atlanta, GA: U.S. Department of Health and Human Services.

Centers for Disease Control and Prevention. 2012b. *Parent Engagement: Strategies for Involving Parents in School Health*. Atlanta, GA: U.S. Department of Health and Human Services.

Centers for Disease Control and Prevention. 2013. *Comprehensive School Physical Activity Programs: A Guide for Schools*. Atlanta, GA: U.S. Department of Health and Human Services.

Centers for Disease Control and Prevention. n.d. *Characteristics of an Effective School Health Curriculum*. Atlanta, GA: U.S. Department of Health and Human Services. www.cdc.gov/healthyyouth/SHER/characteristics/index.htm

Centers for Disease Control and Prevention. 2014a. *School Health Index: A Self-Assessment and Planning Guide. Elementary School Version*. Atlanta, GA: U.S. Department of Health and Human Services.

Centers for Disease Control and Prevention. 2014b. *School Health Index: A Self-Assessment and Planning Guide. Middle School/High School Version*. Atlanta, GA: U.S. Department of Health and Human Services.

Directors of Health Promotion and Education. n.d. *School Employee Wellness—A Guide for Protecting the Assets of Our Nation's Schools*. https://c.ymcdn.com/sites/dhpe.site-ym.com/resource/group/75a95e00-448d-41c5-8226-0d20f29787de/Downloadable_Materials/EntireGuide.pdf

Joint Committee on National Health Education Standards. 2007. *National Health Education Standards: Achieving Excellence* (2nd ed.). Atlanta, GA: American Cancer Society.

Lounsbery, M.A.F., McKenzie, T.L., Morrow, J.R., Holt, K.A., & Budnar, R.G. 2013. School Physical Activity Policy Assessment (SPAPA): Test-Retest Reliabilities. *Journal of Physical Activity and Health*, 10, 496–503.

Meyer L., & Chiang, R.J. 2012. *Fit, Healthy, Ready to Learn: A School Health Policy Guide*. Chapter I: Policies to Promote Safety and Prevent Violence. Arlington, VA: National Association of State Boards of Education.

National Association for Sport and Physical Education. 2004. *National Standards for Physical Education*. Arlington, VA: National Association for Sport and Physical Education.

National Association for Sport and Physical Education. 2013. *High Quality Physical Education: How Does Your Program Rate?* Arlington, VA: National Association for Sport and Physical Education.

National School Boards Association. 2012. *Safe at School and Ready to Learn: A Comprehensive Policy Guide for Protecting Students With Life-threatening Food Allergies*. Washington, DC: National School Board Association.

Nihiser, A.J., Lee, S.M., Wechsler, H., McKenna, M., Odom, E., Reinold, C., Thompson, D., & Grummer-Strawn, L. 2007. Body Mass Index Measurement in Schools. *Journal of School Health*, *77*, 651–71.

Pearlman D.N., Dowling, E., Bayuk, C., Cullinen, K., & Thacher, A.K. 2005. From Concept to Practice: Using the School Health Index to Create Healthy School Environments in Rhode Island Elementary Schools. *Preventing Chronic Disease*, *2*(Nov) [serial online]. www.cdc.gov/pcd/issues/2005/nov/05_0070.htm

Schwartz, M.B., Lund, A.E., Grow, M., McDonnell, E., Probart, C., Samuelson, A., & Lytle, L. 2009. A Comprehensive Coding System to Measure the Quality of School Wellness Policies. *Journal of the American Dietetic Association*, *109*, 1256–62.

Staten, L.K., Teufel-Shone, N.I., Steinfelt, V.E., Ortega, N., Halverson, K., Flores, C. et al. 2005. The School Health Index as an Impetus for Change. *Preventing Chronic Disease*, *2*(1) [serial online]. www.cdc.gov/pcd/issues/2005/jan/04_0076.htm

Index

Note: The italicized *f* and *t* following page numbers refer to figures and tables, respectively. **Boldface** page numbers refer to glossary terms.

H

I

J

K

About the Editors

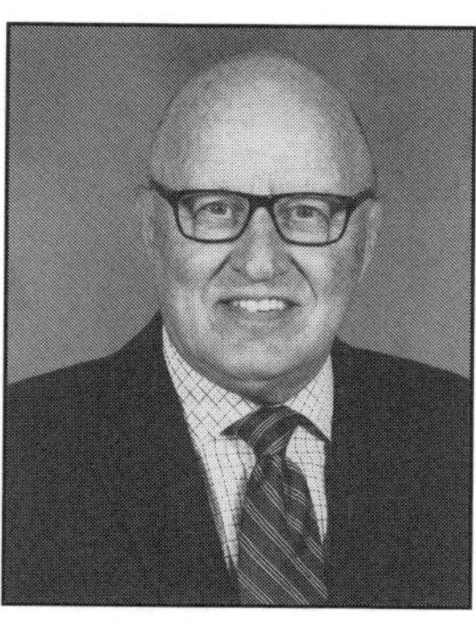

David A. Birch, PhD, MCHES, is professor and chair of the Department of Health Science at the University of Alabama. He is president-elect of the Society for Public Health Education (SOPHE) and is past president of the American Association for Health Education (AAHE). He has served on the board of directors of AAHE, the American School Health Association (ASHA), the National Association of Health Education Centers (NAHEC), and the board of trustees of the Society for Public Health Education (SOPHE). Dr. Birch is cochair of the National Implementation Task Force for Accreditation in Health Education, a member of the Governing Council of the American Public Health Association, and a member of the board of directors of the Foundation for the Advancement for Health Education. He is chair of the editorial board of the Journal of School Health and a member of the editorial boards of Pedagogy in Health Promotion: The Scholarship of Teaching and Learning and the American Journal of Health Studies. Dr. Birch is a charter fellow of AAHE and a fellow of ASHA. He has received the Eta Sigma Gamma Honor Award (2015), the SOPHE Presidential Citation (2012), the ASHA Outstanding Researcher Award (2010), AAHE Professional Service Award (2008), AAHE Presidential Citation (2008, 2012, and 2013), and ASHA Distinguished Service Award (1996). He was the 2008 Ann E. Nolte Scholar in Health Education at Illinois State University and a 2000 Robert D. Russell Scholar at Southern Illinois University at Carbondale. As a faculty member at Indiana University, Dr. Birch received the Trustee's Teaching Award and the Teaching Excellence Recognition Award. His research interests include professional preparation, professional leadership, and the Whole School, Whole Community, Whole Child model.

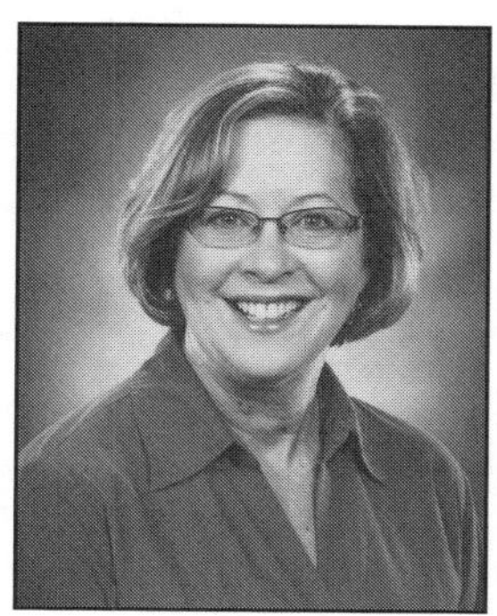

Donna M. Videto, PhD, MCHES, is a professor of health at SUNY College at Cortland. She is a national leader in school health and has published articles on health education in several journals, written chapters in four books, and coauthored a book on assessment in health education. She has also made numerous presentations across the United States on health education and was given the 2012 New York AHPERD Amazing People Award for outstanding contributions and commitment to professional excellence. She became an American Association for Health Education fellow in 2012, and she has received several awards for her teaching. Videto is a member of the American School Health Association and the Society for Public Health Education.

About the Contributors

Diane Allensworth began her career in school health in 1966 as a school nurse after returning from serving in a public health project in the Peace Corps in Panama. She taught health education at Kent State University from 1976 to 1995. She has promoted a coordinated school health program detailed in the *Journal of School Health* in 1987. In 1997 Allensworth was writer and editor of the Institute of Medicine's report *Schools and Health: Our Nation's Investment*. She has written numerous books, including *Healthy Students 2000: An Agenda for Continuous Improvement in America's Schools*. In 2010, she co-edited, with Carl Fertman, *Health Promotion Programs: From Theory to Practice*.

While on faculty at Kent State University, she began her work with the American School Health Association as the associate executive director for sponsored programs, where she secured more than $3 million in funding. In 1997 she became chief of the Program Development Services Branch in the Division of Adolescent School Health for the CDC. In 2006 Dr. Allensworth was the associate director for education in the Division of Partnerships and Strategic Alliances. She has more than 30 publications in peer-reviewed journals and made more than 200 presentations worldwide.

Lisa K. Angermeier, PhD, MCHES, is a clinical assistant professor of health education in the department of kinesiology at Indiana University–Purdue University Indianapolis. Dr. Angermeier earned a PhD in health behavior from Indiana University. She is a fellow of the American School Health Association and a master certified health education specialist. She has been closely involved with the development of coordinated school health programs in Indiana, where she was a facilitator for the Indianapolis Public Schools' CSHP team and a former member of the Michiana Core Team.

Lisa Cohen Barrios has been chief of the Research Application and Evaluation Branch in the Division of Adolescent and School Health (DASH) at the U.S. Centers for Disease Control and Prevention (CDC) since April 2004. In this position, Dr. Barrios directs synthesis and translation of research and evaluation activities that provide health professionals the tools for improving sexual health and preventing HIV, other STDs, and teen pregnancy. Dr. Barrios joined CDC in 1997 as the DASH health scientist responsible for developing, implementing, and managing research synthesis activities and research application tools for prevention of injury and violence. Dr. Barrios is the lead author on CDC's School Health Guidelines to Prevent Unintentional Injuries and Violence and a major contributor to the CDC's School Health Index and Health Education Curriculum Analysis Tool. She has published more than 35 peer-reviewed articles related to childhood injury and violence prevention, adolescent health, and school health. Dr. Barrios received a doctorate of public health in health behavior and health education from the University of North Carolina School of Public Health, a master of science degree in behavioral sciences from the Harvard School of Public Health, and a bachelor's degree in psychology from the University of Rochester.

Bonni C. Hodges, PhD, is professor and chair of the health department at SUNY Cortland. Dr. Hodges also is primary investigator and co-director of the School Health System Change Project. She is the primary author of assessment and planning in health programs and numerous scholarly papers on school and community health education. In her two decades in health education and promotion, she has presented her work at national and international conferences. She is a 2009 recipient of the SUNY Chancellor's Award for Excellence in Faculty Service; a 2005 recipient of the SUNY Chancellor's Research and Scholarship Recognition Award; and a 2006, 2009, 2010, and 2011 recipient of a SUNY Cortland Excellence in Research and Scholarship Award. Dr. Hodges received her PhD in health education with concentrations in adolescent health and research and evaluation from the University of Maryland at College Park.

Sarah M. Lee is the team lead for the research application and evaluation team in the School Health Branch of the Division of Population Health at the Centers for Disease Control and Prevention. The team is focused on prevention of chronic disease in schools, including promotion of physical activity and healthy eating and prevention of tobacco use. She provides scientific expertise and leadership on numerous documents, resources, surveillance studies, and CDC school health programs related to youth physical activity and obesity prevention. Her research interests include school policies and environmental influences on physical activity among youth, physical activity assessment, dissemination and diffusion of school health tools and resources, and the coordinated school health model applied to designing effective programs. Sarah is the lead author on CDC's Physical Education Curriculum Analysis Tool (PECAT) and CDC's Guidelines for Schools to Promote Lifelong Healthy Eating and Physical Activity Among Young People. Additionally, she has published more than 30 peer-reviewed manuscripts related to youth physical activity, prevention of childhood obesity, and evidence-based strategies for schools to implement policies and programs related to both of these topics. Sarah earned her PhD in exercise and wellness education from Arizona State University.

Dr. Jeremy Lyon is superintendent of the Frisco Independent School District, one of the fastest-growing school districts in the United States. Since 1986 Dr. Lyon has served in public education as a teacher, coach, principal, and superintendent. He received his bachelor of science degree from Texas A&M University and his doctoral degree in school administration from the University of Texas at Austin. He was a fellow of the Cooperative Superintendent program at UT. Dr. Lyon received the Nolan Estes Leadership Ascension Award in 2009 from the University of Texas Department of Education. In 2012, he received the Superintendent's School Health Leadership Award from the American School Health Association. Dr. Lyon is the first school superintendent in the country to serve on an affiliate board of the American Heart Association. He is passionate about health and wellness issues affecting children and staff.

Qshequilla P. Mitchell, PhD, MPH, is a postdoctoral fellow at the University of Alabama's Center for the Prevention of Youth Behavior Problems. Dr. Mitchell received her PhD in health education and promotion at the University of Alabama and a master's of public health degree in health care, organization, and policy from the University of Alabama at Birmingham. She has research experience in childhood obesity, adolescent risk behavior in high-poverty neighborhoods, and child oral health. Her line of research focuses on the racial and ethnic health disparities in adolescent health outcomes among youth from rural areas.

Angelia M. Paschal, PhD, is an associate professor of health education and health promotion at the University of Alabama in Tuscaloosa, where she works in the department of health science. Her research focuses on eliminating health disparities in disadvantaged children and other underserved populations. She has taught courses in program planning and evaluation, cultural competency, and health disparities, among other topics. Dr. Paschal earned her bachelor's and master's degrees in psychology and educational psychology from the University of Mississippi. She earned her doctoral degree in sociology at Kent State University.

Hannah M. Priest is a doctoral candidate of health education and promotion and graduate assistant in the department of health science at the University of Alabama. She holds a BS in physical education and an MAED in health education from East Carolina University. Ms. Priest is a former health and physical education teacher. She became a certified health education specialist in 2013. Her research focuses on adolescent and young adult health with an emphasis on sexual health promotion. Ms. Priest is an active member of several professional health organizations, including the Society for Public Health Education, American Public Health Association, and Eta Sigma Gamma.

Sean Slade, MEd, is the director of whole child programs at ASCD, a global educational leadership organization. At ASCD he directs the Whole Child unit, ensuring that their philosophy is integrated into other units, including professional development, publications, and policy. To leverage the influence and reach of ASCD, Sean has engaged in and developed ongoing relationships with key international organizations, including OECD, UNESCO, IUHPE, and UNICEF.

He is a key member of several leadership committees for the ASCD. He serves on steering committees for numerous organizations, including International Alliance for Child and Adolescent Mental Health and Schools and the Let's Move in School initiative.

Sean has delivered several keynote speeches and presentations worldwide. In more than two decades in education he has been a teacher, head of a department, educational researcher, and senior education officer. He has taught, trained, and administered educational projects and promoted educational reform in the United States and abroad. He has written extensively on topics related to the whole child, health, and well-being. Sean writes blogs for *Washington Post*'s The Answer Sheet as well as ASCD's Inservice and Whole Child blogs.

Robert F. Valois, MS, PhD, MPH, FASHA, FAAHB, FAAHE, is a professor of health promotion, education, and behavior in the Arnold School of Public Health and holds an adjunct appointment in family and preventive medicine in the School of Medicine at the University of South Carolina. Dr. Valois holds a BS degree in health science from the SUNY College at Brockport. His MS degree in school health and PhD in community health with a minor in educational psychology and program evaluation are from the University of Illinois at Urbana-Champaign. Dr. Valois completed his post-doctoral fellowship, a U.S. Public Health Service traineeship, and the MPH degree in health behavior at the University of Alabama Medical Center School of Public Health in Birmingham. Dr. Valois was the director of corporate health promotion for Carle Clinic in Urbana, Illinois, and held faculty positions at Eastern Illinois University, the University of Illinois, and the University of Texas. Dr. Valois' research is focused on child, adolescent, and school health; adolescent health-risk behaviors; adolescent quality of life and life satisfaction; smoking cessation; and program evaluation. He has published peer-reviewed journals and an ASCD monograph, The Healthy School Communities Model: Aligning Health and Education in the School Setting. He was an evaluator for the Healthy School Communities Project funded by ASCD and for the Mariner Project for coordinated school health in South Carolina funded by the U.S. Department of Education. Dr. Valois is a consultant to the Healthy Kids program of the California Department of Education and Health and the Center for Health Promoting Schools at the National Department of Health of Taiwan.

Michele Wallen, PhD, is an associate professor in the department of health education and promotion at East Carolina University (ECU). Her professional career began as a teacher in North Carolina public high schools. Before joining the faculty at ECU, she worked as a health education consultant for the North Carolina Department of Public Instruction. Michele earned her BA at the University of North Carolina at Chapel Hill and her MPH and PhD at the University of North Carolina at Greensboro. Michele works to advance health education initiatives in schools and has worked on numerous projects to support the preparation and development of health education teachers.